PET Imaging in Pediatric Patients

Editors

HONGMING ZHUANG
ABASS ALAVI

PET CLINICS

www.pet.theclinics.com

Consulting Editor
ABASS ALAVI

July 2020 • Volume 15 • Number 3

ELSEVIER

1600 John F. Kennedy Boulevard ● Suite 1800 ● Philadelphia, Pennsylvania, 19103-2899

http://www.pet.theclinics.com

PET CLINICS Volume 15, Number 3
July 2020 ISSN 1556-8598, ISBN-13: 978-0-323-73379-3

Editor: John Vassallo (j.vassallo@elsevier.com)
Developmental Editor: Casey Potter

PET Clinics (ISSN 1556-8598) is published quarterly by Elsevier Inc., 360 Park Avenue South, New York, NY 10010-1710. Months of issue are January, April, July, and October. Periodicals postage paid at New York, NY, and additional mailing offices. Subscription prices per year are $247.00 (US individuals), $422.00 (US institutions), $100.00 (US students), $279.00 (Canadian individuals), $475.00 (Canadian institutions), $100.00 (Canadian students), $275.00 (foreign individuals), $475.00 (foreign institutions), and $140.00 (foreign students). To receive student and resident rate, orders must be accompanied by name of affiliated institution, date of term, and the signature of program/residency coordinator on institution letterhead. Orders will be billed at individual rate until proof of status is received. Foreign air speed delivery is included in all Clinics subscription prices. All prices are subject to change without notice. POSTMASTER: Send address changes to PET Clinics, Elsevier Health Sciences Division, Subscription Customer Service, 3251 Riverport Lane, Maryland Heights, MO 63043. **Customer Service: 1-800-654-2452 (U.S. and Canada); 314-447-8871 (outside U.S. and Canada). Fax: 314-447-8029. E-mail: journalscustomerservice-usa@elsevier.com (for print support); journalsonlinesupport-usa@elsevier.com (for online support).**

Reprints. For copies of 100 or more of articles in this publication, please contact the Commercial Reprints Department, Elsevier Inc., 360 Park Avenue South, New York, NY 10010-1710. Tel.: 212-633-3874; Fax: 212-633-3820; E-mail: reprints@elsevier.com.

PET Clinics is covered in MEDLINE/PubMed (Index Medicus).

Contributors

CONSULTING EDITOR

ABASS ALAVI, MD, MD (Hon), PhD (Hon), DSc (Hon)
Professor of Radiology, Division of Nuclear Medicine, Department of Radiology, Hospital of the University of Pennsylvania, Perelman School of Medicine, University of Pennsylvania, Philadelphia, Pennsylvania, USA; Department of Pediatric Hematology-Oncology, University of California, Davis, Sacramento, California, USA

EDITORS

HONGMING ZHUANG, MD, PhD, FACNM
Professor of Radiology, Chief, Division of Nuclear Medicine, Department of Radiology, The Children's Hospital of Philadelphia, Perelman School of Medicine, University of Pennsylvania, Philadelphia, Pennsylvania, USA

ABASS ALAVI, MD, MD (Hon), PhD (Hon), DSc (Hon)
Professor of Radiology, Division of Nuclear Medicine, Department of Radiology, Hospital of the University of Pennsylvania, Perelman School of Medicine, University of Pennsylvania, Philadelphia, Pennsylvania, USA; Department of Pediatric Hematology-Oncology, University of California, Davis, Sacramento, California, USA

AUTHORS

ABASS ALAVI, MD, MD (Hon), PhD (Hon), DSc (Hon)
Professor of Radiology, Division of Nuclear Medicine, Department of Radiology, Hospital of the University of Pennsylvania, Perelman School of Medicine, University of Pennsylvania, Philadelphia, Pennsylvania, USA; Department of Pediatric Hematology-Oncology, University of California, Davis, Sacramento, California, USA

RAMSEY D. BADAWI, PhD
Chief, Division of Nuclear Medicine, Co-Director, EXPLORER Molecular Imaging

Center ,Vice-chair for Research, Department of Radiology and Department of Biomedical Engineering, University of California, Davis, Sacramento, California, USA

WICHANA CHAMROONRAT, MD
Division of Nuclear Medicine, Department of Diagnostic and Therapeutic Radiology, Faculty of Medicine Ramathibodi Hospital, Mahidol University, Bangkok, Thailand

DIVA D. DE LEON, MD, MSCE
Chief, Division of Endocrinology and Diabetes, Director, Congenital Hyperinsulinism Center,

The Children's Hospital of Philadelphia, Professor of Pediatrics, Perelman School of Medicine, University of Pennsylvania, Philadelphia, Pennsylvania, USA

KEVIN W. EDWARDS, BSRT (N)(R), CNMT (RS,PET)
Nuclear Medicine and PET Team Leader, Radiology/Nuclear Medicine, The Children's Hospital of Philadelphia, Philadelphia, Pennsylvania, USA

JENNIFER GILLMAN, MD, MSCI
Department of Radiology, Hospital of the University of Pennsylvania, Philadelphia, Pennsylvania, USA

DOUGLAS J. HARRISON, MD, MS
Associate Professor of Pediatrics, University of Texas MD Anderson Cancer Center, Houston, Texas, USA

MIGUEL HERNANDEZ PAMPALONI, MD, PhD
Associate Professor of Radiology and Medicine (Cardiology), UCSF Nuclear Medicine Chief, San Francisco, California, USA

SINA HOUSHMAND, MD
Department of Radiology, University of Pittsburgh, Pittsburgh, Pennsylvania, USA

LI HUO, MD, PhD
Department of Nuclear Medicine, Peking Union Medical College Hospital, Chinese Academy of Medical Sciences and Peking Union Medical College, Beijing Key Laboratory of Molecular Targeted Diagnosis and Therapy in Nuclear Medicine, Beijing, China

HEDIEH KHALATBARI, MD, MBA
Assistant Professor of Radiology, University of Washington School of Medicine, Seattle Children's Hospital, Seattle, Washington, USA

DENNISE MAGILL, MS
Senior Medical Physicist, Environmental Health and Radiation Safety, University of Pennsylvania, Philadelphia, Pennsylvania, USA

MARCIO MALOGOLOWKIN, MD
Professor of Pediatrics, Chief, Division of Pediatric Hematology-Oncology, UC Davis

Children's Hospital, UC Davis Comprehensive Cancer Center, University of California, Davis, Sacramento, California, USA

LORENZO NARDO, MD, PhD
Assistant professor of radiology, Department of Radiology, University of California, Davis, Sacramento, California, USA

MARGUERITE T. PARISI, MD, MS
Professor of Radiology and Adjunct Professor of Pediatrics, University of Washington School of Medicine, Seattle Children's Hospital, Seattle, Washington, USA

SANDRA SAADE-LEMUS, MD
Postdoctoral Research Fellow, Radiology Department, Children's Hospital of Philadelphia, Philadelphia, Pennsylvania, USA

JEFFREY P. SCHMALL, PhD
Department of Radiology, University of California, Davis, Sacramento, California, MI Clinical Collaboration Manager, United Imaging Healthcare of America, Houston, TX, USA

SABAH SERVAES, MD
Attending Radiologist, Radiology Department, Children's Hospital of Philadelphia, Associate Professor of Clinical Radiology, Perelman School of Medicine, University of Pennsylvania, Philadelphia, Pennsylvania, USA

BARRY L. SHULKIN, MD, MBA
Adjunct Professor of Radiology, University of Tennessee Health Science Center, Diagnostic Imaging, St. Jude Children's Research Hospital, Memphis, Tennessee, USA

LISA J. STATES, MD
Attending Radiologist, Director, Section of Oncologic Imaging, Radiology Department, Children's Hospital of Philadelphia, Associate Professor of Clinical Radiology, Perelman School of Medicine, University of Pennsylvania, Philadelphia, Pennsylvania, USA

AMOL TAKALKAR, MD, MS, MBA, FACNM
Medical Director, Center for Molecular Imaging and Therapy, Biomedical Research Foundation of Northwest Louisiana, Associate Director of Research, Professor, Department of Radiology, Louisiana State University Health Sciences System Shreveport, Shreveport, Louisiana, USA

SARA R. TEIXEIRA, MD, PhD
Postdoctoral Research Fellow, Radiology
Department, Children's Hospital of
Philadelphia, Philadelphia, Pennsylvania, USA

ARASTOO VOSSOUGH, MD, PhD
Attending Neuroradiologist, Radiology
Department, Children's Hospital of
Philadelphia, Associate Professor of
Radiology, Perelman School of Medicine,
University of Pennsylvania, Philadelphia,
Pennsylvania, USA

XUEZHU WANG, MD
Department of Nuclear Medicine, Peking Union
Medical College Hospital, Chinese Academy of
Medical Sciences and Peking Union Medical
College, Beijing Key Laboratory of Molecular
Targeted Diagnosis and Therapy in Nuclear
Medicine, Beijing, China

ZHE WEN, MD, PhD
Vice Chairwoman and Associate Professor,
Department of Nuclear Medicine, Beijing
Shijitan Hospital, Capital Medical University,
Beijing, China

THOMAS J. WERNER, MSE
Department of Radiology, University of
Pennsylvania, Philadelphia, Pennsylvania, USA

YAN-FENG XU, MD, PhD
Physician, Nuclear Medicine
Department, Beijing Friendship
Hospital, Capital Medical University,
Beijing, China

JI-GANG YANG, MD, PhD
Physician, Nuclear Medicine Department,
Beijing Friendship Hospital, Capital Medical
University, Beijing, China

HABIB ZAIDI, PhD, PD
Division of Nuclear Medicine and Molecular
Imaging, Geneva University Hospital, Geneva,
Switzerland

LIN ZHANG, MD
Associate Professor, Department of
Radiology, Xiamen Children's Hospital,
Xiamen Branch Hospital, Children's
Hospital, FUDAN University, Xiamen, Fujian,
China

HONGMING ZHUANG, MD, PhD, FACNM
Professor of Radiology, Chief, Division of
Nuclear Medicine, Department of
Radiology, The Children's Hospital of
Philadelphia, Perelman School of Medicine,
University of Pennsylvania, Philadelphia,
Pennsylvania, USA

Contents

[18]F-fluorodeoxyglucose (FDG) PET/computed tomography (CT) is an efficient method of diagnosing, staging, treatment evaluation, and recurrence monitoring of pediatric diseases. FDG has some limitations, but other PET/CT tracers have shown promising roles in evaluation of pathologies in pediatric patients. FDG is the most commonly used PET tracer but can accumulate in different types of infection and inflammation. In recent years, more non-FDG tracers have shown utility in evaluating pediatric disease. This article reviews currently available literature on the clinical application of non-FDG PET tracers in the application in the pediatric population.

Add "improving" before "detection"? PET/MR is beneficial particularly in pediatric patients who undergo recurrent imaging, such as those with cancer or chronic inflammatory disease. PET/MR has advantages compared with PET/computed tomography, including decreased radiation exposure and superior characterization of soft tissue. Ongoing challenges include reducing examination duration and costs and detection of pulmonary lesions. Accepted clinical applications of PET/MR in pediatric patients are evaluation of epileptic foci and diagnosis, staging, and follow-up of solid tumors. PET/MR also may have a role in diagnosis and management of infectious and inflammatory conditions relevant to the pediatric population, including osteomyelitis and Crohn disease.

Total-body (TB) PET/computed tomography (CT) provides a substantial gain in the physical sensitivity of PET, leading to vastly improved image quality or can enable imaging applications that are either not possible with conventional PET or suffer from poor signal-to-noise. The paradigm-shifting promise of TB-PET/CT lies in its capability to perform dynamic, delayed, and low-dose imaging, which have the potential to increase the range of diseases and disorders that can be investigated or managed using PET. Here we discuss the use of TB-PET/CT and describe protocols that take advantage of this unique innovation applied to the needs of the pediatric population.

The progress made in hybrid PET imaging during the past decades has significantly expanded the role of this modality in both clinical and research applications. Semi-quantitative PET/CT has been the workhorse of clinical PET/CT due to its simplicity and availability. In addition to semi-quantitative PET/CT, volumetric PET and global metabolic activity have recently shown promise in a more accurate assessment of various diseases. PET/CT has been widely used in pediatric oncologic and non-oncologic diseases. Here we have highlighted few of the pitfalls in the quantitative PET/CT and their potential remedies which have potential in PET/CT evaluation of pediatric diseases.

It is good for the nuclear medicine technologist to be aware of the normal variants and the appearance of a good-quality scan. The primary responsibility as a nuclear medicine technologist is to provide an optimal quality scan that maximizes the reading physician's ability to correctly interpret while using current radiation safety practices as the best possible experience is created for patients and families. Combining the radiation safety aspects (nuclear) with how care is provided (medicine) and the use of the most recent equipment (technology) is what defines a nuclear medicine technologist.

PET/computed tomography (CT) is a common hybrid imaging modality utilized in a variety of diagnostic imaging applications in pediatrics. This literature review focuses on the current state of pediatric patient radiation safety by exploring topics related to radiation risk and controversy, advances in imaging technology, and available clinical resources including those from Image Gently and the Society of Nuclear Medicine and Molecular Imaging.

Although fluorodeoxyglucose PET/MR imaging is a promising new modality, there is not yet enough data to support its routine use for staging or surveillance of children with lymphoma. PET/MR imaging protocols are still under development, and its availability globally is limited. The cost-benefit of using PET/MR imaging has not yet been established, especially because annual post-treatment surveillance imaging with fluorodeoxyglucose PET is not necessary in most patients with lymphoma. Further research into the use of PET/MR imaging in pediatric oncology patients is needed with continued collaborations among institutions.

Post-transplant lymphoproliferative disease is a well-known complication in transplant recipients. Evaluating the extent and stage of disease is important for management and follow-up. As a combination of anatomic and functional imaging, PET/CT is a sensitive and specific tool to stage and detect occult disease compared with conventional imaging. PET/CT also has a role in monitoring treatment response. Although PET/CT has been shown to be potentially useful in adults, evidence in children is insufficient. This review provides an overview of the use of PET/CT in post-transplant lymphoproliferative disease, especially in pediatric patients.

Neuroblastoma is one of the most common pediatric malignant tumors. Functional imaging plays an important role in the diagnosis, staging, and therapy response monitoring of neuroblastoma. Although metaiodobenzylguanidine scan with single-photon emission computed tomography/computed tomography remains the mainstay in functional imaging of the neuroblastomas, PET/CT has begun to show increased utility in this clinical setting.

The role of ^{18}F-fluorodeoxyglucose positron emission tomography/computed tomography ([18]F -FDG PET/CT) continues to develop. The literature supports a role for PET/CT in the staging and surveillance of certain specific pediatric sarcoma subtypes; however, the data are less clear regarding whether PET/CT can be used as a biomarker for prognostication. Despite the interest in using this imaging modality in the management of pediatric sarcomas, most studies are limited by retrospective design and small sample size. Additional data are necessary to fully understand how best to use ^{18}F-FDG PET/CT in pediatric sarcoma management.

Congenital hyperinsulinism (HI) is the most common cause of persistent hypoglycemia in neonates and infants. Several genetic mutations have been identified and are associated with 2 distinct histopathologic forms of disease: diffuse and focal. Targeted clinical evaluation to distinguish medically treatable disease from disease requiring surgical management can prevent life-threatening complications. Detection and localization of a surgically curable focal lesion using PET imaging with 18-F-L 3,4-dihydroxyphenylalanine ([18F]-FDOPA) has become standard of care. This article provides guidelines for the selection of patients who can benefit from [18F]-FDOPA-PET/computed tomography and protocols and tips used to diagnose a focal lesion of HI.

Fever in children is common. If it persists and its cause cannot be identified in a reasonable time, along with laboratory and conventional imaging investigations, it is defined as fever of unknown origin (FUO). 18F-fluorodeoxyglucose (FDG) PET/computed tomography (CT) is well established in the evaluation of malignancy, which is a possible cause of FUO. FDG often locates inflammatory and infectious

PET CLINICS

SERIES OF RELATED INTEREST

Advances in Clinical Radiology
Available at: Advancesinclinicalradiology.com
MRI Clinics of North America
Available at: MRI.theclinics.com
Neuroimaging Clinics of North America
Available at: Neuroimaging.theclinics.com
Radiologic Clinics of North America
Available at: Radiologic.theclinics.com

THE CLINICS ARE AVAILABLE ONLINE!
Access your subscription at:
www.theclinics.com

PROGRAM OBJECTIVE

The goal of the *PET Clinics* is to keep practicing radiologists and radiology residents up to date with current clinical practice in positron emission tomography by providing timely articles reviewing the state of the art in patient care.

TARGET AUDIENCE

Practicing radiologists, radiology residents, and other health care professionals who provide patient care utilizing radiologic findings.

LEARNING OBJECTIVES

Upon completion of this activity, participants will be able to:

1. Review select imaging modalities that may be used for the diagnosis, staging, response to treatment, and monitoring the course of various disease states and detecting recurrence in several malignancies.
2. Discuss how PET-CT-MRI enhances the role of medical imaging in children and leads to effective therapeutic interventions and successful outcomes in this population.
3. Recognize benefits and advances of select PET-CT-MRI modalities to assess and diagnose a variety of benign and malignant disorders, detecting and characterizing soft tissue abnormalities, and managing infectious and inflammatory disorders.

ACCREDITATION

The Elsevier Office of Continuing Medical Education (EOCME) is accredited by the Accreditation Council for Continuing Medical Education (ACCME) to provide continuing medical education for physicians.

The EOCME designates this journal-based CME activity for a maximum of 13 *AMA PRA Category 1 Credit*(s)™. Physicians should claim only the credit commensurate with the extent of their participation in the activity.

All other health care professionals requesting continuing education credit for this enduring material will be issued a certificate of participation.

DISCLOSURE OF CONFLICTS OF INTEREST

The EOCME assesses conflict of interest with its instructors, faculty, planners, and other individuals who are in a position to control the content of CME activities. All relevant conflicts of interest that are identified are thoroughly vetted by EOCME for fair balance, scientific objectivity, and patient care recommendations. EOCME is committed to providing its learners with CME activities that promote improvements or quality in healthcare and not a specific proprietary business or a commercial interest.

The planning committee, staff, authors and editors listed below have identified no financial relationships or relationships to products or devices they or their spouse/life partner have with commercial interest related to the content of this CME activity:

Abass Alavi, MD, MD (Hon), PhD (Hon), DSc (Hon); Wichana Chamroonrat, MD; Ramsey D. Badawi, PhD; Kevin W. Edwards, BSRT (N)(R), CNMT (RS,PET); Jennifer Gillman, MD, MSCI; Douglas J. Harrison, MD, MS; Miguel Hernandez Pampolini, MD, PhD; Sina Houshmand, MD; Li Huo, MD, PhD; Marilu Kelly, MSN, RN, CNE, CHCP; Hedieh Khalatbari, MD, MBA; Dennise Magill, MS; Lorenzo Nardo, MD, PhD; Marcio Malogolowkin, MD; Marguerite T. Parisi, MD, MS; Sandra Saade-Lemus, MD; Jeffrey P. Schmall, PhD; Sabah Servaes, MD; Barry L. Shulkin, MD, MBA; Lisa J. States, MD; Amol Takalkar, MD, MS, MBA, FACNM; Sara R. Teixeira, MD, PhD; John Vassallo; Vignesh Viswanathan; Arastoo Vossough, MD, PhD; Xuezhu Wang, MD; Zhe Wen, MD, PhD; Thomas J. Werner, MSE; Yan-feng Xu, MD, PhD; Ji-gang Yang, MD, PhD; Habib Zaidi, PhD, PD; Lin Zhang, MD; Hongming Zhuang, MD, PhD, FACNM.

The planning committee, staff, authors and editors listed below have identified financial relationships or relationships to products or devices they or their spouse/life partner have with commercial interest related to the content of this CME activity:

Diva D. De Leon, MD, MSCE: consultant/advisor for Novartis AG and ProSciento; consultant/advisor and research support from Zealand Pharma A/S and Crinetics Pharmaceuticals.

UNAPPROVED/OFF-LABEL USE DISCLOSURE

The EOCME requires CME faculty to disclose to the participants:

1. When products or procedures being discussed are off-label, unlabelled, experimental, and/or investigational (not US Food and Drug Administration [FDA] approved); and
2. Any limitations on the information presented, such as data that are preliminary or that represent ongoing research, interim analyses, and/or unsupported opinions. Faculty may discuss information about pharmaceutical agents that is outside of FDA-approved labelling. This information is intended solely for CME and is not intended to promote off-label use of these medications. If you have any questions, contact the medical affairs department of the manufacturer for the most recent prescribing information.

TO ENROLL

To enroll in the *PET Clinics* Continuing Medical Education program, call customer service at 1-800-654-2452 or sign up online at http://www.theclinics.com/home/cme. The CME program is available to subscribers for an additional annual fee of USD 235.00.

METHOD OF PARTICIPATION

In order to claim credit, participants must complete the following:

1. Complete enrolment as indicated above.
2. Read the activity.
3. Complete the CME Test and Evaluation. Participants must achieve a score of 70% on the test. All CME Tests and Evaluations must be completed online.

CME INQUIRIES/SPECIAL NEEDS

For all CME inquiries or special needs, please contact elsevierCME@elsevier.com.

Preface
Evolving Role of PET in Pediatric Disorders

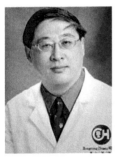
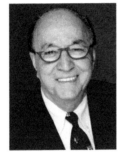

Hongming Zhuang, MD, PhD   Abass Alavi, MD, MD (Hon), PhD (Hon), DSc (Hon)

Editors

All along, performing imaging studies in children has posed significant challenges to practicing radiologists and technical staff, and this has limited their routine use in certain settings. Such limitations have deprived pediatric patients from the benefits of certain very powerful and useful imaging techniques. Many pediatric imaging studies are performed with some degree of sedation and at times under complete anesthesia. Up until 3 to 4 decades ago, radiologic imaging in children was primarily confined to planar x-ray radiography and to some limited extent to ultrasonography. Obviously, the introduction of tomographic techniques in the 1970s and the 1980s substantially enhanced the role of medical imaging in medicine. These modalities have played a critical role in the management of many serious diseases and disorders in both the adult and the pediatric populations. Over the years both x-ray computed tomography (X-CT) and MR imaging have been adopted as essential tools in both adult and pediatric medicine, and this has enhanced the impact of many invasive and noninvasive procedures/interventions. In recent years, concerns have been raised about the safety of X-CT as a routine diagnostic test, particularly in the pediatric population. Some epidemiologic studies have shown a high incidence of malignancy following exposure to significant radiation doses from modern X-CT instruments. This has led to a source of concern about the role of this imaging technique on a routine ba-

sis in pediatrics. Therefore, MR imaging has gained significant popularity as a safe imaging modality in recent years despite its limitations in assessing certain pediatric pathologic conditions. During the past few years, some concerns also have been raised about the toxicity of MR imaging contrast agents in adults as well as in children. Particularly, the retention of such agents in organs like the brain and elsewhere may potentially prove to be harmful.

PET was introduced as an imaging modality in the 1970s and was used as a powerful investigational tool at major research institutions. PET imaging for the first time allowed imaging normal function and disease activity at the molecular and cellular levels. During the 1980s and 1990s, such molecular studies were performed by using PET alone as a single instrument. However, the introduction of PET-CT in 2001 substantially enhanced of the role of this imaging technique during the ensuing 2 decades. PET-CT has been increasingly used in the adult population for the management of many serious diseases and disorders. In fact, imaging with this modality is the fastest growing domain in radiology and is expected to become the study of choice for certain disorders in the coming years. PET-CT as a single modality allows generating structural and molecular images with a single data acquisition.

Currently, most specialized pediatric hospitals provide PET-CT imaging on a routine and daily

PET Clin 15 (2020) xv–xvii
https://doi.org/10.1016/j.cpet.2020.05.001
1556-8598/20/© 2020 Published by Elsevier Inc.

basis. This is particularly true for institutions that are major referral centers for serious diseases and disorders in children. The impact of PET-CT has been particularly recognized in the management of patients with a variety of malignancies. PET is routinely used for diagnosis, staging, assessing response to treatment, monitoring the course of the disease, and detecting recurrence in many malignancies. It is expected that the unparalleled impact of PET in the adult cancer population will be soon replicated in children. The majority of adult malignancies assessed by PET-CT includes solid tumors in organs such as the lungs, head and neck, breasts, prostate, colon, and other miscellaneous organs. In contrast, pediatric studies are mostly confined to imaging sarcomas, brain tumors, or hematologic malignancies, such as lymphomas and leukemias. PET has proven to be essential for the management of patients with lymphoma and their optimal management on a routine basis. We believe that in the future, patients with other hematologic malignancies, such as leukemias, will be assessed with these techniques because of their importance in detecting and characterizing of the disease process at the molecular and cellular levels. This approach will also play an important role in introducing novel therapeutic interventions in hematologic malignancies and assessing the efficacy of the modern cell-based treatment modalities.

PET imaging, particularly with fluodeoxyglucose (FDG) as the main and routinely available radiotracer, has been extensively tested and validated as an effective modality for managing patients with infectious and inflammatory disorders. Since such diseases and disorders are also frequently encountered in the pediatric population, there is a high probability of adopting PET in children to detect and manage inflammatory disorders in the near future. Musculoskeletal infections could be the main domains for these applications. Also, FDG-PET is frequently used to assess patients with fever of unknown origin (and occult infections) to determine the location and its underlying causes, such as cancer and inflammation.

PET is increasingly used for the diagnosis and follow-up of many neurologic diseases in adults, and we foresee a similar trend for this modality in the field of pediatric neurology. FDG-PET is often utilized to detect the epileptogenic trigger points before surgical intervention in children and adult patients with seizure disorders.

During the past 2 decades, PET imaging with fluorodopa (FDOPA) has proven to be essential for the management of patients with hyperinsulinism. This approach has allowed distinguishing focal lesions from the diffuse process in the pancreas due to this disease. FDOPA-PET imaging has truly revolutionized the management of patients with this serious and disabling disorder. Before the introduction of this approach, patients with hyperinsulinism were subjected to hours of dangerous diagnostic procedures, while FDOPA-PET has allowed such diagnosis to be made within 20 to 30 minutes. Furthermore, the time required to perform surgery to treat this disease has decreased from 8 hours to less than 60 minutes based on the results from this imaging technique. Furthermore, the rate of successful outcome is frequently higher if surgery is performed following the results from FDOPA-PET.

While PET-CT played a major role in enhancing the impact of this modality in the day-to-day practice of medicine, the introduction of PET-MR imaging over the past decade has opened a new era in both adult and pediatric imaging. MR imaging has been extensively used to examine children for a variety of benign and malignant disorders. In particular, MR imaging has been of great value in detecting and characterizing soft tissue abnormalities. Efforts have been made to avoid CT scans because of the substantial radiation dose from this modality in the pediatric population. This has led to frequent applications of MR imaging in children. Similarly, PET-MR imaging is an attractive modality for assessing domains where MR imaging alone has made an impact over the past decades. This applies to disorders of the brain and the cardiovascular and musculoskeletal systems. Therefore, it is expected that combined hybrid PET-MR imaging will play a major role in the optimal management of pediatric diseases. We should emphasize that PET tracers may obviate administering MR imaging contrast agents that are implicated as being toxic in pediatric patients. This may support PET-MR imaging as the modality of choice in managing many pediatrics maladies.

The recent advances in PET imaging include the development of total-body instruments that can image the entire body with 1 data acquisition. This revolutionary approach greatly reduces the imaging time compared with that of conventional PET-CT instruments with a limited field of view. Prototype instruments that have been introduced to the field allow imaging the entire body of adults in only several minutes. This invention not only allows for shorter imaging times but also can be successfully performed with substantially smaller doses of the intended radiopharmaceuticals. Both of these benefits support the use of total-body PET imaging in children. For example, the pediatric population can be examined without sedation or general anesthesia, which is typically induced during most imaging techniques in children. Furthermore, the radiation dose, which is of major concern in this population, will be substantially reduced with this approach. It is expected that total-body PET machines designed specifically for applications in children will have a shorter field of view that is in the range of 80 to 100 cm, and this will accommodate the majority of the pediatric population. This will also reduce the cost of manufacturing such instruments for pediatric applications.

Overall, we believe that PET-CT-MR imaging will substantially enhance the role of medical imaging in children and therefore lead to more effective therapeutic interventions and successful outcomes in this population.

Hongming Zhuang, MD, PhD
Division of Nuclear Medicine
Department of Radiology
The Children's Hospital of Philadelphia
34th Street and Civic Center Boulevard
Philadelphia, PA 19104, USA

Abass Alavi, MD, MD (Hon), PhD (Hon), DSc (Hon)
Division of Nuclear Medicine
Department of Radiology
Hospital of the University of Pennsylvania
3400 Spruce Street
Philadelphia, PA 19104, USA

E-mail addresses:
zhuang@email.chop.edu (H. Zhuang)
Abass.Alavi@pennmedicine.upenn.edu (A. Alavi)

Non-^{18}F-Fluorodeoxyglucos PET Tracers in Pediatric Disease

Xuezhu Wang, MD[a,b], Li Huo, MD, PhD[a,b],*

KEYWORDS

• Pediatric disease • PET • New tracer

KEY POINTS

- ^{18}F-fluoro-L-dihydroxyphenylalanine (^{18}) PET has demonstrated a higher sensitivity and accuracy than MIBG scintigraphy but no difference in specificity. It has advantages of detecting soft tissue recurrence and bone marrow involvement.
- 18F-MIBG analogs (including 4-[18F]fluoro-3-iodobenzylguanidine (18F-FIBG), meta-[18F]fluoro-benzylguanidine(18F-MFBG), para-[18F]Fluorobenzylguanidine (18F-PFBG), 18FN-[3-bromo-4-(3-fluoro-propoxy)-benzyl]-guanidine, and (18F-LMI1195) have high sensitivity and specificity for neuroblastoma (NB) lesions and their metastases. Preclinical studies have confirmed that the biological distribution of NB models in vitro and in vivo is similar to that of MIBG.
- ^{18}F-MIBG analogs (including ^{18}F-FIBG, ^{18}F-MFBG, ^{18}F-PFBG, and LMI1195) have high sensitivity and specificity for neuroblastoma (NB) lesions and their metastases. Preclinical studies have confirmed that the biological distribution of NB models in vitro and in vivo is similar to that of MIBG.
- ^{18}F-DOPA is superior to ^{18}F-Fluorodeoxyglucos in diagnosis of brain tumors, especially in diagnosis of low-grade brain tumors, differential diagnosis of recurrent tumors, and scar formation after radiotherapy. It also can select lesions more suitable for biopsies.
- ^{18}F-fluoro-ethyl-tyrosine (^{18}F-FET) PET is more sensitive than MR spectroscopy in providing biopsy sites, which provides information for subsequent treatment. The combination of ^{18}F-FET PET and MR imaging after surgery is highly specific for distinguishing residual disease or injury after radiotherapy, which also provides sufficient information for determining whether to choose clinical reoperation.

LYMPHOMA

Children and adolescents with lymphoma frequently have better outcomes than adults. ^{18}F-fluorodeoxyglucose (^{18}F-Fluorodeoxyglucos) currently remains the most commonly used PET tracer in the evaluation of pediatric lymphoma, but ^{18}F-^{18}F-Fluorodeoxyglucos has its limitation especially in infection and inflammation.[1–25] ^{18}F-Fluorodeoxyglucos contributes to distinguishing low risk of progress from high risk of recurrence.[26] It was found that PET/computed tomography (CT) was significantly superior to bone marrow biopsies in detecting bone marrow infiltration in children and adolescents with lymphomas.[27,28] In patients who have finished therapy, ^{18}F-Fluorodeoxyglucos PET can evaluate the residual lesions of patients more accurately, especially in patients with Hodgkin lymphoma, which can directly affect management.[29,30] Nevertheless, other PET tracers were investigated to supplement ^{18}F-Fluorodeoxyglucos due to the nonspecific nature of ^{18}F-Fluorodeoxyglucos.

[a] Department of Nuclear Medicine, Peking Union Medical College Hospital, Chinese Academy of Medical Sciences & Peking Union Medical College, Beijing, 100730, China; [b] Beijing Key Laboratory of Molecular Targeted Diagnosis and Therapy in Nuclear Medicine, Beijing, 100730, China
* Corresponding author.
E-mail address: Huoli@pumch.cn

PET Clin 15 (2020) 241–251
https://doi.org/10.1016/j.cpet.2020.03.013
1556-8598/20/© 2020 Elsevier Inc. All rights reserved.

[11]C-methionine

Methionine (MET) is a naturally occurring essential amino acid critical not only for making protein but also for phospholipid synthesis through intermediate compounds. Some evidence has shown that the increased uptake of MET mainly reflected the amino acid transport activity and thus affected protein synthesis indirectly.[31] Imaging with ^{11}C-MET is as follows: it may be transported through the L-amino acid transport system on the endothelial cell membrane and participate in the synthesis of proteins or transform into S-adenosylmethionine. Many investigators have shown potential utility of ^{11}C-MET PET/CT in the evaluation of lymphoma.[32–34] Due to low background of ^{11}C-MET in brain in comparison to ^{18}F-Fluorodeoxyglucos, ^{11}C-MET PET/CT imaging is more suitable for the assessment of lymphomas in the brain.[35,36] On the other hand, normal intense ^{11}C-MET uptake in the pancreas and liver reduced sensitivity for disease detection in these regions. In an investigation of direct comparison between ^{11}C-MET and ^{18}F-Fluorodeoxyglucos in 18 pediatric patients, it was found that the utility of ^{11}C-MET PET/CT in the abdomen is limited due to high uptake in normal structures[37] although another investigation indicated that ^{11}C-MET and ^{18}F-Fluorodeoxyglucos PET were equally effective in detecting lesions.[38] It is controversial whether or not ^{11}C-MET can distinguish well and poorly differentiated lymphomas.[39]

[18]F-fluorothymidine

[18]F-fluorothymidine (^{18}F-FLT) is a thymidine analog with uptake that reflects cellular proliferation through the activity of thymidine kinase 1, an enzyme that is highly expressed during the synthesis phase of cell cycle. Its products are not involved in DNA synthesis but aggregate only in cells. When the tumor cells proliferate, a large amount of DNA synthesis requires the upregulation of thymidine kinase 1. As a result, there is increased FLT accumulation in tumor cells.[40]

The literature regarding FLT PET/CT in the pediatric population is relatively limited. An FLT standardized uptake value (SUV) cutoff of 3.0 was reported to be able to accurately discriminate between indolent and aggressive lymphoma in adults.[41] Other investigators, however, have suggested higher FLT SUV cutoffs. Some investigators report good sensitivity and specificity (81% and 71%, respectively) for distinguishing indolent from aggressive lymphoma using an FLT SUV cutoff greater than 10.[42] In 8 pediatric lymphoma patients with equivocal ^{18}F-Fluorodeoxyglucos PET/CT findings, Costantini and colleagues[43] found

that FLT PET/CT was useful to reach more definite diagnosis.

NEUROBLASTOMA

MIBG scintigraphy with [123/131]I-labeled MIBG, including single-photon emission CT (SPECT)/CT, is a well-established method in the accurate diagnosis and staging of neuroblastoma (NB).[44–56] NB is the most common extracranial solid tumor in children and adolescents, accounting for approximately 8% of children's diseases. Adrenal gland was the most common primary site (40%), followed by abdominal sympathetic ganglion (25%), chest sympathetic ganglion (15%), cervical sympathetic ganglion (5%), and pelvic sympathetic ganglion (5%),[57] whereas NB rarely occurs in the central nervous system or autonomic nervous system. Up to 70% of NBs present with distant metastases at the diagnosis, leading to a poor prognosis.[58] NB often is evaluated by CT, MR imaging, [123/131]I-MIBG, and PET (containing ^{18}F-Fluorodeoxyglucos and other tracers[58,59]) in order to choose the appropriate treatment (**Table 1**).

^{18}F-MIBG Analogs

[123/131]I-MIBG imaging has high sensitivity and specificity for NB primary lesions and metastases ones. It has been widely used in the diagnosis and initial treatment of NB, and the results from MIBG imaging are important in guiding appropriate therapy.[60] MIBG SPECT has many limitations, however, including 2 days' imaging protocol, less ideal image quality, and significantly longer imaging time, which might require sedation or even anesthesia. For these reasons, positron tracers using MIBG analogs were investigated. The most promising is ^{18}F-MFBG. In a preliminary study, ^{18}F-MFBG PET/CT imaging was performed in 10 patients (including 5 with NB and 5 with pheochromocytoma/paraganglioma) by Pandit-Taskar and colleagues,[61] which showed excellent target ratio of bone and soft tissue lesions at 1 hour to 2 hours after injection. The sensitivity in the detecting lesions of ^{18}F-MFBG PET/CT was higher than ^{123}I-MIBG. The results indicated that ^{18}F-MFBG had great potential in imaging neuroendocrine tumors, especially NB. More evidence is needed, however, before this new PET tracer can be widely accepted in the evaluation of NB.

Catecholamine Analogs

[18]F-fluoro- L-dihydroxyphenylalanine (^{18}F-DOPA) is a precursor analog of catecholamine metabolic pathway, which enters the cell via the amino acid

Table 1
Summary of advantages and limitations of PET tracers for neuroblastoma

PET Tracer	Advantages	Limitations
^{18}F-DOPA	• High sensitivity and accuracy • In detecting soft tissue recurrence and bone marrow manifestations, especially when the size of the lesion is <15 mm • In the detection of head and neck metastases	Poor yield of the standard synthesis reactions
[11]C-HED	High sensitivity	• Short half-life • In discovery of liver lesions because of high physiologic uptake
^{18}F-MIBG analogs	High sensitivity and specificity	Little research
[68]Ga- somatostatin analogs	To select suitable persons for radionuclide therapy	No satisfactory effect Not widely used

transport system on the cell membrane, and it stores in the vesicle of the cell after decarboxylated to ^{18}F-dopamine by aromatic acid decarboxylase.[62] Two studies compared the diagnostic performance of ^{18}F-DOPA and ^{123}I-MIBG in NB.[63,64] ^{18}F-DOPA PET demonstrated a higher sensitivity (DOPA, 90%, vs MIBG, 56%) and accuracy (DOPA, 90%, vs MIBG, 57%) (P<.001) than ^{123}I-MIBG scintigraphy. There was no significant difference, however, in specificity (DOPA, 75%, vs MIBG, 62%).[63] Piccardo and colleagues[64] found that ^{18}F-DOPA had advantages in comparison to ^{123}I-MIBG in detecting soft tissue recurrence and bone marrow manifestations,[65] especially when the size of the lesion was less than 1.5 cm. The sensitivity on ^{18}F-DOPA was 84% (vs MIBG, 34%; P<.001) and 96% (vs MIBG, 71%; P<.001) respectively. ^{18}F-DOPA changed the clinical decision of 32% patients in this study. The tumor accumulation of ^{18}F-DOPA significantly correlated with the level of urinary catecholamine.[63] In addition, positivity of the post-therapeutic ^{18}F-DOPA study is the only risk factor associated with disease progression.[66]

Piccardo and colleagues[67] also explored the relationship between the uptake of ^{18}F-DOPA or ^{123}I-MIBG and prognosis (including age, stage, MYCN amplification, and the time of initial recurrence after diagnosis). In order to facilitate the evaluation of the imaging value of ^{18}F-DOPA, a new concept of systemic metabolic load score (whole-body metabolic burden [WBMB]) was proposed, which increased the range and uptake of soft tissue metastases compared with ^{123}I-MIBG score.[68] The results showed that ^{18}F-DOPA WBMB score greater than 7.5 and ^{123}I-MIBG score greater than 3 had higher risks of disease

progress and higher mortality, and the 2 imaging scores were positively correlated. The results of multivariate analysis suggested that the relationship between ^{18}F-DOPA WBMB score and nonprogressive survival was more relevant than compared with ^{123}I-MIBG (hazard ratio 17 vs 37, respectively).

Another research compared ^{18}F-DOPA PET/CT with CT/MR imaging. ^{18}F-DOPA also had higher sensitivity, specificity, negative predictive value, positive predictive value, and accuracy (90.6%, 90%, 73.5%, 96.9%, and 90.5%, respectively, vs 47.5%, 27.5%, 13.1%, 69.5%, and 43%, respectively; P<.001).[69] There was no difference in the detection of primary lesions. ^{18}F-DOPA had more advantages, however, in detecting bone marrow, lymph nodes, and soft tissue involvement whereas CT/MR imaging was more accurate in the detection of liver metastases. ^{18}F-DOPA PET/CT was more valuable in the detection of head and neck metastases in NB.[70,71] ^{18}F-DOPA is a promising positron tracer.[63,64,67,69–71]

Other catecholamines tracers, including ^{11}C-metahydroxyephridrine (^{11}C-HED), also were reported. Franzius and colleagues[72] performed ^{11}C-HED and ^{123}I-MIBG imaging in 14 children (including 6 with NB, 5 with pheochromocytoma, 1 with ganglioma, and 2 with paraganglioma). The results showed that ^{11}C-HED had a higher sensitivity (99%; soft tissue, 76.2%, and bone, 23.7%) with high target ratio compared with MIBG (93%, 74.6%, and 25.3%, respectively). The half-life of carbon 11 is very short, however, which affected the preparation process and clinical utility. In addition, the high physiologic uptake in the liver restricted the accuracy to discover liver lesions.[73,74]

[68]Ga-Somatostatin Analogs

Somatostatin receptor (SSTR) imaging has been used widely in diagnosis and treatment of neuro-endocrine tumors.[75] SSTR, in particular, SSTR1 and SSTR2, was overexpressed in NB cells.[76] Although SSTR scintigraphy using non-PET tracers has been used to evaluate NB,[77,78] the effect is not as good as with ^{123}I-MIBG. In recent years, the application value of ^{68}Ga-labeled SSTR imaging in NB has been tried by many investigators. A study involving 11 children with metastatic pheochromocytoma and NB found that ^{68}Ga-DOTATOC showed slightly better diagnostic sensitivity than ^{123}I-MIBG (97.2% vs 90.7%), and it also laid a foundation for subsequent radiation therapy.[79] Gains and colleagues[80] performed ^{68}Ga-DOTATATE imaging in 8 patients with recurrent or refractory NB in order to select suitable patients for ^{177}Lu-DOTATATE treatment. Kong and colleagues[81] also used ^{68}Ga-DOTATATE positivity as a way to select patients for ^{177}Lu-DOTATATE therapy in 8 patients with NB.

OTHER SOMATOSTATIN RECEPTOR–RICH TUMORS

There are many types of SSTR-rich tumors that can be evaluated by ^{68}Ga-DOTATATE PET/CT. In addition to NB, there exist gastroenteropancreatic tumors, multiple endocrine neoplasia types 1 and 2, von Hippel-Lindau disease, pheochromocytoma/paragangliomas, medullary thyroid carcinoma, and mesenchymal tumors causing tumor-induced osteomalacia. Functional imaging of neuroendocrine tumors is used for diagnosis and initial staging, assessing for recurrence, and response to therapy and ^{68}Ga-DOTATATE PET/CT has been used widely in adult patient populations in the evaluation of different SSTR-rich neoplasms.[75,82–93] SSTR-rich neoplasms are not adult-specific and also can occur in children. Goel and colleagues[94] performed ^{68}Ga-DOTATATE PET/CT imaging in 30 pediatric patients compared with CT scans to evaluate the ability in the detection of bone metastases in pediatric neuroendocrine tumors. They reported that ^{68}Ga-DOTATATE could detect bone metastases at a significantly higher rate (P = .0039) than the CT examination. Karageorgiadis and colleagues[95] found that ^{68}Ga-DOTATATE PET/CT imaging was helpful in localizing adrenocorticotropic hormone and corticotropin-releasing hormone cosecreting tumors in children and adolescents causing Cushing syndrome. ^{68}Ga-DOTATATE PET/CT also can be utilized in pediatric patients who are suspected of having pheochromocytoma (**Fig. 1**) because

DOTATATE PET/CT is known to be more sensitive the MIBG imaging[96] and also is superior to ^{18}F-Fluorodeoxyglucos PET/CT and anatomic imaging in the evaluation of succinate dehydrogenase mutation–related pheochromocytoma and paraganglioma in the pediatric patients.[97]

BRAIN TUMOR

Central nervous system tumor includes tumor of brain and spinal cord. Primary central nervous system malignant tumor is the second most common malignant tumor in children (followed by hematological disease), and it is the most common cause of cancer death in children.[98] It is difficult to distinguish tumor from benign change by conventional imaging, especially in distinguishing postoperative change or tumor remnant caused by operation, as well as tumor recurrence or normal tissue injury after radiotherapy. ^{18}F-Fluorodeoxyglucos PET combined with CT/MR imaging organically combines anatomic morphology and functional metabolism, which can locate and characterize the lesion more accurately. The high uptake of ^{18}F-Fluorodeoxyglucos in normal brain tissue, however, affected the accuracy of ^{18}F-Fluorodeoxyglucos PET in distinguishing tumor recurrence, residual lesions and normal tissue. For this reason, new PET tracers constantly are being explored to overcome the shortcomings.

[18]F-fluoro-ʟ-dihydroxyphenylalanine

^{18}F-DOPA is superior to ^{18}F-Fluorodeoxyglucos in the diagnosis of brain tumors, especially in diagnosis of low-grade brain tumors, differential diagnosis of recurrent tumors, and scar formation after radiotherapy. One study included 27 patients with suspected supratentorial brain tissue infiltration (21 lesions were gliomas and the remaining 6 lesions were nontumor lesions), which showed that MR spectroscopy and ^{18}F-DOPA had similar specificity (83%), but MR spectroscopy had higher diagnostic sensitivity (95% vs 76%, respectively). The level of ^{18}F-DOPA uptake correlated with progression-free survival and overall survival whereas the results of MR spectroscopy did not.[99] In 1 study, 13 patients with supratentorial astrocytoma (including 5 with low-grade gliomas)[100] underwent ^{18}F-DOPA PET/MR imaging. The investigators discovered that ^{18}F-DOPA uptake was correlated with tumor grade and progression-free survival. Lesions with high accumulation of DOPA suggested high heterogeneity in tumors. Two tumors were PET positive but not enhanced on MR imaging.[100] ^{18}F-DOPA PET/MR imaging could attribute to select lesions that were more suitable for biopsies. More importantly,

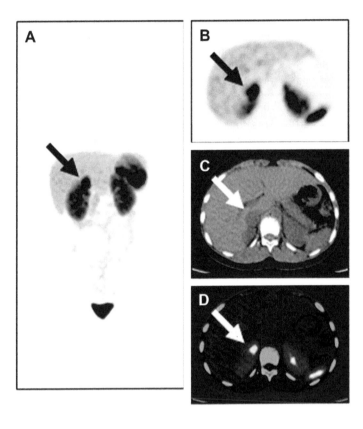

Fig. 1. An 11-year-old boy with intractable hypertension underwent ^{68}Ga-DOTATATE PET/CT for likely pheochromocytoma suggested by laboratory examination. The maximum intensity projection image (A) showed a right suprarenal activity (arrow). On the axial images of the PET (B), CT (C), and fusion (D) images, this activity was located in a 3-cm hypodense right adrenal lesion (arrows), consistent with right adrenal pheochromocytoma.

5 of the children changed their clinical decisions based on ^{18}F-DOPA PET/MR imaging. Four patients with low ^{18}F-DOPA uptake were observed conservatively, avoiding unnecessary surgery or radiotherapy and chemotherapy. PET/MR imaging had higher accuracy than PET/CT, which could highly predict dorsal striatum involvement.[101]

Amino Acids

Based on the results of a retrospective study of 26 children, which showed that the tumor/brain background uptake ratio was 1.7, ^{18}F-fluoro-ethyl-tyrosine (^{18}F-FET) PET has potential to accurately discriminate tumor tissue from nontumor tissue. The accuracy rate of using ^{18}F-FET PET to evaluate brain tumor was 77%, and the positive predictive value was 88%.[102] It was reported that FET PET was more sensitive than MR spectroscopy in providing the correct sites for biopsies, which led to additional information for subsequent treatment.[103] A prospective study showed that the specificity of postoperative combined ^{18}F-FET PET and MR imaging in differentiating residual lesions or postradiotherapy injuries was 100% (compared with 75% of MR imaging alone), which also provided sufficient material for clinical reoperation.[104]

The concentration of ^{11}C-MET in glioma may be related to the increase of protein synthesis, the destruction of blood-brain barrier, and the increase of vascular density. Many studies have explored the value of amino acid imaging agents in evaluating the grading of brain tumors. Utriainen and colleagues[105] performed ^{11}C-MET and ^{18}F-Fluorodeoxyglucos imaging in 27 patients with glioma, most of whom (19/27) were astrocytoma or glial neuroma. The result showed that the accumulation of both ^{18}F-Fluorodeoxyglucos and MET was significantly higher in high-grade than in low-grade tumors. The accumulation of both tracers was associated positively with age. In addition, the Cox proportional hazards regression model suggested that the increased uptake of ^{18}F-Fluorodeoxyglucos and MET was related to the progress of the disease.

BONE AND SOFT TISSUE SARCOMAS

Bone and soft tissue sarcomas account for approximately 10% of malignant diseases in the pediatric population.[106] The most common primary bone tumors are osteosarcoma and Ewing sarcomas. Imaging examinations, including ^{99m}Tc-methylene diphosphonate (MDP), MR imaging, CT, and ^{18}F-Fluorodeoxyglucos PET/CT, are used to determine tumor location, tumor size, bone destruction, periosteal new bone, and tumor margin. Many studies revealed that ^{18}F-sodium fluoride (NaF) PET/CT is significantly superior to ^{99m}Tc-MDP in the detection of osteolytic lesions in the adult population.[107–109] In addition, Jackson and colleagues[110] recruited 21 adult patients with soft tissue and osteosarcoma (13 of whom had metastases) and performed ^{18}F-NaF and ^{18}F-Fluorodeoxyglucos imaging, which showed that ^{18}F-NaF was more suitable for detecting osteogenic lesions, whereas ^{18}F-Fluorodeoxyglucos was more accurate for osteolytic lesions. The potential application of ^{18}F-NaF in the pediatric populations, however, was reported only sparsely.[111,112] The results of further investigation likely will support for the application of ^{18}F-NaF in children.

NONTUMOR DISEASE
Congenital Hyperinsulinemia

Congenital hyperinsulinemia is a common cause of persistent hypoglycemia in neonates and infants, mainly owing to excessive insulin secretion caused by pancreatic β-cell disorder, resulting in severe intractable hypoglycemia.[113] There are 2 distinct types of pancreatic β-cell hyperplasia, focal and diffuse. The 2 different types have different management approach. Accurate localization of focal lesion is paramount in successful treatment in focal form of congenital hyperinsulinemia. Islets have been shown to ingest levodopa and then convert to dopamine. Based on this principle, ^{18}F-DOPA had been successfully used in this setting with high accuracy.[114–116]

Type 1 Diabetes Mellitus

Type 1 diabetes mellitus commonly occurs in childhood and is characterized by a decrease in the number of β cells in the islets of Langerhans of the pancreas due to autoimmune reactions leading to a deficit in subsequent insulin secretion. Therefore, a measurement of the β-cell mass in vivo can improve the monitoring of the therapeutic effect.[117] One study showed that [11]C-(+)-4-propyl-9-hydroxynaphthoxazine (PHNO) can be used as a potential marker to detect β-cell mass.[118] In patients with type 1 diabetes mellitus, there is focally or diffuse decrease of pancreatic PHNO activity.[118] For this reason, PHNO PET/CT could potentially evolve to a PET tracer to evaluate diabetes in children.

Urinary Disorders

Renal scintigraphy is one of the most commonly performed nuclear medicine studies in pediatric patients.[119–123] The quality of the dynamic images acquired using a gamma camera, however, is significantly inferior to that of PET images. 2-deoxy-2-^{18}F-Fluorosorbitol (^{18}F-FDS) has shown favorable renal kinetics in both animal models[124] and humans,[125] with cortical transit and excretion of urine better visualized on PET/CT images.[125] Due to its simple 1-step radiosynthesis via the most frequently used PET radiotracer ^{18}F-Fluorodeoxyglucos, ^{18}F-FDS can be easily available at any PET facility with radiochemistry ability.[126] It is likely that FDS soon will win widespread acceptance in pediatric renal imaging.

SUMMARY

PET/CT is of great value in the diagnosis, staging, therapy evaluation, and recurrence monitoring of many different pediatric diseases (mainly malignant tumors). ^{18}F-Fluorodeoxyglucos, as an indispensable part of imaging modality, is well-established. Many non-^{18}F-Fluorodeoxyglucos tracers, however, which are used in adult populations, also have great potential in pediatric populations. Non-^{18}F-Fluorodeoxyglucos tracers specific to children and adolescents deserve further clinical exploration.

DISCLOSURE

The authors have nothing to disclose.

REFERENCES

1. Toriihara A, Arai A, Nakadate M, et al. FDG-PET/CT findings of chronic active Epstein-Barr virus infection. Leuk Lymphoma 2018;59:1470–3.
2. Kouijzer IJE, Mulders-Manders CM, Bleeker-Rovers CP, et al. Fever of unknown origin: the value of FDG-PET/CT. Semin Nucl Med 2018;48:100–7.
3. Zhuang H, Alavi A. 18-fluorodeoxyglucose positron emission tomographic imaging in the detection and monitoring of infection and inflammation. Semin Nucl Med 2002;32:47–59.
4. Alavi A, Zhuang H. Finding infection–help from PET. Lancet 2001;358:1386.
5. Foret T, Dhomps A, Dauwalder O, et al. FDG PET/CT of Gardnerella vaginalis infection. Clin Nucl Med 2019;44:660–2.
6. Pijl JP, Glaudemans A, Slart R, et al. FDG-PET/CT for detecting an infection focus in patients with bloodstream infection: factors affecting diagnostic yield. Clin Nucl Med 2019;44:99–106.
7. Ran P, Liang X, Zhang Y, et al. FDG PET/CT in a case of bilateral tuberculous epididymo-orchitis. Clin Nucl Med 2019;44:757–60.

8. Altinyay ME, Alharthi A, Alassiri AH, et al. 18F-FDG hypermetabolism in spinal cord schistosomiasis. Clin Nucl Med 2016;41:211–3.

9. Deroose CM, Van Weehaeghe D, Tousseyn T, et al. Diffuse 18F-FDG muscle uptake in trichinella spiralis infection. Clin Nucl Med 2016;41:55–6.

10. Lawal I, Sathekge M. F-18 FDG PET/CT imaging of cardiac and vascular inflammation and infection. Br Med Bull 2016;120:55–74.

11. Hess S, Alavi A, Basu S. PET-based Personalized management of infectious and inflammatory disorders. PET Clin 2016;11:351–61.

12. Son SH, Jeong SY, Lee SW, et al. Primary aspergillosis of the sphenoid sinus observed on bone SPECT/CT. Clin Nucl Med 2018;43:141–3.

13. Xiao Z, Dong A, Wang Y. FDG PET/CT in a case of human african trypanosomiasis (sleeping sickness). Clin Nucl Med 2018;43:619–22.

14. Xiu Y, Zhang J, Shi H. Duodenum cryptococcosis mimicking primary duodenum cancer on PET/CT imaging. Clin Nucl Med 2018;43:335–6.

15. Yu JQ, Kumar R, Xiu Y, et al. Diffuse FDG uptake in the lungs in aspiration pneumonia on positron emission tomographic imaging. Clin Nucl Med 2004;29:567–8.

16. Zhuang H, Chacko TK, Hickeson M, et al. Persistent non-specific FDG uptake on PET imaging following hip arthroplasty. Eur J Nucl Med Mol Imaging 2002;29:1328–33.

17. Basu S, Zhuang H, Alavi A. FDG PET and PET/CT imaging in complicated diabetic foot. PET Clin 2012;7:151–60.

18. Dioguardi P, Gaddam SR, Zhuang H, et al. FDG PET assessment of osteomyelitis: a review. PET Clin 2012;7:161–79.

19. Saboury B, Ziai P, Parsons M, et al. Promising roles of PET in management of arthroplasty-associated infection. PET Clin 2012;7:139–50.

20. Roengvoraphoj O, Pazos-Escudero M, Eze C, et al. 18FDG-PET/CT for the visualization of inflammatory component of radiation-induced lung injury after stereotactic radiotherapy. Clin Nucl Med 2018;43: e87–8.

21. Zhuang H, Duarte PS, Pourdehnad M, et al. The promising role of 18F-FDG PET in detecting infected lower limb prosthesis implants. J Nucl Med 2001;42:44–8.

22. Shao D, Deng YT, Shao FQ, et al. 18F-FDG PET/CT imaging findings of leprosy. Clin Nucl Med 2020 May;;45(5):e236–8.

23. London K, Cross S, Onikul E, et al. 18F-FDG PET/ CT in paediatric lymphoma: comparison with conventional imaging. Eur J Nucl Med Mol Imaging 2011;38:274–84.

24. Cheng G, Servaes S, Zhuang H. Value of (18)F-fluoro-2-deoxy-D-glucose positron emission tomography/computed tomography scan versus diagnostic contrast computed tomography in initial staging of pediatric patients with lymphoma. Leuk Lymphoma 2013;54:737–42.

25. Cheng G, Servaes S, Alavi A, et al. FDG PET and PET/CT in the management of pediatric lymphoma patients. PET Clin 2008;3:621–34.

26. Shankar A, Fiumara F, Pinkerton R. Role of FDG PET in the management of childhood lymphomas - case proven or is the jury still out? Eur J Cancer 2008;44:663–73.

27. Badr S, Kotb M, Elahmadawy MA, et al. Predictive value of FDG PET/CT versus bone marrow biopsy in pediatric lymphoma. Clin Nucl Med 2018;43:e428–38.

28. Cheng G, Chen W, Chamroonrat W, et al. Biopsy versus FDG PET/CT in the initial evaluation of bone marrow involvement in pediatric lymphoma patients. Eur J Nucl Med Mol Imaging 2011;38:1469–76.

29. Canellos GP. Residual mass in lymphoma may not be residual disease. J Clin Oncol 1988;6:931–3.

30. Hill M, Cunningham D, MacVicar D, et al. Role of magnetic resonance imaging in predicting relapse in residual masses after treatment of lymphoma. J Clin Oncol 1993;11:2273–8.

31. Miyazawa H, Arai T, Iio M, et al. PET imaging of non-small-cell lung carcinoma with carbon-11-methionine: relationship between radioactivity uptake and flow-cytometric parameters. J Nucl Med 1993;34:1886–91.

32. Leskinen-Kallio S, Minn H, Joensuu H. PET and [11C]methionine in assessment of response in non-Hodgkin lymphoma. Lancet 1990;336:1188.

33. Annunziata S, Cuccaro A, Caldarella C, et al. 11C-methionine-avid plasmablastic lymphoma. Clin Nucl Med 2017;42:872–3.

34. Annunziata S, Cuccaro A, Rizzo A, et al. Bronchial mucosa-associated lymphoid tissue lymphoma staged by 11C-Methionine. Clin Nucl Med 2018; 43:e276–7.

35. Jang SJ, Lee KH, Lee JY, et al. 11)C-methionine PET/CT and MRI of primary central nervous system diffuse large B-cell lymphoma before and after high-dose methotrexate. Clin Nucl Med 2012;37: e241–4.

36. Ahn SY, Kwon SY, Jung SH, et al. Prognostic significance of Interim 11C-methionine PET/CT in primary central nervous system lymphoma. Clin Nucl Med 2018;43:e259–64.

37. Kaste SC, Snyder SE, Metzger ML, et al. Comparison of ^{11}C-methionine and ^{18}F-FDG PET/CT for staging and follow-up of pediatric lymphoma. J Nucl Med 2017;58:419–24.

38. Leskinen-Kallio S, Ruotsalainen U, Nagren K, et al. Uptake of carbon-11-methionine and fluorodeoxyglucose in non-Hodgkin's lymphoma: a PET study. J Nucl Med 1991;32:1211–8.

39. Nuutinen J, Leskinen S, Lindholm P, et al. Use of carbon-11 methionine positron emission

tomography to assess malignancy grade and predict survival in patients with lymphomas. Eur J Nucl Med 1998;25:729–35.

40. Reske SN, Deisenhofer S. Is 3'-deoxy-3'-18F-fluorothymidine a better marker for tumour response than 18F-fluorodeoxyglucose? Eur J Nucl Med Mol Imaging 2006;33:38–43.

41. Buck AK, Bommer M, Stilgenbauer S, et al. Molecular imaging of proliferation in malignant lymphoma. Cancer Res 2006;66:11055–61.

42. Schöder H, Noy A, Go nen M, et al. Intensity of 18Fluorodeoxyglucose uptake in positron emission tomography distinguishes between indolent and aggressive Non-Hodgkin's lymphoma. J Clin Oncol 2005;23:4643–51.

43. Costantini DL, Vali R, McQuattie S, et al. A pilot study of 18F-FLT PET/CT in pediatric lymphoma. Int J Mol Imaging 2016;2016:6045894.

44. Bar-Sever Z, Biassoni L, Shulkin B, et al. Guidelines on nuclear medicine imaging in neuroblastoma. Eur J Nucl Med Mol Imaging 2018;45:2009–24.

45. Liu B, Servaes S, Zhuang H. SPECT/CT MIBG imaging is crucial in the follow-up of the patients with high-risk neuroblastoma. Clin Nucl Med 2018;43:232–8.

46. Wen Z, Zhuang H. Renal metastasis from neuroblastoma shown on MIBG imaging. Clin Nucl Med 2020;45:87–9.

47. Liu B, Zhuang H, Servaes S. Comparison of [123I] MIBG and [131I]MIBG for imaging of neuroblastoma and other neural crest tumors. Q J Nucl Med Mol Imaging 2013;57:21–8.

48. Rogasch JMM, Amthauer H, Furth C, et al. I-123-MIBG scintigraphy in patients with neuroblastoma. Nuklearmedizin 2018;57:35–9.

49. Theerakulpisut D, Raruenrom Y, Wongsurawat N, et al. Value of SPECT/CT in diagnostic I-131 MIBG Scintigraphy in patients with neuroblastoma. Nucl Med Mol Imaging 2018;52:350–8.

50. Villani MF, D'Andrea ML, Castellano A, et al. Unusual presentation of relapse in neuroblastoma: pancreatic metastases detected by 123I-MIBG scintigraphy. Clin Nucl Med 2017;42:610–1.

51. Zheng K, Zhuang H. Acrometastasis of neuroblastoma to the great toe revealed by MIBG scan. Clin Nucl Med 2017;42:397–400.

52. Xie P, Shao F, Zhuang H. Primary neuroblastoma involving spinal canal. Clin Nucl Med 2016;41:986–8.

53. Zhao X, Zhuang H. Variable MIBG activity in the same renal cyst. Clin Nucl Med 2017;42:887–9.

54. Pirson AS, Krug B, Tuerlinckx D, et al. Additional value of I-123 MIBG SPECT in neuroblastoma. Clin Nucl Med 2005;30:100–1.

55. Yang J, Codreanu I, Servaes S, et al. Persistent intense MIBG activity in the liver caused by prior radiation. Clin Nucl Med 2014;39:926–30.

56. Nadel HR. SPECT/CT in pediatric patient management. Eur J Nucl Med Mol Imaging 2014;41(Suppl 1):S104–14.

57. Belgaumi AF, Kauffman WM, Jenkins JJ, et al. Blindness in children with neuroblastoma. Cancer 1997;80:1997–2004.

58. DuBois SG, Matthay KK. Radiolabeled metaiodobenzylguanidine for the treatment of neuroblastoma. Nucl Med Biol 2008;35:S35–48.

59. Taggart D, Dubois S, Matthay KK. Radiolabeled metaiodobenzylguanidine for imaging and therapy of neuroblastoma. Q J Nucl Med Mol Imaging 2008;52:403–18.

60. Newman EA, Abdessalam S, Aldrink JH, et al. Update on neuroblastoma. J Pediatr Surg 2019;54:383–9.

61. Pandit-Taskar N, Zanzonico P, Staton KD, et al. Biodistribution and dosimetry of 18F-Meta-Fluorobenzylguanidine: a first-in-human PET/CT imaging study of patients with neuroendocrine malignancies. J Nucl Med 2018;59:147–53.

62. Minn H, Kauhanen S, Seppanen M, et al. 18F-FDOPA: a multiple-target molecule. J Nucl Med 2009;50:1915–8.

63. Lu MY, Liu YL, Chang H-H, et al. Characterization of neuroblastic tumors using 18F-FDOPA PET. J Nucl Med 2013;54:42–9.

64. Piccardo A, Lopci E, Conte M, et al. Comparison of 18F-dopa PET/CT and 123I-MIBG scintigraphy in stage 3 and 4 neuroblastoma: a pilot study. Eur J Nucl Med Mol Imaging 2012;39:57–71.

65. Piccardo A, Lopci E, Conte M, et al. Bone and lymph node metastases from neuroblastoma detected by 18F-DOPA-PET/CT and confirmed by posttherapy 131I-MIBG but negative on diagnostic 123I-MIBG scan. Clin Nucl Med 2014;39:e80–3.

66. Piccardo A, Morana G, Puntoni M, et al. Diagnosis, treatment response, and prognosis: the role of (18) F-DOPA PET/CT in children affected by neuroblastoma in comparison with (123)I-mIBG scan: the first prospective study. J Nucl Med 2020;61:367–74.

67. Piccardo A, Puntoni M, Lopci E, et al. Prognostic value of 18F-DOPA PET/CT at the time of recurrence in patients affected by neuroblastoma. Eur J Nucl Med Mol Imaging 2014;41:1046–56.

68. Matthay KK, Shulkin B, Ladenstein R, et al. Criteria for evaluation of disease extent by 123I-metaiodobenzylguanidine scans in neuroblastoma: a report for the international neuroblastoma risk Group (INRG) Task Force. Br J Cancer 2010;102:1319–26.

69. Lopci E, Piccardo A, Nanni C, et al. 18F-DOPA PET/CT in neuroblastoma: comparison of conventional imaging with CT/MR. Clin Nucl Med 2012;37:e73–8.

70. Liu YL, Lu MY, Chang HH, et al. Diagnostic FDG and FDOPA positron emission tomography scans distinguish the genomic type and treatment outcome of neuroblastoma. Oncotarget 2016;7:18774–86.

71. Piccardo A, Morana G, Massollo M, et al. Brain metastasis from neuroblastoma depicted by ^{18}F-DOPA PET/CT. Nucl Med Mol Imaging 2015;49:241–2.

72. Franzius C, Hermann K, Weckesser M, et al. Whole-body PET/CT with ^{11}C-meta-hydroxyephedrine in tumors of the sympathetic nervous system: feasibility study and comparison with ^{123}I-MIBG SPECT/CT. J Nucl Med 2006;47:1635–42.

73. Piccardo A, Lopci E, Conte M, et al. PET/CT imaging in neuroblastoma. Q J Nucl Med Mol Imaging 2013;57:29–39.

74. Shulkin BL, Wieland DM, Baro ME, et al. PET hydroxyephedrine imaging of neuroblastoma. J Nucl Med 1996;37:16–21.

75. Bozkurt MF, Virgolini I, Balogova S, et al. Guideline for PET/CT imaging of neuroendocrine neoplasms with ^{68}Ga-DOTA-conjugated somatostatin receptor targeting peptides and ^{18}F-DOPA. Eur J Nucl Med Mol Imaging 2017;44:1588–601.

76. Albers AR, O'Dorisio MS, Balster DA, et al. Somatostatin receptor gene expression in neuroblastoma. Regul Pept 2000;88:61–73.

77. Kropp J, Hofmann M, Bihl H. Comparison of MIBG and pentetreotide scintigraphy in children with neuroblastoma. Is the expression of somatostatin receptors a prognostic factor? Anticancer Res 1997;17:1583.

78. Shalaby-Rana E, Majd M, Andrich MP, et al. In-111 pentetreotide scintigraphy in patients with neuroblastoma: comparison with 1-131 MIBG, N-Myc oncogene amplification, and patient outcome. Clin Nucl Med 1997;22:315–9.

79. Kroiss A, Putzer D, Uprimny C, et al. Functional imaging in phaeochromocytoma and neuroblastoma with ^{68}Ga-DOTA-Tyr 3-octreotide positron emission tomography and ^{123}I-metaiodobenzylguanidine. Eur J Nucl Med Mol Imaging 2011;38:865–73.

80. Gains JE, Bomanji JB, Fersht NL, et al. ^{177}Lu-DOTATATE molecular radiotherapy for childhood neuroblastoma. J Nucl Med 2011;52:1041–7.

81. Kong G, Hofman MS, Murray WK, et al. Initial experience with Gallium-68 DOTA-Octreotate PET/CT and peptide receptor radionuclide therapy for pediatric patients with refractory metastatic neuroblastoma. J Pediatr Hematol Oncol 2016;38:87–96.

82. Archier A, Varoquaux A, Garrigue P, et al. Prospective comparison of (68)Ga-DOTATATE and (18)F-FDOPA PET/CT in patients with various pheochromocytomas and paragangliomas with emphasis on sporadic cases. Eur J Nucl Med Mol Imaging 2016;43:1248–57.

83. Barrio M, Czernin J, Fanti S, et al. The impact of somatostatin receptor-directed PET/CT on the management of patients with neuroendocrine tumor: a systematic review and meta-analysis. J Nucl Med 2017;58:756–61.

84. Banezhad F, Kiamanesh Z, Emami F, et al. 68Ga DOTATATE PET/CT versus 18F-FDG PET/CT for detecting intramedullary hemangioblastoma in a patient with Von Hippel-Lindau disease. Clin Nucl Med 2019;44:e385–7.

85. Zhang J, Zhu Z, Zhong D, et al. 68Ga DOTATATE PET/CT is an accurate imaging modality in the detection of culprit tumors causing osteomalacia. Clin Nucl Med 2015;40:642–6.

86. Ding J, Hu G, Wang L, et al. Increased activity due to fractures does not significantly affect the accuracy of 68Ga-DOTATATE PET/CT in the detection of culprit tumor in the evaluation of tumor-induced osteomalacia. Clin Nucl Med 2018;43:880–6.

87. Diwaker C, Shah RK, Patil V, et al. 68Ga-DOTATATE PET/CT of ectopic cushing syndrome due to appendicular carcinoid. Clin Nucl Med 2019;44:881–2.

88. Wen Z, Edwards KW, States LJ, et al. Heat-damaged red blood cell scintigraphy in helping interpretation of 68Ga-DOTATATE PET/CT. Clin Nucl Med 2019;44:927–8.

89. Lu Y. Imaging characteristics of coexisting primary pulmonary carcinoid tumor and multiple myeloma on 18F-FDG and 68Ga-DOTATATE PET/CT. Clin Nucl Med 2019;44:914–5.

90. Yamaga LYI, Cunha ML, Campos Neto GC, et al. 68)Ga-DOTATATE PET/CT in recurrent medullary thyroid carcinoma: a lesion-by-lesion comparison with (111)In-octreotide SPECT/CT and conventional imaging. Eur J Nucl Med Mol Imaging 2017;44:1695–701.

91. Nockel P, Babic B, Millo C, et al. Localization of Insulinoma using 68Ga-DOTATATE PET/CT scan. J Clin Endocrinol Metab 2017;102:195–9.

92. Jing H, Li F, Wang L, et al. Comparison of the 68Ga-DOTATATA PET/CT, FDG PET/CT, and MIBG SPECT/CT in the evaluation of suspected primary pheochromocytomas and paragangliomas. Clin Nucl Med 2017;42:525–9.

93. Haug AR, Cindea-Drimus R, Auernhammer CJ, et al. Neuroendocrine tumor recurrence: diagnosis with 68Ga-DOTATATE PET/CT. Radiology 2014;270:517–25.

94. Goel R, Shukla J, Bansal D, et al. ^{68}Ga-DOTATATE positron emission tomography/computed tomography scan in the detection of bone metastases in pediatric neuroendocrine tumors. Indian J Nucl Med 2014;29:13–7.

95. Karageorgiadis AS, Papadakis GZ, Biro J, et al. Ectopic adrenocorticotropic hormone and corticotropin-releasing hormone co-secreting tumors in children and adolescents causing cushing syndrome: a diagnostic dilemma and

how to solve it. J Clin Endocrinol Metab 2015;100: 141–8.

96. Jha A, de Luna K, Balili CA, et al. Clinical, diagnostic, and treatment characteristics of SDHA-related metastatic pheochromocytoma and paraganglioma. Front Oncol 2019;9:53.

97. Jha A, Ling A, Millo C, et al. Superiority of (68)Ga-DOTATATE over (18)F-FDG and anatomic imaging in the detection of succinate dehydrogenase mutation (SDHx)-related pheochromocytoma and paraganglioma in the pediatric population. Eur J Nucl Med Mol Imaging 2018;45:787–97.

98. Linabery AM, Ross JA. Trends in childhood cancer incidence in the US (1992-2004). Cancer 2008; 112:416–32.

99. Morana G, Piccardo A, Puntoni M, et al. Diagnostic and prognostic value of 18F-DOPA PET and 1H-MR spectroscopy in pediatric supratentorial infiltrative gliomas: a comparative study. Neuro Oncol 2015; 17:1637–47.

100. Morana G, Piccardo A, Milanaccio C, et al. Value of ^{18}F-3,4-dihydroxyphenylalanine PET/MR image fusion in pediatric supratentorial infiltrative astrocytomas: a prospective pilot study. J Nucl Med 2014; 55:718–23.

101. Morana G, Puntoni M, Garre ML, et al. Ability of ^{18}F-DOPA PET/CT and fused ^{18}F-DOPA PET/MRI to assess striatal involvement in paediatric glioma. Eur J Nucl Med Mol Imaging 2016;43:1664–72.

102. Dunkl V, Cleff C, Stoffels G, et al. NI-19 the use of dynamic O-(2-^{18}F]fluoroethyl)-L-tyrosine-PET in the clinical evaluation of brain tumors in children and adolescents. Neuro Oncol 2014;16:v142.

103. Messing-Junger AM, Floeth FW, Pauleit D, et al. Multimodal target point assessment for stereotactic biopsy with diffuse bithalamic in children astrocytomas. Childs Nerv Syst 2002;18:445–9.

104. Marner L, Nysom K, Sehested A, et al. Early postoperative ^{18}F-FET PET/MRI for pediatric brain and spinal cord tumors. J Nucl Med 2019;60: 1053–8.

105. Utriainen M, Metsahonkala L, Salmi TT, et al. Metabolic characterization of childhood brain tumors: comparison of ^{18}F-fluorodeoxyglucose and ^{11}C-methionine positron emission tomography. Cancer 2002;95:1376–86.

106. Siegel RL, Miller KD, Jemal A. Cancer statistics, 2019. CA Cancer J Clin 2019;69:7–34.

107. Even-Sapir E, Metser U, Flusser G, et al. Assessment of malignant skeletal disease: initial experience with ^{18}F-fluoride PET/CT and comparison between ^{18}F-fluoride PET and ^{18}F-fluoride PET/CT. J Nucl Med 2004;45:272–8.

108. Iagaru A, Mittra E, Mosci C, et al. Combined ^{18}F-fluoride and ^{18}F-FDG PET/CT scanning for evaluation of malignancy: results of an international multicenter trial. J Nucl Med 2013;54:176–83.

109. Bortot DC, Amorim BARJ, Oki GC, et al. ^{18}F-Fluoride PET/CT is highly effective for excluding bone metastases even in patients with equivocal bone scintigraphy. Eur J Nucl Med Mol Imaging 2012; 39:1730–6.

110. Jackson T, Mosci C, von Eyben R, et al. Combined ^{18}F-NaF and ^{18}F-FDG PET/CT in the evaluation of sarcoma patients. Clin Nucl Med 2015;40: 720–4.

111. Usmani S, Marafi F, Rasheed R, et al. Targeted therapy with anaplastic lymphoma kinase inhibitor (Alectinib) in adolescent metastatic non-small cell lung carcinoma: 18F-NaF PET/CT in response evaluation. Clin Nucl Med 2018;43:752–4.

112. Drubach LA. Pediatric bone scanning: clinical indication of (18)F NaF PET/CT. PET Clin 2012;7: 293–301.

113. Pellicano R, De Angelis C, Resegotti A, et al. Zollinger-Ellison syndrome in 2006: concepts from a clinical point of view. Panminerva Med 2006;48: 33–40.

114. Mohnike K, Blankenstein O, Christesen HT, et al. Proposal for a standardized protocol for ^{18}F-DOPA-PET (PET/CT) in congenital hyperinsulinism. Horm Res 2006;66:40–2.

115. Hardy OT, Hernandez-Pampaloni M, Saffer JR, et al. Accuracy of [18F]fluorodopa positron emission tomography for diagnosing and localizing focal congenital hyperinsulinism. J Clin Endocrinol Metab 2007;92:4706–11.

116. Cherubini V, Bagalini LS, Ianilli A, et al. Rapid genetic analysis, imaging with 18F-DOPA-PET/CT scan and laparoscopic surgery in congenital hyperinsulinism. J Pediatr Endocrinol Metab 2010; 23:171–7.

117. Steele C, Hagopian WA, Gitelman S, et al. Insulin secretion in type 1 diabetes. Diabetes 2004;53: 426–33.

118. Bini J, Naganawa M, Nabulsi N, et al. Evaluation of PET brain radioligands for imaging pancreatic beta-cell mass: potential utility of [11]C-(+)-PHNO. J Nucl Med 2018;59:1249–54.

119. Kandur Y, Salan A, Guler AG, et al. Diuretic renography in hydronephrosis: a retrospective single-center study. Int Urol Nephrol 2018;50:1199–204.

120. Sfakianakis GN, Carmona AJ, Sharma A, et al. Diuretic MAG3 scintirenography in children with HIV nephropathy: diffuse parenchymal dysfunction. J Nucl Med 2000;41:1037–42.

121. Othman S, Al-Hawas A, Al-Maqtari R. Renal cortical imaging in children: 99mTc MAG3 versus 99mTc DMSA. Clin Nucl Med 2012;37:351–5.

122. Arena S, Chimenz R, Antonelli E, et al. A long-term follow-up in conservative management of unilateral ureteropelvic junction obstruction with poor drainage and good renal function. Eur J Pediatr 2018;177:1761–5.

123. Liu B, Kaplan SL, Zhuang H. Suspected urine leak in a pediatric renal transplant patient with prune belly syndrome. Clin Nucl Med 2016;41:257–8.

124. Werner RA, Wakabayashi H, Chen X, et al. Functional renal imaging with 2-Deoxy-2-(18)F-Fluorosorbitol PET in rat models of renal disorders. J Nucl Med 2018;59:828–32.

125. Werner RA, Ordonez AA, Sanchez-Bautista J, et al. Novel functional renal PET imaging with 18F-FDS in human subjects. Clin Nucl Med 2019;44:410–1.

126. Werner RA, Chen X, Lapa C, et al. The next era of renal radionuclide imaging: novel PET radiotracers. Eur J Nucl Med Mol Imaging 2019;46: 1773–86.

Emerging Roles of PET/MR in the Pediatric Hospital

Sandra Saade-Lemus, MD[a,c], Sara R. Teixeira, MD, PhD[a], Arastoo Vossough, MD, PhD[a,b], Sabah Servaes, MD[a,b,c], Lisa J. States, MD[a,b,c],*

KEYWORDS

- PET/MR imaging • Pediatrics • Oncology • Radiation dose

KEY POINTS

- PET/MR is increasingly available in pediatric hospitals.
- The main clinical applications of PET/MR are in oncology and epilepsy imaging.
- Emerging applications in pediatric imaging are infectious disease, inflammatory conditions, and neuropsychiatric development.
- PET/MR currently is not replacing PET/computed tomography: each modality has advantages and limitations.
- Improvement of scan time is an ongoing challenge.

INTRODUCTION

PET/MR imaging currently is available in more than 100 sites worldwide.[1] Beyond research applications, potential clinical applications of the modality have expanded in both adult and pediatric imaging to assess oncologic, inflammatory, and infectious conditions. This hybrid modality combines the high soft tissue resolution and characterization of MR, especially valuable in the assessment of brain, liver, pelvis, and musculoskeletal conditions, with the metabolic information provided by PET.

PET/MR repeatedly has shown comparable image quality and strong correlation of standardized uptake value (SUV) measurements with PET/computed tomography (CT).[2] In addition, PET/MR has shown a reduction in radiation dose compared with PET/CT as well as the possibility of radiotracer dose reduction without compromising diagnostic image quality.[3] Given the concern of increased susceptibility to ionizing radiation in children and adolescents, the clinical value of PET/MR has been studied in pediatric conditions, especially when there is a need for patients to undergo multiple imaging scans, such as in oncology.[3,4] Nonetheless, PET/MR still needs to be explored for the multicapability of MR imaging—high tissue contrast and anatomic, functional, and even molecular characterization of tissues.[5]

PET/MR began to be used clinically in 2010, and consensus recommendations on adult 18F-fluorodeoxyglucose (18F-FDG) PET/MR whole-body staging in oncology have been published, emphasizing the need for adequate patient preparation to reduce tracer uptake in normal tissue, for identification of artifacts, and for standardized imaging protocols.[6,7] Nonetheless, protocols for the pediatric population have continued to be variable according to each institution, with no standardized acquisition protocol for children[1] (see **Table 1** for the protocol the authors use).

This review describes the existent PET/MR studies performed in children for oncologic and nononcologic conditions, emphasizing the need for multi-institutional collaborations to achieve greater cohort numbers in specific conditions,

[a] Radiology Department, Children's Hospital of Philadelphia, 3401 Civic Center Boulevard, Philadelphia, PA 19104, USA; [b] Perelman School of Medicine, University of Pennsylvania, Philadelphia, PA, 19104, USA; [c] Section of Oncologic Imaging, Radiology Department, Children's Hospital of Philadelphia, 3401 Civic Center Boulevard, Philadelphia, PA 19104, USA
* Corresponding author.
E-mail address: states@email.chop.edu

PET Clin 15 (2020) 253–269
https://doi.org/10.1016/j.cpet.2020.03.005
1556-8598/20/© 2020 Elsevier Inc. All rights reserved.

Table 1
Sample PET/MR protocol from The Children's Hospital of Philadelphia (GE Signa PET/MR)

MR Imaging Component

Sequence	Plane	Repetition Time (msec)	Echo Time (msec)	Inversion Time (msec)	Matrix	Section Thickness (mm)	Section Gap (mm)
Whole-body localizer	3 planes	Minimum	80	TI	288 × 160	10	5
MRAC	Axial	4	1.6	N/A	256 × 128	5.2	2.6
3D T1 LAVA-Flex	Axial	4	Minimum	N/A	288 × 224	4	0
2D T2 Dixon	*Axial*	*2*	*15*	*NA*	*256 × 256*	*VARIABLE 4–5*	*0*
DWI	Axial	5500	Minimum	249	128 × 160	0	0
Additional sequences:							
T2 FRFSE	Axial	Non-gated	80	N/A	320 × 224	4	0.4
Spinal STIR	Cor	2000–6500	42	190	320 × 224	3	0

PET Component

Sequence	Acquisition Time per Bed Position	Iterative Reconstruction Algorithm	No. of Iterations	No. of Subsets	Axial Field of View (mm)	Voxel Size (mm3)	Image Grid
PET	3–4	VUE Point FX	2	28	600	9.69	192 * 192

Abbreviations: CHOP, children's hospital of philadelphia; mse, millisecond; Cor, coronal; MRAC, magnetic resonance-based attenuation correction; N/A, non applicable; 3D, three dimensional; T1, T1-weighted; LAVA, liver acquisition with volume acquisition; DWI, diffusion-weighted imaging; T2, T2-weighted; FRFSE, fast relaxation fast spin echo sequence; STIR, short-TI inversion recovery; PET, positron emission tomography; VUE Point FX, GE Healthcare time-of-flight.

and discusses the relevance of PET/MR and potential controversy surrounding it replacing PET/CT. Additionally, potential applications of PET/MR in the near future are outlined.

Studies have been carried out to compare simultaneous PET/MR with sequential PET/MR with software image fusion, and PET/CT, demonstrating equivalent diagnostic accuracy as well as improved delineation of many lesions with PET/MR.[8–11] The staffing, planning, and cost challenges of implementing PET/MR on the pediatric hospital are described elsewhere.[12]

PET/MR IN PEDIATRIC NEUROIMAGING

The first simultaneous clinical PET/MR was tailored to imaging of the brain.[13] Use of MR is widespread in brain imaging due to the high soft tissue resolution and functional capabilities of this modality, and it is natural to combine PET and MR imaging for evaluation of brain disease. 18F-FDG is the most widely used Food and Drug Administration–approved radiotracer used for pediatric brain imaging. There is high normal 18F-FDG uptake of the normal brain parenchyma,

however, which may limit the utility in many instances. This has prompted investigational use of different radiotracers to better identify brain lesions, particularly for tumor evaluations.[14]

MR acquisition in PET/MR brain imaging protocols usually includes a T1-weighted Dixon sequence for PET attenuation correction in combination with CT-based atlas or an attenuation correction map generated from zero echo time images. Standard MR sequences otherwise are performed, with selective addition of advanced imaging sequences tailored to the disease and clinical questions. Perfusion-weighted imaging, MR spectroscopy, functional MR imaging, and diffusion tensor imaging can provide complementary information for further evaluation and management planning of brain tumors, whereas including high-resolution isotropic T1-weighted imaging, coronal T2-weighted imaging, and fluid-attenuation inversion recovery may facilitate imaging of epileptic foci.[15]

Epilepsy

Diagnosis of epileptic lesions using MR imaging only may be challenging in the pediatric population, where common etiologies, such as some forms of cortical dysplasia, may not be evident.[16] PET, on the other hand, may be helpful in showing epileptogenic zones, such as cortical dysplasia using 18F-FDG, by demonstrating lesions as areas of hypometabolism[17–19] (**Fig. 1**).

The diagnostic accuracy of PET/MR has shown to be at least comparable to that of PET/CT for localization of seizure focus in pediatric patients.[20] There is evidence of relative high sensitivity of PET and PET/MR in detecting cortical dysplasia in patients with nonlesional MR imaging.[19,21–23] Relatedly, Salamon and colleagues[24] described the benefit of using PET/MR to identify these lesions in addition to providing high anatomic resolution that allows delineation of the lesion to aid in presurgical planning.

Rubi and colleagues[21] evaluated the use of fused 18F-FDG PET and MR imaging in 31 children with medically intractable epilepsy and brain MR imaging deemed as normal or nonlesional who underwent presurgical evaluation. They demonstrated that stand-alone PET and PET/MR both had good concordance in diagnostic accuracy of epileptogenic zones in pediatric patients with nonlesional epilepsy. This included PET/MR concordance evaluation not only with PET alone but also with electroencephalography and postsurgical pathology and outcomes. The investigators used PET/MR fusion images, obtained from PET/CT PET information and brain MR imaging. A similar study using hybrid PET/MR imaging would be highly valuable.

In these times of stereotactic neuronavigation guided surgery, the anatomic resolution provided by the MR component in PET/MR is crucial in evaluating potentially resectable epileptogenic areas. It is highly relevant to try to define the anatomic boundaries of the hypometabolic area to improve effective resection and decrease recurrence of seizures. PET/MR also can show extensive hypometabolic regions or involvement of eloquent areas, helping in identifying patients who may not fully benefit from surgery.[25]

Neuro-oncology

Central nervous system neoplasms are the most common and among the highest mortality solid tumors in pediatric patients. The first study comparing the feasibility of PET/MR with PET/CT was performed in the setting of central nervous system tumors.[26] Although 18F-FDG-PET is still used uncommonly for preoperative characterization of brain masses, it is utilized more commonly in posttreatment evaluation of brain tumors, such as assessment of radiation necrosis versus tumor

progression or trying to distinguish true progression versus pseudoprogression. Nevertheless, new PET tracers are currently used to increase accuracy by overcoming the limitation imposed by normal high glucose uptake in the brain and for molecular and functional characterization of tumors.[27] They include tracers to serve as markers of tumor amino acid transport and protein synthesis (such as 11C-methionine, 18F-fluoroethyltyrosine [18F-FET], and 18F-fluorodopa), markers of tumor proliferation rate (18F-fluorothymidine), and markers of tumor oxygen metabolism (18F-fluoromisonidazole).[28] Although these newer radiotracers increasingly are used in adults with brain tumors, there is a paucity of evidence in the pediatric population. Pirotte and colleagues[29] found value in the use of 11C-methionine PET or 18F-FDG PET in 20 children during the early postoperative period in order to guide management and second-look surgery. Marner and colleagues[30] evaluated the use of 18F-FET–PET/MR in the early postoperative assessment of brain and spinal cord tumors in pediatric patients. The study included low-grade gliomas, such as pilocytic astrocytomas and spinal gangliogliomas, among others. 18F-FET–PET/MR images not only had high diagnostic accuracy but also aided in identifying additional residual tumor sites.[30]

PET/MR IN PEDIATRIC BODY IMAGING
Solid Tumor Disease

Patients with oncologic disease usually are assessed with sequential scanning, including local MR imaging, PET or PET/CT, whole-body MR imaging, and chest CT.[4] PET/MR has shown promising results in differentiating tumor recurrence from tissue changes secondary to radiation therapy.[3] 18F-FDG is the most widely used tracer in pediatric body oncology because most tumors have increased glucose utilization compared with surrounding healthy cells.[31–33] In addition, it can be used to distinguish benign from malignant disease (**Fig. 2**).

Histiocytosis
Overproduction of histiocytes, a type of white blood cells, causes diseases of varying severity and prognosis categorized as pediatric histiocytic disorders, with more than 100 subtypes described.[34] Langerhans cell histiocytosis (LCH), the most common subtype, presents with multiorgan disease and can occur at any age but affects younger children, in particular, with a median age at diagnosis of 3 years.[35] LCH and less common subtypes, such as Rosai-Dorfman disease, also known as sinus histiocytosis with massive

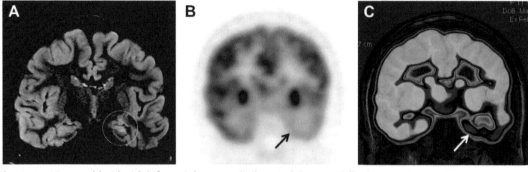

Fig. 1. An 11-year-old girl with left mesial temporal sclerosis. (*A*) Coronal fluid attenuation inversion recovery image shows small left hippocampus with associated T2-weighted hyperintensity (*circle*). (*B*) Coronal 18F-FDG–PET and (*C*) PET/MR fused image show significant hypometabolism in the region of the medial and inferomedial left temporal lobe (*arrows*).

lymphadenopathy, and Erdheim-Chester disease, have been evaluated with 18F-FDG–PET/CT.[36-38] PET and PET/CT show increased characterization of disease and treatment response compared with the multimodal approach used before hybrid imaging, including radiographic skeletal surveys, MR imaging, and CT.[39,40]

Given the decreased radiation dose possible with 18F-FDG–PET/MR, the modality has been demonstrated as a feasible alternative to PET/CT by Sher and colleagues[41] at Texas Children's Hospital (Houston, Texas). The study included 9 patients with a mean age of 6.2 years with LCH or Rosai-Dorfman disease referred to PET/CT. A total of 17 scans were included, accounting for subjects with multiple examinations, with most of them undergoing PET/MR first after the radiotracer injection, followed by PET/CT, with constant time per bed position for the 2 modalities in all examinations to decrease variability. Most subjects had bone and lymph nodes as primary tumor site and the most common indication for the examinations was treatment monitoring.[41] Image quality and identification of active disease were comparable. Differing workflow and attenuation correction algorithms did not have a significant impact on SUV measurements and these were strongly correlated for both modalities.[41] This study opens the door for further investigation of PET/MR as an alternative for the assessment of patients with histiocytosis with comparable diagnostic performance and less radiation, specifically in children who undergo repeated imaging and are highly susceptible to radiation.

In addition, compromise of liver, spleen, and bone marrow is associated with increased

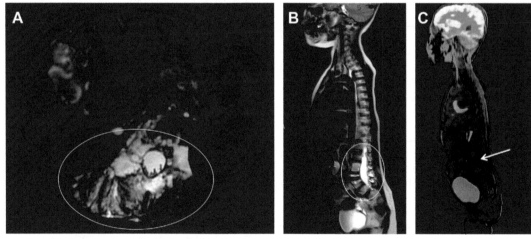

Fig. 2. An 8-year-old boy with Gorham-Stout disease with worsening pain in lumbar region concerning for malignancy. (*A*) Axial T2-weighted with fat saturation and (*B*) sagittal T2-weighted MR image show lymphangiomatosis involving the paraspinal musculature and lumbar vertebrae (*circles*). (*C*) Sagittal Dixon T1-weighted water-only fused PET/MR image shows no hypermetabolic activity in the lumbar spine lesion (*arrow*).

mortality in LCH[42] and the high soft tissue contrast and variety of tailored sequences provided by MR imaging offer diagnostic benefit. Thus, the efforts to transition to PET/MR in the diagnosis and treatment monitoring of this disease can be useful especially in cases of high-risk LCH.

Melanoma

Even though melanoma usually presents at ages 55 to 64 and is uncommon in children, it is the second most common cancer in adolescents and the most common cancer in young adults, and is part of the presentation of genetic syndromes, such as Wiskott-Aldrich and xeroderma pigmentosa.[43]

The optimal imaging modality for malignant melanoma is still undetermined. Imaging work-up of melanoma varies depending on cutaneous or noncutaneous presentation, with different techniques providing complementary information and differing effectiveness in disease evaluation, such as multiphoton microscopy, high-frequency ultrasonography, PET, and MR for cutaneous melanoma.[44] For noncutaneous disease, ultrasound has shown high sensitivity and high specificity for regional lymph nodes, whereas PET/CT has shown the most sensitive and specific imaging modality for distant metastases. PET and CT have proved useful in the assessment of occult metastasis in those with advanced melanoma, namely stages III and IV, and in patients with palpable lymph nodes to determine need for surgery.[45]

Nonetheless, in a cohort of 21 pediatric patients with a median age of 14 years (range 3.2–22.1 years) with cutaneous melanoma, a median of 8 PET/CT scans per patient were performed, and based on disease severity patients could undergo PET/CT up to every 2 months.[46] The study showed an average of 108.8 mSv accumulated ionizing radiation over 35 months when combining all imaging modalities, including PET/CT and dedicated CT scans of chest, abdomen, and pelvis. The accumulated radiation exposure with repeated imaging in this population opens the possibility for PET/MR to be used as an alternative in cutaneous and noncutaneous melanoma in pediatric patients.

Neuroblastoma

Neuroblastoma is the most common extracranial malignancy in pediatric patients.[47] Most neuroblastomas arise in the retroperitoneum; thus, PET/MR with the high anatomic resolution and characterization of soft tissue may be helpful in early detection of these tumors.

For neuroblastoma, 123I-metaiodobenzylguanidine (123I-MIBG) imaging is preferred to 18F-FDG

due to higher specificity.[48] 18F-FDG is less specific; however, it has a role in the evaluation of MIBG-nonavid tumors and is indicated for staging, evaluation of treatment response, follow-up, and differentiating residual disease from post-therapeutic changes.[49] Thus, 18F-FDG–PET/MR can be an alternative to PET/CT in cases of indeterminate, poor, or absent take-up of MIBG.[50] Gallium 68 (Ga-68) dotatate also has been shown to have uptake in neuroblastoma, due to the presence of somatostatin receptor type 2, and can provide an alternative diagnostic agent for MIBG-nonavid neuroblastoma and has the added benefit of a complementary therapeutic agent, Lutetium (Lu-177) dotatate (Lutathera).[51] A promising investigational radiotracer is 18F-MFBG, a PET analog of I123MIBG, which has improved imaging characteristics with higher resolution compared with 123I-MIBG single-photon emission CT/CT.[52] As with 18F-FDG, PET/MR can be substituted for PET/CT.

Sarcoma

Sarcomas encompass 10% to 13% of pediatric malignancies.[53] Rhabdomyosarcoma occurs mostly in young children and nonrhabdomyosarcomas present in infants and adolescents[54] (**Fig. 3**). Because the most common site of metastasis is the lung, imaging work-up includes chest imaging. PET/MR has shown comparable to conventional techniques of CT and MR in the initial staging of sarcoma in adults.[55]

Similarly, 18F-FDG–PET has clinical value in the initial staging of children with soft tissue sarcoma, as demonstrated by Elmanzalawy and colleagues,[56] at the Hospital for Sick Children in Toronto, Canada, comparing the diagnostic value of this modality only with CT and MR imaging in 26 patients. Further investigations of PET/MR in pediatric sarcoma are necessary; nonetheless, Hirsch and colleagues[4] included 2 children with soft tissue sarcoma and 1 with Ewing sarcoma for analysis, where PET/MR showed a technical success rate of 100%. However, study cohorts addressing the role of PET/MR in pediatric sarcoma are scarce and still necessary.

Lymphoma

All pediatric lymphomas have a high metabolism and have been shown 18F-FDG-avid, benefitting especially from imaging assessment with PET.[57] Negative imaging findings in both Hodgkin lymphoma and non-Hodgkin lymphoma are reliable indicators of favorable clinical outcome and determine treatment. Thus, 18F-FDG–PET/CT has been used in staging evaluations of lymphoma in children, and study of the diagnostic performance of

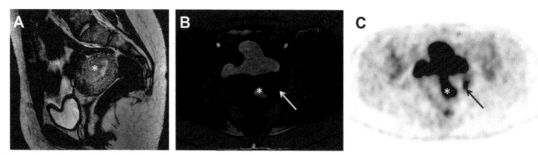

Fig. 3. A 15-year-old girl referred for initial imaging evaluation of a uterine rhabdomyosarcoma. (*A*) Sagittal T2-weighted MR image shows an irregular mass infiltrating the uterine wall and occupying the uterine cavity (*asterisk*). (*B*) Fused PET/MR Dixon T1-weighted water-only image and (*C*) axial attenuation corrected PET image show hypermetabolic activity in the uterine endometrial cavity (*asterisk*) corresponding to mass (*asterisk*) seen on pelvic MR imaging. There also is a common left iliac lymph node concerning for metastatic disease (*arrows*).

PET/MR has garnered attention in pediatric lymphoma over the past years[58–60] (**Figs. 4–6**).

In the initial clinical experience of PET/MR in children at the University Hospital Leipzig, Germany, Hirsch and colleagues[4] evaluated 6 children with lymphoma, including 2 in whom the interpretation of PET/MR scans resulted in restaging of disease. In malignant lymph nodes specifically, 18F-FDG–PET/MR has shown comparable or superior diagnostic sensitivity compared with PET/

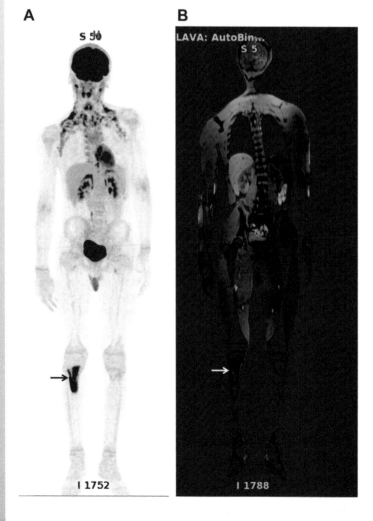

Fig. 4. A 12-year-old boy with diffuse large B-cell lymphoma. One month of right knee pain without improvement after treatment of osteomyelitis suggested on radiographs (not shown). Biopsy confirmed primary diffuse large B-cell lymphoma of the tibia. (*A*) Maximum intensity projection and (*B*) coronal 18F-FDG–PET/MR Dixon T1-weighted water-only fused image show a hypermetabolic lesion in the right proximal tibia (*arrows*) with no metastatic disease. Note brown fat activation along neck, supraclavicular, axillary, costovertebral junction, and supra-adrenal regions.

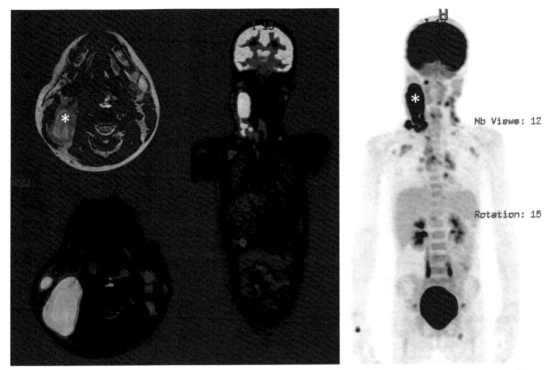

Fig. 5. A 9-year-old girl with ataxia telangiectasia and right neck mass proved to be diffuse large B-cell lymphoma. Axial T2-weighted MR image shows a heterogeneous, increased T2-weighted signal right neck mass (asterisk) lateral to carotid sheath and multiple bilateral cervical lymph nodes. Axial and coronal 18F-FDG–PET/MR Dixon T2-weighted water-only fused image shows a large right hypermetabolic conglomerate lymph node mass with associated right-sided hypermetabolic cervical adenopathy and bilateral supraclavicular adenopathy. Hypermetabolic adenopathy also is seen in the right paratracheal mediastinum, retropectoral. Maximum intensity projection shows additional hypermetabolic lymph adenopathy in the left retropectoral, subcarinal, azygoesophageal recess and bilateral hila, peripancreatic, bilateral iliac, and left inguinal region.

CT in adult patients.[61] Hirsch and colleagues'[4] initial experience shows the complementary information provided by each modality, with the case of 1 child being upstaged when borderline nodes as observed on MR showed increased uptake suspicious of malignancy, whereas studies in adults have shown the MR component to be useful in cases of low or equivocal uptake of 18F-FDG in the tumor tissue in lymphoma.[61]

Sher and colleagues[58] evaluated 25 children with a mean age of 14.6 years (SD 3.9) undergoing PET/CT and sequential PET/MR scans after one 18F-FDG radiotracer injection. There was no difference in disease staging between modalities, and a strong correlation was shown between SUV measurements with each.[58] In addition, Ponisio and colleagues[59] showed PET/MR clinically feasible and comparable to PET/CT in 8 children with a mean age of 15.3 years. SUVs showed a statistically significant correlation between modalities, even more so in highly 18F-FDG-avid lesions, as well as a significant decrease of 39% in average radiation exposure compared with low-dose PET/CT.[59] This study emphasizes only 1 of the main

advantages of PET/MR imaging over PET/CT—reduce ionizing radiation exposure in children undergoing multiple examinations.

Neurofibromatosis type 1

Patients with neurofibromatosis type 1 develop a variety of multisystem manifestations, including central and peripheral nervous system tumors. A subset of patients develops widespread plexiform neurofibromas in the body. There is an approximately 10% lifetime risk of transformation to malignant peripheral nerve sheath tumors (MPNSTs) in these plexiform neurofibromas (**Fig. 7**). MR imaging detection of MPNSTs often can be challenging given the variable imaging appearance. Abnormally rapid interval growth and development of necrosis are some of the potential warning signs, but these are variable and not very specific. 18F-FDG-PET/MR imaging can be helpful in evaluation of lesions suspicious for MPNSTs using either specific SUV thresholds or dynamic PET.[62,63] Use of newer tracers and diffusion imaging on PET/MR may provide increased accuracy for this entity.

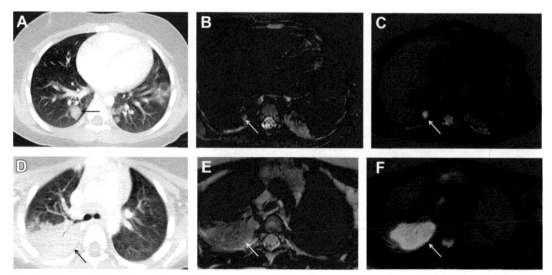

Fig. 6. A 3-year-old boy 9 months post–liver transplant with progressing pneumonia without improvement after 1 month of treatment. Biopsy confirmed post-transplant lymphoproliferative disorder. Axial CT (*left column*) and axial short-TI inversion recovery images (*middle column*) show consolidation and lung nodule in the right lower lobe (*arrows*) and left upper lobe. Fused PET/MR images (*right column*) show hypermetabolic activity within these areas. Left lower lobe lesions on CT were located within atelectasis. The inflammatory process in the lingula has mild FDG uptake. Also noted is activity in the retrosternal anterior mediastinum and right paratracheal region. Axillary lymph nodes do not have increased activity.

Infectious and Inflammatory Conditions

Osteomyelitis

When conventional methods fail to localize infection, PET/MR may play an important role in cases of osteomyelitis, commonly of hematogenous origin in the pediatric population.[64] In a study of 6 children with confirmed osteomyelitis and prolonged use of antibiotics, 18F-PET/CT was proved superior to MR imaging alone to differentiate reparative tissue from persistent foci of osteomyelitis.[65] The same investigators point out that PET/MR imaging could be an alternative in pediatric patients, due to ionizing radiation exposure. Another group showed that PET/CT helped diagnose osteomyelitis in a child with occult bacterial infection.[66] MR imaging has become the imaging choice for diagnosing osteomyelitis with a level of evidence A2.[67] Therefore, PET/MR imaging is expected to exceed PET/CT in this setting, given the higher sensitivity of MR imaging compared with CT alone to detect foci of osteomyelitis, depict abnormal inflammatory bone conditions, and accurately show the extent of disease to soft tissues (**Figs. 8** and **9**).

Inflammatory bowel disease

Intestinal peristalsis may result in miss-registration artifacts in sequential acquisition of images; thus, simultaneous PET/MR not only improves the evaluation of bowel wall thickening but also may reduce artifacts due to motion and peristalsis.[68]

Patients with Crohn disease typically are young and incidence in children is increasing.[69,70] These patients undergo multiple scans throughout their lifetimes and thus benefit from the reduction in radiation dose associated with performing PET/MR instead of PET/CT. Preoperative PET/MR enterography has been shown accurate for assessing Crohn disease lesions, with a higher clinical impact than its PET/CT counterpart.[71,72]

Catalano and colleagues[73] recently evaluated the diagnostic performance of PET/MR in 19 subjects who underwent abdominal surgery. The image was PET/MR enterography, with patients drinking polyethylene glycol–based negative oral solution 2 hours before imaging, and 18F-FDG, with a mean dose of 4.44 MBq/kg, was injected intravenously. The investigators used an integrated PET/MR system (Biograph mMR, Siemens, Harleysville, PA). After evaluating 105 bowel segments and comparing imaging results with intraoperative findings as the standard of reference, PET/MR showed greater diagnostic accuracy than either PET or MR alone.[73]

DISCUSSION

PET/MR increasingly is used in assessment of pediatric patients with varied oncologic and nononcologic indications due to advantages, such as decreased radiation exposure and higher soft tissue contrast resolution. In addition, longer

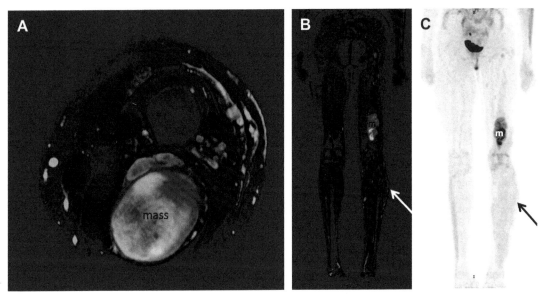

Fig. 7. A 15-year-old boy with neurofibromatosis and a fast-growing left thigh mass consistent with MPNST. (*A*) Axial and (*B*) coronal fused PET/MR short-TI inversion recovery images and (*C*) coronal maximum intensity projection show a hypermetabolic posterior thigh mass (m). Other increased T2-weighted signal plexiform neurofibromas (*arrows*) do not show increased 18F-FDG uptake.

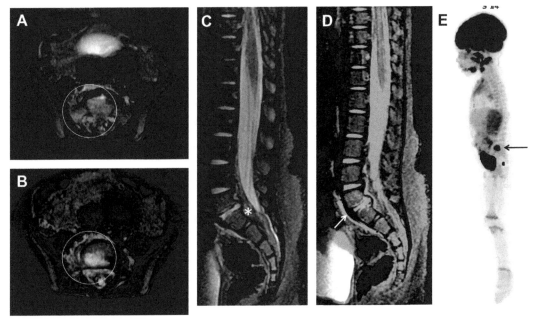

Fig. 8. An 18-month-old girl with spondylodiscitis due to presumed Kingella kingae presented with history of limp. Negative I123-MIBG scan and biopsy excluded a neoplastic process. (*A*) Axial and (*C*) sagittal short-TI inversion recovery images show a hyperintense lesion in the S1 vertebral body (*circle* on A) extending to the adjacent soft tissues, L5-S1 neural foramen and right-sided epidural space (*asterisk*). (*B*) Axial PET/MR water only fused image showing hypermetabolic focus (*circle*) and (*D*) sagittal PET/MR water only fused image shows hypermetabolic process involving the L5/S1 disc space (*arrow*) and adjacent vertebral bodies (*circle* on B) consistent with spondylodiscitis. (*E*) 3-Dimensional sagittal maximum intensity projection depicts the hypermetabolic focus (*arrow*) at the level of the lumbosacral junction.

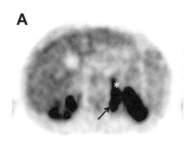
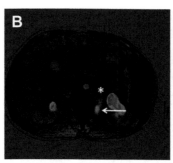
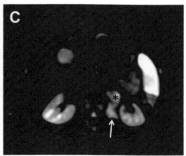

Fig. 9. A 10-year-old boy with HIV infection presents with back pain and retroperitoneal lymphadenopathy. PET/MR was performed for identification of lymph nodes for biopsy to exclude lymphoma. Biopsy confirmed mycobacterial infection. (*A*) Axial attenuation corrected PET image and (*B*) axial PET/MR Dixon T1-weighted water-only fused image depict a hypermetabolic FDG-avid process in the left psoas muscle (*asterisk* and *arrow*). (*C*) MR DWI with b value of 800 shows better depiction of the lesion (*asterisk* and *white arrow*) due to restricted diffusion. Enlarged lymph nodes at the mesenteric root (*not shown*) also were seen better on the DWIs.

acquisition times of the modality allow for reduced dosage of injected radiotracers, opening the door for further reduced radiation.[74]

The main challenge of pediatric PET/MR is that evidence so far is being produced by few single institutions; therefore, collaboration and pooling of data evaluation for various clinical indications are necessary. Time-efficient protocols have been designed and vary in each institution.[75] The use of shorter protocols for the evaluation of specific diseases, such as lymphoma, or specific time points needs to be further validated. Currently, lymphomas and sarcomas are the most common tumors that are referred for PET/CT, which naturally means PET/MR is being first explored further in these conditions.[76–78]

Added Value of Diffusion-weighted Imaging Sequences

It is important to determine in which cases addition of diffusion-weighted imaging (diffusion-weighted imaging) sequences to PET/MR imaging adds clinical value. Diffusion often can act as an ideal screening tool for reviewing cases. The axial diffusion trace image can be viewed to assess restricted diffusion in soft tissue lesions, lymph nodes, and bone marrow. Neurofibromas also are easier to visually detect using diffusion images.

The use of quantitative apparent diffusion coefficient (ADC) values to evaluate response to treatment and presence of necrosis in patients undergoing chemotherapy has been studied for more than a decade in pediatric patients. Necrotic areas are confirmed by macroscopic examination showing higher ADC values in adolescents with osteosarcoma.[79] More recently, Demir and colleagues[80] showed statistically significant variations in ADC in 15 pediatric patients with

abdominopelvic neuroblastomas. In addition, ADC values also can guide follow-up assessments and prognosis in brain gliomas, sarcomas, lymphoma, and abdominal solid tumors.[81–83] Furthermore, as proposed by Rakheja and colleagues,[84] ratios of both measurements (SUV and ADC) at times may be useful as a prognostic biomarker.

diffusion-weighted imaging also has been described as an alternative to 18F-FDG-PET to assess for malignancy in pulmonary nodules, with Mori and colleagues[85] finding fewer false-positive results with this modality. Thus, diffusion-weighted imaging sequences may be used in PET/MR examinations in the future to complement evaluation of lung nodules.

Will PET/MR Replace PET/Computed Tomography?

In understanding that modality choice varies depending on condition, the contributions of each component must be known.[86] The benefit of decreased radiation is important especially in populations, such as children, with certain cancer predisposition syndromes[87] (**Figs. 10** and **11**). Nonetheless, each modality has advantages and limitations specific to the clinical condition, and the authors do not foresee PET/MR replacing PET/CT altogether in the near future.

In general, although PET/MR is better in detecting liver metastases, PET/CT has been found better in detection of pulmonary metastases.[88] Nonetheless, Chandarana and colleagues[89] compared maximum SUV values of pulmonary nodules using PET/CT and PET/MR and found a strong correlation of uptake measurements between the 2 modalities. In addition, the MR component may increase characterization of lung adjacent structures and identify invasion of

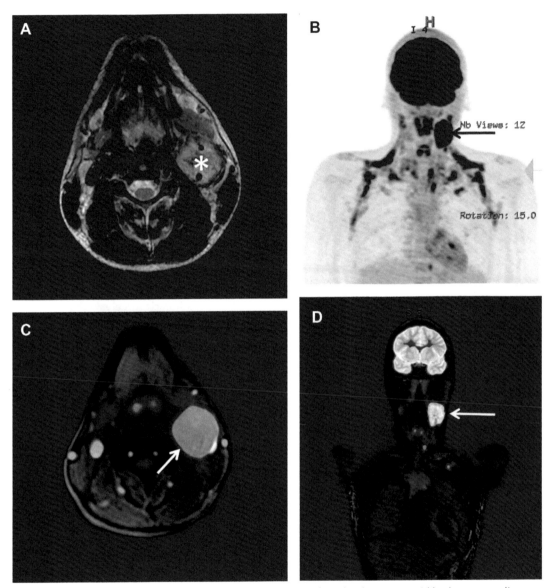

Fig. 10. A 16-year-old boy with family history of paraganglioma found to have a carotid body paraganglioma on whole-body MR imaging, which led to PET/MR. (*A*) Axial T2-weighted MR image demonstrates a left neck mass at the carotid bifurcation (*asterisk*) with hyperintense signal. Both vessels are encased by the mass and remain patent. (*B*) Coronal 3-dimensional maximum intensity projection and (*C*) axial and (*D*) coronal fused PET/MR Dixon T1-weighted water-only images show marked hypermetabolism in the left neck mass (*arrows*). Other foci represent brown fat activation, tonsils and adenoids, vocal cords, and gastroesophageal junction.

mediastinum or chest wall.[90] Furthermore, a recent meta-analysis showed the diagnostic accuracy of diffusion-weighted imaging MR is comparable or superior to 18F-FDG–PET/CT.[91] PET/MR is useful in assessment not only of lung nodules but also in inflammatory processes, such as pneumonia (see **Fig. 10**). Nevertheless, further research is needed to compare both technologies in different conditions directly in order to better define their particular advantages.

See **Box 1** for the widely used clinical application of each component along with its advantages, limitations, and current challenges.

PET/MR SUVs have a strong correlation with PET/CT but can be relatively underestimated in comparison, although without necessarily compromising lesion detection.[41,58] These differences can be attributed to inaccurate segmentation by PET/MR on the attenuation-correction algorithm. Thus, further research is warranted to

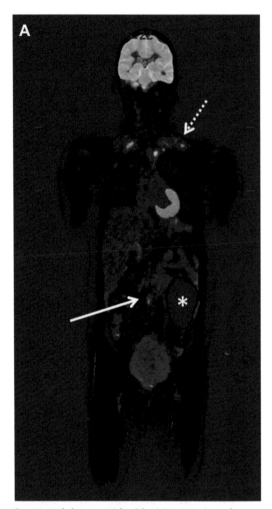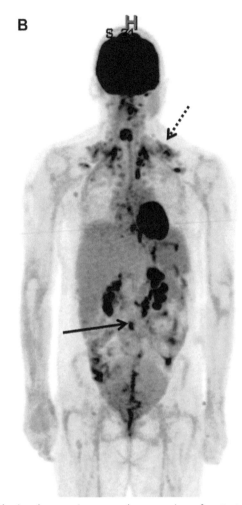

Fig. 11. Adolescent girl with Li-Fraumeni syndrome and colonic adenocarcinoma and progression of metastatic disease. (*A*) Coronal fused PET/MR and (*B*) 3-dimensional maximum intensity projection show an FDG-avid left supraclavicular lymph node (*dashed arrows*) and periaortic lymph nodes (*non-dashed arrows*), which are stable in comparison with previous studies (*not shown*). Left colon dilatation proximal to the postoperative site is seen on the MR image (*asterisk*).

optimize attenuation-correction sequences in PET/MR.[6] More recently, deep learning–based methods for PET/MR attenuation correction have proved successful and accurate, including for pediatric patients.

The cost of PET/MR is an important consideration for many pediatric hospitals. Software-based solutions resulting in PET/MR image coregistration can be an alternative when cost is prohibitive.[96]

Future Perspectives

The authors envision a growing number uses of PET/MR. Virtually, indications for PET/MR will be similar to those for PET/CT, especially in cases of MR imaging as the gold standard diagnostic and staging imaging modality. Moreover, the functional and molecular capabilities of MR imaging pave the road to a broader use of PET/MR in different scenarios and evaluation of novel treatments. There are upcoming novel applications that need to be further explored in detail for clinical value. Coregistration of PET and MR imaging and adding diffusion tensor imaging to the protocol in children with tuberous sclerosis has been shown to improve preoperative assessment in distinguishing epileptogenic sites.[97] In neuro-oncology, diffusion-weighted imaging already has proved useful in depicting focal relapse in embryonal tumors.[98] Arterial spin labeling MR imaging also may increase accuracy in the detection of hypoperfusion areas in cases of stroke or other vascular diseases, such as moyamoya.[99]

Functional connectivity is potentially characterized using receptor studies and simultaneous PET/MR in memory and pathologic conditions, such as pain.[100] Altogether, PET/MR offers promising results in assessment of brain connectivity, function, flow, and physiologic and pathologic adaptation.[100] Musculoskeletal tumors also can benefit from the simultaneous combination of PET/MR. diffusion-weighted imaging derivative metrics are comparable with SUV and can be used to assess areas of necrosis after treatment.[101,102]

Chronic Recurrent Multifocal Osteomyelitis

Chronic recurrent multifocal osteomyelitis, also known as chronic nonbacterial osteomyelitis, is an autoinflammatory disease that affects children and adults. Main clinical manifestations are local signs of inflammation presented in up to 50% of pediatric patients.[103] Chronic recurrent multifocal osteomyelitis is characterized by sterile abscess and multifocal bone lesions. Whole-body MR imaging frequently is applied to depict extension of the disease and aid in patient care approach.[103,104] Bone biopsies often are

performed and antibiotic therapy frequently is used due to delayed diagnosis. Complications, such as bone fractures, in children can be observed in up to 33.3% of patients.[103] MR imaging has been shown superior to scintigraphy in detecting silent lesions and monitoring therapeutic response.[105] Likewise, combining the whole-body MR imaging capability of PET/MR imaging with the functional information of the PET component potentially can improve ascertainment of the prognosis and direct patient-centered treatment in these children.

In summary, as discussed previously, inflammatory bowel disease, differentiation between infection and neoplastic process, detection of epileptogenic foci, and surveillance of response to treatment are a few of the promising areas in which PET/MR may play a central role.

SUMMARY

The establishment of an evidence-based clinical role for PET/MR is in progress and increasingly growing in emergent applications, such as inflammation, infection, and certain oncologic disease with undetermined imaging work-up, such as pediatric melanoma. PET/MR is increasingly available in pediatric hospitals and used mostly in pediatric patients with solid tumor disease or epilepsy. Thus far, cost-effectiveness of the modality remains a valid concern that needs tailoring in each different health care system. Large clinical studies evaluating feasibility, diagnostic performance, and impact on management are necessary and welcome. PET/MR offers valuable information and may replace PET/CT in several indications, although the authors do not expect complete replacement of PET/CT in pediatrics in the short term. Choosing between the 2 modalities will require knowledge of specific needs of disease evaluation and modality. Future challenges are to demonstrate better characterization of pulmonary tissue with the modality, reducing costs and time of scanning to improve cost-efficiency, and exploring the reduction of radiotracer dose to decrease even further radiation exposure in children and adolescents.

DISCLOSURE

The authors have nothing to disclose.

REFERENCES

1. Bailey DL, Pichler BJ, Guckel B, et al. Combined PET/MRI: from Status Quo to Status Go. Summary Report of the Fifth International Workshop on PET/MR Imaging. Mol Imaging Biol. United States 2016. Tubingen, Germany, February 15–19, 2016. p. 637–50.
2. Varoquaux A, Rager O, Poncet A, et al. Detection and quantification of focal uptake in head and neck tumours: (18)F-FDG PET/MR versus PET/CT. Eur J Nucl Med Mol Imaging 2014;41:462–75.
3. Schafer JF, Gatidis S, Schmidt H, et al. Simultaneous whole-body PET/MR imaging in comparison to PET/CT in pediatric oncology: initial results. Radiology 2014;273:220–31.
4. Hirsch FW, Sattler B, Sorge I, et al. PET/MR in children. Initial clinical experience in paediatric oncology using an integrated PET/MR scanner. Pediatr Radiol 2013;43:860–75.
5. Beyer T, Hacker M, Goh V. PET/MRI-knocking on the doors of the rich and famous. Br J Radiol 2017;90:20170347.
6. Umutlu L, Beyer T, Grueneisen JS, et al. Whole-body [18F]-FDG-PET/MRI for oncology: a consensus recommendation. Nuklearmedizin 2019;58:68–76.
7. Rosenkrantz AB, Friedman K, Chandarana H, et al. Current status of hybrid PET/MRI in oncologic imaging. AJR Am J Roentgenol 2016;206:162–72.
8. Spick C, Herrmann K, Czernin J. 18F-FDG PET/CT and PET/MRI perform equally well in cancer: evidence from studies on more than 2,300 patients. J Nucl Med 2016;57:420–30.
9. Czernin J, Ta L, Herrmann K. Does PET/MR imaging improve cancer assessments? Literature evidence from more than 900 patients. J Nucl Med 2014;55:59s–62s.
10. Bailey DL, Pichler BJ, Gückel B, et al. Combined PET/MRI: global warming-summary report of the 6th International Workshop on PET/MRI, March 27-29, 2017, Tübingen, Germany. Mol Imaging Biol 2018;20:4–20.
11. Schaarschmidt BM, Grueneisen J, Heusch P, et al. Does 18F-FDG PET/MRI reduce the number of indeterminate abdominal incidentalomas compared with 18F-FDG PET/CT? Nucl Med Commun 2015;36:588–95.
12. Kwatra NS, Lim R, Gee MS, et al. PET/MR imaging:: current updates on pediatric applications. Magn Reson Imaging Clin N Am 2019;27:387–407.
13. Schlemmer HP, Pichler BJ, Schmand M, et al. Simultaneous MR/PET imaging of the human brain: feasibility study. Radiology 2008;248:1028–35.
14. Broski SM, Goenka AH, Kemp BJ, et al. Clinical PET/MRI: 2018 update. AJR Am J Roentgenol 2018;211:295–313.
15. Miller-Thomas MM, Benzinger TL. Neurologic applications of PET/MR imaging. Magn Reson Imaging Clin N Am 2017;25:297–313.
16. Lagae L. Cortical malformations: a frequent cause of epilepsy in children. Eur J Pediatr 2000;159:555–62.
17. Kurian M, Spinelli L, Delavelle J, et al. Multimodality imaging for focus localization in pediatric pharmacoresistant epilepsy. Epileptic Disord 2007;9:20–31.
18. Villanueva V, Carreno M, Herranz Fernandez JL, et al. Surgery and electrical stimulation in epilepsy: selection of candidates and results. Neurologist 2007;13:S29–37.
19. Lerner JT, Salamon N, Hauptman JS, et al. Assessment and surgical outcomes for mild type I and severe type II cortical dysplasia: a critical review and the UCLA experience. Epilepsia 2009;50:1310–35.
20. Paldino MJ, Yang E, Jones JY, et al. Comparison of the diagnostic accuracy of PET/MRI to PET/CT-acquired FDG brain exams for seizure focus detection: a prospective study. Pediatr Radiol 2017;47:1500–7.
21. Rubi S, Setoain X, Donaire A, et al. Validation of 18F-FDG-PET/MRI coregistration in nonlesional refractory childhood epilepsy. Epilepsia 2011;52:2216–24.
22. Chassoux F, Rodrigo S, Semah F, et al. 18F-FDG-PET improves surgical outcome in negative MRI Taylor-type focal cortical dysplasias. Neurology 2010;75:2168–75.

23. Kumar A, Juhasz C, Asano E, et al. Objective detection of epileptic foci by 18F-FDG PET in children undergoing epilepsy surgery. J Nucl Med 2010;51:1901–7.

24. Salamon N, Kung J, Shaw SJ, et al. 18F-FDG-PET/MRI coregistration improves detection of cortical dysplasia in patients with epilepsy. Neurology 2008;71:1594–601.

25. Hader WJ, Mackay M, Otsubo H, et al. Cortical dysplastic lesions in children with intractable epilepsy: role of complete resection. J Neurosurg 2004;100:110–7.

26. Boss A, Bisdas S, Kolb A, et al. Hybrid PET/MRI of intracranial masses: initial experiences and comparison to PET/CT. J Nucl Med 2010;51:1198–205.

27. la Fougere C, Suchorska B, Bartenstein P, et al. Molecular imaging of gliomas with PET: opportunities and limitations. Neuro Oncol 2011;13:806–19.

28. Nikaki A, Angelidis G, Efthimiadou R, et al. (18)F-fluorothymidine PET imaging in gliomas: an update. Ann Nucl Med 2017;31:495–505.

29. Pirotte B, Levivier M, Morelli D, et al. Positron emission tomography for the early postsurgical evaluation of pediatric brain tumors. Childs Nerv Syst 2005;21:294–300.

30. Marner L, Henriksen OM, Lundemann M, et al. Clinical PET/MRI in neurooncology: opportunities and challenges from a single-institution perspective. Clin Transl Imaging 2017;5:135–49.

31. Gambhir SS, Czernin J, Schwimmer J, et al. A tabulated summary of the 18F-FDG PET literature. J Nucl Med 2001;42:1s–93s.

32. Smith TA. 18F-FDG uptake, tumour characteristics and response to therapy: a review. Nucl Med Commun 1998;19:97–105.

33. Kapoor V, McCook BM, Torok FS. An introduction to PET-CT imaging. Radiographics 2004;24:523–43.

34. Emile JF, Abla O, Fraitag S, et al. Revised classification of histiocytoses and neoplasms of the macrophage-dendritic cell lineages. Blood 2016;127:2672–81.

35. Bhatia S, Nesbit ME Jr, Egeler RM, et al. Epidemiologic study of Langerhans cell histiocytosis in children. J Pediatr 1997;130:774–84.

36. Asabella AN, Cimmino A, Altini C, et al. (18)F-FDG positron emission tomography/computed tomography and (99m)Tc-MDP skeletal scintigraphy in a case of Erdheim-Chester disease. Hell J Nucl Med 2011;14:311–2.

37. Garcia-Gomez FJ, Acevedo-Banez I, Martinez-Castillo R, et al. The role of 18FDG, 18FDOPA PET/CT and 99mTc bone scintigraphy imaging in Erdheim-Chester disease. Eur J Radiol 2015;84:1586–92.

38. Shamim SA, Tripathy S, Mukherjee A, et al. (18-)F-FDG PET/CT in localizing additional CNS lesion in a case of Langerhans cell histiocytosis: determining accurate extent of the disease. Indian J Nucl Med 2017;32:162–3.

39. Phillips M, Allen C, Gerson P, et al. Comparison of 18F-FDG-PET scans to conventional radiography and bone scans in management of Langerhans cell histiocytosis. Pediatr Blood Cancer 2009;52:97–101.

40. Kaste SC, Rodriguez-Galindo C, McCarville ME, et al. PET-CT in pediatric Langerhans cell histiocytosis. Pediatr Radiol 2007;37:615–22.

41. Sher AC, Orth R, McClain K, et al. PET/MR in the assessment of pediatric histiocytoses: a comparison to PET/CT. Clin Nucl Med 2017;42:582–8.

42. Gadner H, Grois N, Potschger U, et al. Improved outcome in multisystem Langerhans cell histiocytosis is associated with therapy intensification. Blood 2008;111:2556–62.

43. Kauffmann RM, Chen SL. Workup and staging of malignant melanoma. Surg Clin North Am 2014;94:963–72, vii.

44. Smith L, Macneil S. State of the art in non-invasive imaging of cutaneous melanoma. Skin Res Technol 2011;17:257–69.

45. Niebling MG, Bastiaannet E, Hoekstra OS, et al. Outcome of clinical stage III melanoma patients with 18F-FDG-PET and whole-body CT added to the diagnostic workup. Ann Surg Oncol 2013;20:3098–105.

46. Halalsheh H, Kaste SC, Navid F, et al. The role of routine imaging in pediatric cutaneous melanoma. Pediatr Blood Cancer 2018;65:e27412.

47. Louis CU, Shohet JM. Neuroblastoma: molecular pathogenesis and therapy. Annu Rev Med 2015;66:49–63.

48. Matthay KK, Brisse H, Couanet D, et al. Central nervous system metastases in neuroblastoma: radiologic, clinical, and biologic features in 23 patients. Cancer 2003;98:155–65.

49. Sharp SE, Shulkin BL, Gelfand MJ, et al. 123I-MIBG scintigraphy and 18F-FDG PET in neuroblastoma. J Nucl Med 2009;50:1237–43.

50. Shulkin BL, Hutchinson RJ, Castle VP, et al. Neuroblastoma: positron emission tomography with 2-[fluorine-18]-fluoro-2-deoxy-D-glucose compared with metaiodobenzylguanidine scintigraphy. Radiology 1996;199:743–50.

51. Alexander N, Vali R, Ahmadzadehfar H, et al. Review: the role of radiolabeled DOTA-conjugated peptides for imaging and treatment of childhood neuroblastoma. Curr Radiopharm 2018;11:14–21.

52. Pandit-Taskar N, Zanzonico P, Staton KD, et al. Biodistribution and dosimetry of (18)F-Meta-Fluorobenzylguanidine: a first-in-human PET/CT imaging

study of patients with neuroendocrine malignancies. J Nucl Med 2018;59:147–53.

53. Linabery AM, Ross JA. Childhood and adolescent cancer survival in the US by race and ethnicity for the diagnostic period 1975-1999. Cancer 2008;113:2575–96.

54. Williams RF, Fernandez-Pineda I, Gosain A. Pediatric sarcomas. Surg Clin North Am 2016;96:1107–25.

55. Platzek I, Beuthien-Baumann B, Schramm G, et al. 18F-FDG PET/MR in initial staging of sarcoma: initial experience and comparison with conventional imaging. Clin Imaging 2017;42:126–32.

56. Elmanzalawy A, Vali R, Chavhan GB, et al. The impact of (18)F-FDG PET on initial staging and therapy planning of pediatric soft-tissue sarcoma patients. Pediatr Radiol 2020;50(2):252–60.

57. McCarten KM, Nadel HR, Shulkin BL, et al. Imaging for diagnosis, staging and response assessment of Hodgkin lymphoma and non-Hodgkin lymphoma. Pediatr Radiol 2019;49:1545–64.

58. Sher AC, Seghers V, Paldino MJ, et al. Assessment of sequential PET/MRI in comparison with PET/CT of pediatric lymphoma: a prospective study. AJR Am J Roentgenol 2016;206:623–31.

59. Ponisio MR, McConathy J, Laforest R, et al. Evaluation of diagnostic performance of whole-body simultaneous PET/MRI in pediatric lymphoma. Pediatr Radiol 2016;46:1258–68.

60. Kirchner J, Deuschl C, Schweiger B, et al. Imaging children suffering from lymphoma: an evaluation of different (18)F-FDG PET/MRI protocols compared to whole-body DW-MRI. Eur J Nucl Med Mol Imaging 2017;44:1742–50.

61. Heacock L, Weissbrot J, Raad R, et al. PET/MRI for the evaluation of patients with lymphoma: initial observations. AJR Am J Roentgenol 2015;204:842–8.

62. Tsai LL, Drubach L, Fahey F, et al. [18F]-Fluorodeoxyglucose positron emission tomography in children with neurofibromatosis type 1 and plexiform neurofibromas: correlation with malignant transformation. J Neurooncol 2012;108:469–75.

63. Warbey VS, Ferner RE, Dunn JT, et al. [18F]FDG PET/CT in the diagnosis of malignant peripheral nerve sheath tumours in neurofibromatosis type-1. Eur J Nucl Med Mol Imaging 2009;36:751–7.

64. Gholamrezanezhad A, Basques K, Batouli A, et al. Non-oncologic applications of PET/CT and PET/MR in musculoskeletal, orthopedic, and Rheumatologic imaging: general considerations, techniques, and radiopharmaceuticals. J Nucl Med Technol 2017 [pii:jnmt.117.198663].

65. Warmann SW, Dittmann H, Seitz G, et al. Follow-up of acute osteomyelitis in children: the possible role of PET/CT in selected cases. J Pediatr Surg 2011; Aug;46(8):1550–6.

66. del Rosal T, Goycochea WA, Mendez-Echevarria A, et al. (1)(8)F-FDG PET/CT in the diagnosis of occult bacterial infections in children. Eur J Pediatr 2013;172:1111–5.

67. Liu C, Bayer A, Cosgrove SE, et al. Clinical practice guidelines by the infectious diseases society of America for the treatment of methicillin-resistant Staphylococcus aureus infections in adults and children: executive summary. Clin Infect Dis 2011;52:285–92.

68. Roy P, Lee JK, Sheikh A, et al. Quantitative comparison of misregistration in abdominal and pelvic organs between PET/MRI and PET/CT: effect of mode of acquisition and type of sequence on different organs. AJR Am J Roentgenol 2015;205:1295–305.

69. Malaty HM, Fan X, Opekun AR, et al. Rising incidence of inflammatory bowel disease among children: a 12-year study. J Pediatr Gastroenterol Nutr 2010;50:27–31.

70. Feuerstein JD, Cheifetz AS. Crohn disease: epidemiology, diagnosis, and management. Mayo Clin Proc 2017;92:1088–103.

71. Pellino G, Nicolai E, Catalano OA, et al. PET/MR versus PET/CT imaging: impact on the clinical management of small-bowel Crohn's disease. J Crohns Colitis 2016;10:277–85.

72. Biko DM, Mamula P, Chauvin NA, et al. Colonic strictures in children and young adults with Crohn's disease: recognition on MR enterography. Clin Imaging 2018;48:122–6.

73. Catalano OA, Gee MS, Nicolai E, et al. Evaluation of quantitative PET/MR enterography biomarkers for discrimination of inflammatory strictures from fibrotic strictures in Crohn disease. Radiology 2016;278:792–800.

74. Gatidis S, Schmidt H, la Fougere C, et al. Defining optimal tracer activities in pediatric oncologic whole-body (18)F-FDG-PET/MRI. Eur J Nucl Med Mol Imaging 2016;43:2283–9.

75. Pareek A, Muehe AM, Theruvath AJ, et al. Whole-body PET/MRI of pediatric patients: the details that matter. J Vis Exp 2017.

76. Uslu L, Donig J, Link M, et al. Value of 18F-FDG PET and PET/CT for evaluation of pediatric malignancies. J Nucl Med 2015;56:274–86.

77. Bakhshi S, Radhakrishnan V, Sharma P, et al. Pediatric nonlymphoblastic non-Hodgkin lymphoma: baseline, interim, and posttreatment PET/CT versus contrast-enhanced CT for evaluation–a prospective study. Radiology 2012;262:956–68.

78. Furth C, Steffen IG, Amthauer H, et al. Early and late therapy response assessment with [18F]fluorodeoxyglucose positron emission tomography in pediatric Hodgkin's lymphoma: analysis of a prospective multicenter trial. J Clin Oncol 2009;27:4385–91.

79. Uhl M, Saueressig U, Koehler G, et al. Evaluation of tumour necrosis during chemotherapy with diffusion-weighted MR imaging: preliminary results in osteosarcomas. Pediatr Radiol 2006;36: 1306–11.

80. Demir S, Altinkaya N, Kocer NE, et al. Variations in apparent diffusion coefficient values following chemotherapy in pediatric neuroblastoma. Diagn Interv Radiol 2015;21:184–8.

81. Cuccarini V, Erbetta A, Farinotti M, et al. Advanced MRI may complement histological diagnosis of lower grade gliomas and help in predicting survival. J Neurooncol 2016;126:279–88.

82. Padhani AR, Liu G, Koh DM, et al. Diffusion-weighted magnetic resonance imaging as a cancer biomarker: consensus and recommendations. Neoplasia 2009;11:102–25.

83. Gawande RS, Khurana A, Messing S, et al. Differentiation of normal thymus from anterior mediastinal lymphoma and lymphoma recurrence at pediatric PET/CT. Radiology 2012;262:613–22.

84. Rakheja R, Chandarana H, DeMello L, et al. Correlation between standardized uptake value and apparent diffusion coefficient of neoplastic lesions evaluated with whole-body simultaneous hybrid PET/MRI. AJR Am J Roentgenol 2013;201:1115–9.

85. Mori T, Nomori H, Ikeda K, et al. Diffusion-weighted magnetic resonance imaging for diagnosing malignant pulmonary nodules/masses: comparison with positron emission tomography. J Thorac Oncol 2008;3:358–64.

86. States LJ, Meyer JS. Imaging modalities in pediatric oncology. Radiol Clin North Am 2011;49: 579–88, v.

87. Reid JR, States LJ. Ionizing radiation use and cancer predisposition syndromes in children. J Am Coll Radiol 2018;15:1238–9.

88. Ehman EC, Johnson GB, Villanueva-Meyer JE, et al. PET/MRI: where might it replace PET/CT? J Magn Reson Imaging 2017;46:1247–62.

89. Chandarana H, Heacock L, Rakheja R, et al. Pulmonary nodules in patients with primary malignancy: comparison of hybrid PET/MR and PET/CT imaging. Radiology 2013;268:874–81.

90. Fraum TJ, Fowler KJ, McConathy J, et al. Indeterminate findings on oncologic PET/CT: what difference does PET/MRI make? Nucl Med Mol Imaging 2016;50:292–9.

91. Basso Dias A, Zanon M, Altmayer S, et al. Fluorine 18-FDG PET/CT and diffusion-weighted MRI for malignant versus benign pulmonary lesions: a meta-analysis. Radiology 2019;290:525–34.

92. Hudson MM, Krasin MJ, Kaste SC. PET imaging in pediatric Hodgkin's lymphoma. Pediatr Radiol 2004;34:190–8.

93. Shaaban A, Rezvani M. Ovarian cancer: detection and radiologic staging. Clin Obstet Gynecol 2009;52:73–93.

94. Brenner D, Elliston C, Hall E, et al. Estimated risks of radiation-induced fatal cancer from pediatric CT. AJR Am J Roentgenol 2001;176:289–96.

95. Fricke BL, Donnelly LF, Frush DP, et al. In-plane bismuth breast shields for pediatric CT: effects on radiation dose and image quality using experimental and clinical data. AJR Am J Roentgenol 2003;180: 407–11.

96. Robertson MS, Liu X, Plishker W, et al. Software-based PET-MR image coregistration: combined PET-MRI for the rest of us! Pediatr Radiol 2016; 46:1552–61.

97. Chandra PS, Salamon N, Huang J, et al. 18F-FDG-PET/MRI coregistration and diffusion-tensor imaging distinguish epileptogenic tubers and cortex in patients with tuberous sclerosis complex: a preliminary report. Epilepsia 2006;47:1543–9.

98. Morana G, Alves CA, Tortora D, et al. Added value of diffusion weighted imaging in pediatric central nervous system embryonal tumors surveillance. Oncotarget 2017;8:60401–13.

99. Fan AP, Khalighi MM, Guo J, et al. Identifying hypoperfusion in Moyamoya disease with Arterial spin labeling and an [(15)O]-Water positron emission tomography/magnetic resonance imaging Normative Database. Stroke 2019;50:373–80.

100. Cecchin D, Palombit A, Castellaro M, et al. Brain PET and functional MRI: why simultaneously using hybrid PET/MR systems? Q J Nucl Med Mol Imaging 2017;61:345–59.

101. Lee SY, Jee WH, Yoo IR, et al. Comparison of 3T diffusion-weighted MRI and (18)F-FDG PET/CT in musculoskeletal tumours: quantitative analysis of apparent diffusion coefficients and standardized uptake values. Br J Radiol 2019;92:20181051.

102. Wang J, Sun M, Liu D, et al. Correlation between apparent diffusion coefficient and histopathology subtypes of osteosarcoma after neoadjuvant chemotherapy. Acta Radiol 2017;58:971–6.

103. Skrabl-Baumgartner A, Singer P, Greimel T, et al. Chronic non-bacterial osteomyelitis: a comparative study between children and adults. Pediatr Rheumatol Online J 2019;17:49.

104. Andronikou S, Mendes da Costa T, Hussien M, et al. Radiological diagnosis of chronic recurrent multifocal osteomyelitis using whole-body MRI-based lesion distribution patterns. Clin Radiol 2019;74:737.e3–15.

105. Morbach H, Schneider P, Schwarz T, et al. Comparison of magnetic resonance imaging and 99mTechnetium-labelled methylene diphosphonate bone scintigraphy in the initial assessment of chronic non-bacterial osteomyelitis of childhood and adolescents. Clin Exp Rheumatol 2012;30:578–82.

Potential Roles of Total-Body PET/Computed Tomography in Pediatric Imaging

Lorenzo Nardo, MD, PhD[a], Jeffrey P. Schmall, PhD[a,b],
Thomas J. Werner, MSE[c], Marcio Malogolowkin, MD[d],
Ramsey D. Badawi, PhD[a,e], Abass Alavi, MD, MD (Hon), PhD (Hon), DSc (Hon)[c,*]

KEYWORDS

• Total body • PET • Computed tomography • Pediatrics

KEY POINTS

• Total body PET/computed tomography plays a critical role in reducing radiation exposure in the diagnostic imaging of pediatric malignancy.
• Total body PET/computed tomography enables specific scanning protocols that may improve the detection of tumoral sites.
• Total body PET/computed tomography requires the radiologists to retrain their eyes to accurately interpret images of unpreceded quality.

INTRODUCTION

Following developments in the EXPLORER Consortium, in December 2018 the first total-body (TB) PET/computed tomography (CT) system obtained US Food and Drug Administration (FDA) 510(k) clearance and became commercially available in the United States. The main concept underlying this revolutionary idea was to extend the axial field of view (FOV) of PET from 16 to 30 cm, which had been used in conventional whole-body PET/CT scanners, to 194 cm, an axial length long enough to simultaneously image the entire body.[1] This dramatic increase in the PET system's axial length corresponds to a significant increase in the total detector volume, which now surrounds the entire patient body. The elongated PET geometry and increase in detector volume lead to a substantial increase in the system's signal detection efficiency compared with current conventional PET/CT scanners (approximately 40 times more).[2] This gain has the potential to significantly improve PET imaging procedures in pediatric patients in several ways: (1) reduction of acquisition time (whole-body scan in <1 minute); (2) reduction in administrated activity (as low as one-twentieth of the standard dose); (3) delayed imaging (up to 6 radiotracer half-lives); (4) if using conventional uptake time, scan time, and injected dose regimens, providing reconstructed images with much-improved signal/noise ratio and therefore superior image spatial resolution and quality; (5) an optimized combination of these.[3] Furthermore, TB-PET/CT allows imaging the entire body function at the same time, with a temporal resolution less than 1 second per imaging frame,[4] which has

[a] Department of Radiology, University of California, Davis, ACC building Suite 3100, Sacramento, California 95817, USA; [b] United Imaging Healthcare of America, Houston, TX, USA; [c] Department of Radiology, University of Pennsylvania, Philadelphia, Pennsylvania, USA; [d] Division of Pediatric Hematology-Oncology, UC Davis Children's Hospital UC Davis Comprehensive Cancer Center, University of California, Davis, Sacramento, California 95817, USA; [e] Department Biomedical Engineering, University of California, Davis, Sacramento, California 95817, USA
* Corresponding author.
E-mail address: Abass.Alavi@uphs.upenn.edu

PET Clin 15 (2020) 271–279
https://doi.org/10.1016/j.cpet.2020.03.009

profound advantages for whole-body dynamic imaging applications. This article reviews each of these benefits in turn, but, given its current dominant place in the application of pediatric PET, it starts by separately discussing the potential benefits in oncologic applications.

PEDIATRIC ONCOLOGY

Pediatric patients are frequently diagnosed with malignant diseases that are diffuse in the pattern of involvement. For example, hematologic malignancies such as lymphomas and leukemias, which involve the bone marrow and the associated organs such as the lymph nodes and spleen, account for a large number of pediatric cancers.[5,6] In addition, pediatric solid tumors can metastasize to many different sites and often children must be assessed for disease in several different parts of the body. Therefore, a modality that allows image acquisition of the entire body will provide significant advantages in the management of such patients. Recent developments of data analysis schemes that provide segmentation of the entire skeleton will likely be well suited for analyzing data generated by TB-PET/CT imaging instruments.[6] Such approaches have been adopted for image analysis in patients with multiple myeloma and other adult hematologic diseases that primarily involve the bone marrow throughout the skeleton.[7]

At present, PET/CT with 18F-fluorodeoxyglucose (FDG) is recommended for staging, restaging after neoadjuvant chemotherapy, and follow-up of pediatric bone and soft tissue tumors, including Ewing tumor and osteosarcoma.[8] For tumors such as germinal cell tumors, hepatoblastoma, and brain tumors, conventional FDG-PET/CT can be used to assess for the presence of recurrence. Furthermore, PET/CT with other imaging agents has great potential in theranostic imaging applications, and could have immediate impact in the near future in patients such as the subset of neuroblastomas that show no MIBG (iodine-123 meta-iodobenzylguanidine) uptake but that are candidates for targeted therapy based on diagnostic imaging results; for example, Lutathera and its imaging diagnostic correlate Ga68-labeled DOTA peptide Somatostatin receptor (SSTR).[9,10] In all these cases, the improved image quality that can be provided by TB-PET/CT has the potential to increase test sensitivity and (more speculatively) to improve test specificity by improving anatomic localization or by means of parametric imaging/kinetic modeling.

TB-PET/CT will also bring significant advantages for imaging research applications in pediatric oncology, by offering the potential for significant reductions in radiation dose, by enabling studies that could not be done using conventional PET because of low signal or by improving the data quality in current protocols. In addition, TB-PET/CT imaging protocols using rapid acquisitions may eliminate current logistical barriers in patients who otherwise may require anesthesia to mitigate motion artifacts in long-duration scans.

IMAGING FASTER

The increase in the axial FOV with TB-PET has 2 distinct advantages that could allow significantly shorter imaging times. First, the long cylindrical geometry of TB scanners increases the amount of signal captured by detecting annihilation photons that are emitted with oblique angles. The magnitude of this increase in the scanner's detection efficiency also depends on the patient size and, based on simulation results of an adult-sized phantom, is approximately a 4-fold increase in signal per axial slice. The second advantage of TB-PET compared with conventional PET instruments is straightforward: because of the scanner's extended axial coverage, only a single bed position is needed. To assume that conventional PET scanning requires 2-minute bed positions to produce adequate image quality, a 30-second image acquisition with TB-PET could be sufficient to provide images with an axial slice with roughly matched signal. Recent imaging reconstruction experiments using data obtained in list mode from human subjects have shown that whole-body imaging can be performed in less than 1 minute. The quality of images generated is not significantly different from those of a conventional PET/CT scanner.[3,11]

TB-PET for fast whole-body scanning may eliminate the need for anesthesia in patients able to stay still for short periods but not for the duration of a conventional PET/CT scan. Avoiding anesthesia reduces the risks associated with sedation and intubation, especially for those children that require multiple imaging evaluations during their therapy and disease evaluation. This ability may enable scanning in outside facilities where sedation is not an option. This procedure can be facilitated using the help of a child-life specialist, motivating the children to stay still during acquisition. For such a dedicated short acquisition (in the order of 30–60 seconds), the pediatric protocol needs to include the current dose regimen (eg, 0.1–0.15 mCi/kg up to 8 mCi for FDG). The administered amount of activity may be reduced in proportion to the degree of compliance of the patient to the increased scan time.

LOW-DOSE IMAGING

With the advances made in managing many malignancies, it has been estimated that about 84% of pediatric patients survive their cancers for at least 5 years, compared with only 58% in the mid-1970s.[12] Obviously, the survival mostly depends on the type of cancer and the stage of the disease at diagnosis, but, overall, the prognosis has improved for most patients. By now it is well established that exposing pediatric patients to radiation may lead to increased risk of developing secondary malignancy in the future. However, radiation exposure caused by frequent performance of diagnostic imaging procedures has accelerated over the past 10 years. Several disciplines in medicine have been advocating for moderation of radiation exposure in the pediatric population. In particular, the Image Gently Campaign (https://www.imagegently.org) began in 2008 and has been successful in increasing radiologist awareness of the importance of decreasing the radiation dose to the pediatric population.

Several pediatric cancers (eg, Ewing tumor/osteosarcoma), inflammatory/infectious conditions (eg, chronic granulomatous disease), and hereditary diseases (eg, Li-Fraumeni syndrome) may benefit from PET/CT scans for longitudinal follow-up and screening purposes. For example,

a diagnostic scheme for several clinical trials protocols include 3 to 4 PET/CT scans. One PET/CT scan is usually acquired at staging; a second PET/CT scan is at midtreatment (eg, after second chemotherapy cycle for lymphoma) or after neoadjuvant therapy, and a third PET/CT scan after completion of therapy. Often the child is rescanned a few months or years later when there is high risk of tumor recurrence or when clinical indicators or laboratory test results are suspicious for disease relapse.

Older children and adolescent patients may be able to maintain stillness to the same degree as adults and, for this population, particularly where repeated scanning is indicated, it may be appropriate to use TB-PET/CT with a scan time of, say, 20 minutes but with substantially reduced administered activity. However, the lower limit of injected activity remains to be determined and will almost certainly vary by body habitus; for example, for smaller patients, high spatial resolution is desirable, and this will be negatively affected by the use of less injected activity. Another concern for very low injected activity protocols is the proper administration of the radiotracer, because technologists may be less experienced in the accurate handling of such small amounts of radioactive material.

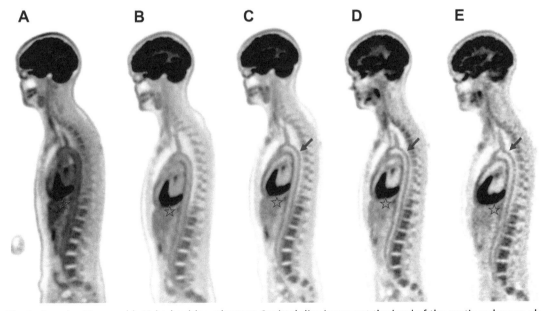

Fig. 1. Female, 41-year-old, 53-kg healthy volunteer. Sagittal slice images at the level of the aortic arch were obtained at 40 minutes (*A*), 90 minutes (*B*), 3 hours (*C*), 6 hours (*D*), and 9 hours (*E*) after injection of 10 mCi of FDG. The aorta shows the decreasing blood pool activity over time, leading to progressively higher signal/noise ratio at the level of the aortic wall (*arrows*) on delayed images. Also brain and liver uptake (*stars*) decreases on delayed images. However, the noise increases on delayed images leading to image quality at 9 hours comparable with image quality of a conventional PET/CT scan obtained at 60 minutes.

If appropriate, such protocols may be coupled with a superlow-dose CT scan for attenuation correction,[13] with the trade-off between low dose and CT image quality being duly noted.

More speculatively, the ability to image with low doses has the potential to broaden the scope with which molecular imaging may be applied. For example, at low doses, the risk/benefit ratio may become much more favorable in musculoskeletal imaging and it is possible to imagine how, say, inflammation imaging could play a role in the management of adolescents and young adults undergoing ligament repair following trauma; there may also be benefits in the management of pediatric patients with autoimmune diseases.

DELAYED IMAGING

The TB-PET geometric sensitivity gain can be used to scan several half-lives after radiotracer administration. Preliminary data acquired at the University of California, Davis (**Fig. 1**) and at the University of Pennsylvania confirmed the feasibility of obtaining diagnostic-quality scans many hours after FDG injection.[11] The possibility of delayed imaging over several half-lives is now a reality and it may provide additional clinically useful information and increase tumor detectability in patients with cancer. Different organs and pathologic entities are characterized by different uptake and washout over time. For FDG, at delayed time points the radiotracer concentration in the background tends to decrease, whereas its update within tumors is shown to increase substantially.[14,15] Therefore, delayed imaging may allow improved detection of small tumors. For example, it is possible to recognize tumor recurrence after radiation therapy in organs that are highly FDG avid, such as the brain. Delayed imaging of the brain has shown substantially reduced

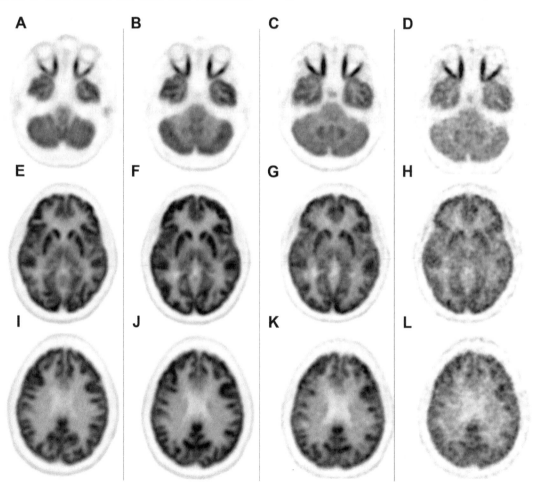

Fig. 2. Healthy volunteer, total body PET/CT 20 minute acquisition at 40 minutes, 3, 6 and 9 hours after administration of 10 mCi of 18F-FGD. Cuts were selected at the orbit level (*A–D*), basal ganglia (*E–H*) and upper aspect of the Lateral ventricles (*I–L*). Brain uptake slowly decreases over time; the increase noise level starts to become clinically evident at 9 hours.

activity compared with a standard scan obtained at 60 minutes after radiotracer injection (**Fig. 2**). This reduced activity may improve detection of recurrent brain tumors. In contrast, inflammatory lesions are often characterized by early washout.[15] Therefore, on delayed images, tumor may appear more prominent, whereas inflammatory changes may be less conspicuous. This difference could allow differentiation of radiation therapy–induced inflammatory changes and tumor recurrence.

The possibility of scanning at delayed time points also opens the door to adopting novel radiotracers that may play a major role in assessing children with benign and malignant disorders. It will facilitate the use of radiotracers with short half-lives, such as those labeled with O-15, C-11, or N-13. TB-PET/CT may also allow detection of activity several weeks after injection of radiotracers with longer half-lives, such as Zr-89.[16]

IMPROVED IMAGE QUALITY

The increase in signal/noise ratio provided by TB-PET improves both the contrast of small structures and the uniformity of large structures (**Fig. 3**). As such, the detection of small and/or low-contrast normal structures as well as disease sites is improved. In our recent experience, we were able to better identify several anatomic structures, such as the spinal cord, the pituitary, and adrenal glands, as well as small soft tissue tumor deposits (**Fig. 4**). The improved resolution gained by this approach opens the door to a more precise quantification of small structures. For example, the uptake in the adrenal glands at 60 minutes in normal patients is often higher than the liver background. On conventional PET/CT scanners (particularly the older models), the adrenals are difficult to resolve and often their level of uptake is underestimated because of the partial volume effect.

The improved uniformity leads to improved assessment of the larger organs. For example, the increase signal/noise ratio decreases the apparent heterogeneity of uptake within the liver and therefore improves the overall performance of FDG-PET in this organ. In our experience with TB-PET/CT, the prevalent random foci of apparent uptake in the liver caused by background noise

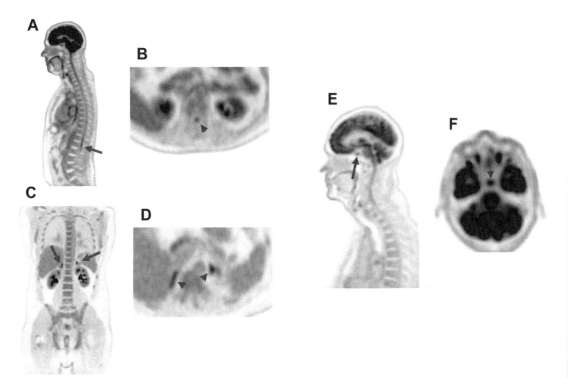

Fig. 3. Several small anatomic structures are nicely shown in these healthy volunteers scanned at 90 minutes after administration of 10 mCi of FDG. The spinal cord (*arrow* and *arrowhead*) is well seen, including the conus medullaris at the level of the upper lumbar spine on both the sagittal images (*A*) and axial images (*B*). The adrenals glands (*arrows* and *arrowheads*) are visualized with uptake higher than liver background in presented coronal (*C*) and axial images (*D*). The pituitary gland (*arrow* and *arrowhead*) has FDG uptake higher than liver background and is visualized in the sagittal (*E*) and in the axial (*F*) images.

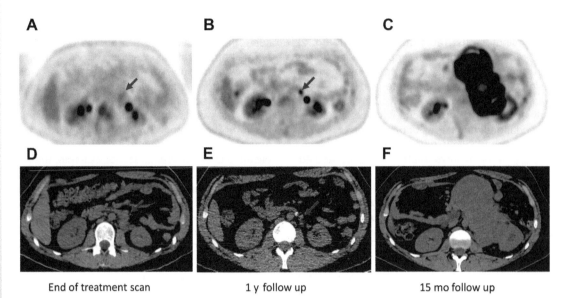

Fig. 4. Pediatric patient with right testicular rhabdomyosarcoma. PET images of the left retroperitoneal mass (*red arrows*) are shown on the top (*A–C*), CT correlated images are seen on the bottom (*D–F*). (*A* and *D*) Images from conventional PET/CT scanner obtained after treatment. Follow-up scan obtained 1 year later using TB-PET/CT (*B, E*) shows decrease in size of retroperitoneal disease but increase focal uptake in this area (*arrows*) without any clinical suspicion of disease recurrence. In this clinical scenario, PET/CT findings not consistent with clinical picture, a close follow-up scan in 3 months was obtained (*C, F*) showing extensive retroperitoneal disease and confirming the prior TB scan of recurrent disease.

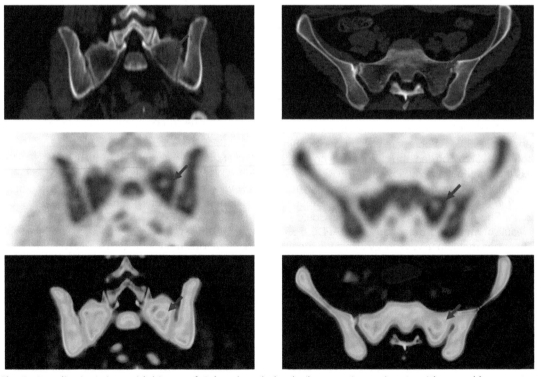

Fig. 5. A pediatric patient with history of right adrenal gland adrenocorticocarcinoma with several bone metastases. First PET/CT was obtained after chemotherapy. A subtle area of lucency surrounded by minimal sclerosis (*arrows*) correlates with area of photopenia on the correlating PET images. These findings probably represent response to treatment. The high spatial resolution and improved signal/noise ratio allow detection of small photopenic regions, which can be often useful for therapy response.

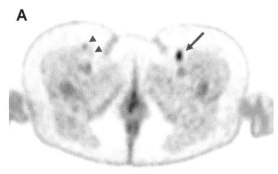
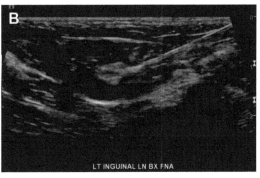

Fig. 6. A 47-year-old woman affected by diffuse large B-cell lymphoma. Axial image through the lower pelvic region was acquired 90 minutes after injection of 5 mCi of FDG (*A*); this image shows focally increased uptake in the left inguinal region (maximal standardized uptake value of 5.4) (*arrow*). In addition, bilateral mildly FDG-avid lymph nodes were noted (*arrowheads*). The highly FDG-avid left inguinal lymph node was shown to be reactive by ultra-sonography and fine-needle aspiration (*B*).

has been low, both decreasing the false-positive/uncertain results and facilitating the detection of small metastases.

An improvement in the known role of FDG-PET/CT in assessing therapy response is also seen using TB-PET/CT. For example, as shown in **Fig. 5**, we were able to detect small photopenic areas within the homogeneously activated bone marrow.

The improved image quality may also redefine the role of PET/CT in the characterization of skeletal lesions. For example, the gold standard for staging of osteosarcoma with suspected bone metastasis is MRI. However, TB-PET/CT may play a major role in this domain in the near future.

A concern is that the ability to detect smaller and less intense foci of uptake may result in reduced specificity, because optimal methods of interpreting such findings have yet to be established (**Fig. 6**). Further experience is needed to clarify this concern.

High-quality, high-resolution TB-PET/CT may be of great value in assessing cardiovascular disorders that involve diffuse segments of the cardiovascular system throughout the body.[17,18] This ability could be particularly relevant in assessing inflammatory vasculitis and in detecting systemic clot formation in the venous system throughout the body.

TOTAL-BODY DYNAMIC IMAGING

TB-PET/CT allows simultaneous full-body coverage for most of the pediatric population and therefore allows TB dynamic imaging. This ability represents the first time that time-activity curves of each part of the body can be obtained at the same time. Necessarily, the application space for this new technique is currently unexplored. However, several potential new uses can

be considered. For example, kinetic modeling with perfusion agents could be used to determine quantitative measures of perfusion throughout the body and this may have value in diseases where multiple organs are involved; for example, Duchenne[19,20] or sickle cell disease.[21]

Time-activity curves could be assessed to determine dosimetry and to predict on-target and off-target effects for theranostics, and possibly also for therapeutics. This use is possible with standard PET/CT but would substantially benefit from TB-PET/CT. Time-activity curves could also be used to perform network analyses for both normal physiologic and pathologic processes, allowing elucidation of physiologic connections between different organs. Such information could be used as a diagnostic tool or to monitor toxicity during chemotherapy or immunotherapy. In metastatic cancer, time-activity curves and parametric images derived using kinetic models could be correlated with therapy response and may prove useful for the separation of responders and nonresponders.

The ability to simultaneously study the kinetic interplay between organs may lead to better understanding of coordination between brain function and other physiologic activities. This understanding could substantially enhance the knowledge of the critical role of the central nervous system in effective function of many organs, including the cardiopulmonary, gastrointestinal, and hematopoietic systems.

GLOBAL DISEASE ASSESSMENT

PET imaging is the only modality that allows assessment of the global disease activity in the entire body system. As such, TB imaging will make it possible to generate a single value that represents the overall ongoing disease process throughout its course at baseline and following therapeutic interventions.[7,22] This possibility potential applies to both benign and malignant disorders and will substantially enhance the role of PET imaging in the day-to-day practice of medicine and research domains in the future. Global disease assessment has been used to assess patients with focal and diffuse disease processes that involve multiple organs.[23–30] In particular, this approach will be of great importance in pediatric patients with hematologic malignancies and diseases that affect the musculoskeletal system, such as metabolic bone disorders and inflammatory bone abnormalities. Therefore, the authors predict that TB-PET/CT will have a major impact on the management of both benign and malignant systemic disorders.[6]

SUMMARY

In the current diagnostic paradigm, the substantial physical sensitivity gain is the main advantage of TB-PET/CT. Therefore, it is up to the imaging community to tailor protocols that take advantage of this unique innovation as it relates to the needs of the pediatric population. However, the paradigm-shifting promise of TB-PET/CT lies in its capability to perform dynamic, delayed, and low-dose imaging, which have the potential to vastly increase the range of diseases and disorders that can be investigated or managed using molecular imaging.

During the coming years, it is expected that pediatric imaging specialists will develop and adopt innovative molecular imaging protocols that will lead to substantial enhancement of the understanding and management of serious and/or chronic diseases in the pediatric population.

ACKNOWLEDGMENTS

The authors acknowledge Dr Yasser Gaber Abdelhafez for help in imaging postprocessing. The authors thank all the EXPLORER team at UC Davis and UPenn. The authors acknowledge Cancer Center Support Grant P30: In Vivo Translational Imaging Shared Resource 5P30CA093373-17. Support for this work was provided in part by the National Cancer Institute under grants R01CA206187 and R01CA249422.

REFERENCES

1. Cherry SR, Jones T, Karp JS, et al. Total-body PET: maximizing sensitivity to create new opportunities for clinical research and patient care. J Nucl Med 2018;59(1):3–12.
2. Poon JK, Dahlbom ML, Moses WW, et al. Optimal whole-body PET scanner configurations for different volumes of LSO scintillator: a simulation study. Phys Med Biol 2012;57(13):4077–94.
3. Badawi RD, Shi H, Hu P, et al. First human imaging studies with the EXPLORER total-body PET scanner. J Nucl Med 2019;60(3):299–303.
4. Zhang X, Cherry SR, Xie Z, et al. Subsecond total-body imaging using ultrasensitive positron emission tomography. Proc Natl Acad Sci U S A 2020;117(5): 2265–7.
5. Kaatsch P. Epidemiology of childhood cancer. Cancer Treat Rev 2010;36(4):277–85.
6. Hoilund-Carlsen PF, Edenbrandt L, Alavi A. Global disease score (GDS) is the name of the game! Eur J Nucl Med Mol Imaging 2019;46(9):1768–72.
7. Raynor WY, Zadeh MZ, Kothekar E, et al. Evolving role of PET-based novel quantitative techniques in the management of hematological malignancies. PET Clin 2019;14(3):331–40.
8. Costelloe CM, Chuang HH, Daw NC. PET/CT of osteosarcoma and ewing sarcoma. Semin Roentgenol 2017;52(4):255–68.
9. Kong G, Hofman MS, Murray WK, et al. Initial experience with gallium-68 DOTA-Octreotate PET/CT and peptide receptor radionuclide therapy for pediatric patients with refractory metastatic neuroblastoma. J Pediatr Hematol Oncol 2016; 38(2):87–96.
10. Hennrich U, Kopka K. Lutathera((R)): the First FDA- and EMA-approved radiopharmaceutical for peptide receptor radionuclide therapy. Pharmaceuticals (Basel) 2019;12(3) [pii:E114].
11. Pantel AR, Viswanath V, Daube-Witherspoon ME, et al. PennPET explorer: human imaging on a whole-body imager. J Nucl Med 2020;61(1): 144–51.
12. Society AC. Cancer facts & figures 2020 2020. Available at: https://www.cancer.org/cancer/cancer-in-children/key-statistics.html#references. Accessed March 04, 2020..
13. Fahey FH, Palmer MR, Strauss KJ, et al. Dosimetry and adequacy of CT-based attenuation correction for pediatric PET: phantom study. Radiology 2007; 243(1):96–104.
14. Basu S, Kung J, Houseni M, et al. Temporal profile of fluorodeoxyglucose uptake in malignant lesions and normal organs over extended time periods in patients with lung carcinoma: implications for its utilization in assessing malignant lesions. Q J Nucl Med Mol Imaging 2009;53(1):9–19.
15. Houshmand S, Salavati A, Hess S, et al. An update on novel quantitative techniques in the context of evolving whole-body PET imaging. PET Clin 2015; 10(1):45–58.

16. Berg E, Gill H, Marik J, et al. Total-body PET and highly stable chelators together enable meaningful (89)Zr-antibody PET studies up to 30 days after injection. J Nucl Med 2020;61(3):453–60.

17. Beheshti M, Saboury B, Mehta NN, et al. Detection and global quantification of cardiovascular molecular calcification by fluoro18-fluoride positron emission tomography/computed tomography–a novel concept. Hell J Nucl Med 2011;14(2):114–20.

18. Schmall JP, Karp JS, Alavi A. The potential role of total body PET imaging in assessment of atherosclerosis. PET Clin 2019;14(2):245–50.

19. Doorenweerd N, Dumas EM, Ghariq E, et al. Decreased cerebral perfusion in Duchenne muscular dystrophy patients. Neuromuscul Disord 2017;27(1):29–37.

20. Quinlivan RM, Lewis P, Marsden P, et al. Cardiac function, metabolism and perfusion in Duchenne and Becker muscular dystrophy. Neuromuscul Disord 1996;6(4):237–46.

21. Nath KA, Katusic ZS, Gladwin MT. The perfusion paradox and vascular instability in sickle cell disease. Microcirculation 2004;11(2):179–93.

22. Raynor WY, Al-Zaghal A, Zadeh MZ, et al. Metastatic seeding attacks bone marrow, not bone: rectifying ongoing misconceptions. PET Clin 2019;14(1):135–44.

23. Basu S, Zaidi H, Salavati A, et al. FDG PET/CT methodology for evaluation of treatment response in lymphoma: from "graded visual analysis" and "semiquantitative SUVmax" to global disease burden assessment. Eur J Nucl Med Mol Imaging 2014;41(11):2158–60.

24. Marin-Oyaga VA, Salavati A, Houshmand S, et al. Feasibility and performance of an adaptive contrast-oriented FDG PET/CT quantification technique for global disease assessment of malignant pleural mesothelioma and a brief review of the literature. Hell J Nucl Med 2015;18(1):11–8.

25. Fardin S, Gholami S, Samimi S, et al. Global quantitative techniques for positron emission tomographic assessment of disease activity in cutaneous T-cell lymphoma and response to treatment. JAMA Dermatol 2016;152(1):103–5.

26. Peter J, Houshmand S, Werner TJ, et al. Applications of global quantitative 18F-FDG-PET analysis in temporal lobe epilepsy. Nucl Med Commun 2016;37(3):223–30.

27. Saboury B, Parsons MA, Moghbel M, et al. Quantification of aging effects upon global knee inflammation by 18F-FDG-PET. Nucl Med Commun 2016;37(3):254–8.

28. Khosravi M, Peter J, Wintering NA, et al. 18F-FDG is a superior indicator of cognitive performance compared to 18F-florbetapir in alzheimer's disease and mild cognitive impairment evaluation: a global quantitative analysis. J Alzheimers Dis 2019;70(4):1197–207.

29. Raynor WY, Jonnakuti VS, Zirakchian Zadeh M, et al. Comparison of methods of quantifying global synovial metabolic activity with FDG-PET/CT in rheumatoid arthritis. Int J Rheum Dis 2019;22(12):2191–8.

30. Seraj SM, Ayubcha C, Zadeh MZ, et al. The evolving role of PET-based novel quantitative techniques in the interventional radiology procedures of the liver. PET Clin 2019;14(4):419–25.

Potential Applications of PET-Based Novel Quantitative Techniques in Pediatric Diseases and Disorders

Abass Alavi, MD, MD (Hon), PhD (Hon), DSc (Hon)[a],*, Sina Houshmand, MD[b],
Thomas J. Werner, MSE[a], Habib Zaidi, PhD, PD[c]

KEYWORDS

- PET • Pediatrics • Quantitative imaging

KEY POINTS

- Hybrid PET imaging has significantly expanded the applications of this imaging modality.
- Semi-quantitative PET/CT imaging has been the predominant technique for assessment of PET images due to its simplicity and practicality.
- Respiratory motion has degrading effect on quantitative PET and its correction improves the image accuracy.
- By combining the metabolic and volumetric information from the PET images, global metabolic activity has been shown to be a better predictor of disease.

INTRODUCTION

The progress made in hybrid PET imaging during the last few decades has significantly expanded the role of this modality in both clinical and research applications.[1–3] When computed tomography (CT) and magnetic resonance imaging are combined with PET imaging, structure and function are mapped in one image, and the quantitative accuracy of the data is improved. The role of PET/CT pediatric oncological and non-oncological disorders has been widely discussed in the literature.[4,5] In this correspondence, we will briefly review different quantitative techniques which could potentially improve PET/CT imaging of the pediatric diseases.

SIMPLIFIED PET QUANTIFICATION OF UPTAKE THROUGH STANDARDIZED UPTAKE VALUES

In an ideal setting, PET quantification should adopt tracer kinetic models. However, this approach has substantial limitations because it requires dynamic data acquisition and continuous arterial blood sampling. Therefore, over the past 2 decades, a simple semiquantitative method has been adopted. This method is practical and can be done in the clinic.

Standardized uptake value (SUV) was developed to measure radiotracer concentration in a specified region of interest at various time points after the injection of the compound.[6] Validation studies show a linear correlation between SUV and kinetic modeling.[7–9]

[a] Department of Radiology, Hospital of the University of Pennsylvania, 3400 Spruce Street, Philadelphia, PA 19104, USA; [b] Department of Radiology, University of Pittsburgh, 200 Lothrop St, Pittsburgh, PA 15213, USA; [c] Department of Radiology, University of Pittsburgh, 200 Lothrop St, Pittsburgh, PA 15213, USA
* Corresponding author.
E-mail address: abass.alavi@pennmedicine.upenn.edu

PET Clin 15 (2020) 281–284
https://doi.org/10.1016/j.cpet.2020.03.010
1556-8598/20/© 2020 Elsevier Inc. All rights reserved.

SUVs are expressed as maximum SUV (SUV_{max}), representing the single highest voxel/pixel in a defined region/volume of interest, or as mean SUV (SUV_{mean}), which provides the average SUV in all voxels/pixels in the assigned location or volume of interest. The specific factors that can influence the accuracy of SUV assessment include extravasation at the site of administration of radiotracer, residual activity in the syringe, and discrepancy between the time recorded in the dose calibrator and the PET acquisition and injection times.[10,11] High blood glucose levels lead to suboptimal SUV measurements.

ADVERSE EFFECT OF RESPIRATORY MOTION ON QUANTITATIVE PET DATA

Respiratory motion is a major factor adversely affecting the accuracy of PET measurements. This factor is most significant when the structure of interest is in the chest or upper abdomen. Correction for misalignment between PET and CT scans caused by respiratory motion has been challenging and is therefore an area of current investigations.[12,13]

PARTIAL VOLUME EFFECT AND ITS IMPACT ON PET QUANTIFICATION

Partial volume effect (PVE) is caused by the suboptimal spatial resolution of PET and results in degradation of the images generated and also underestimation of the true levels of the administered compound at the targeted sites. Respiratory or cardiac motions lead to pronounced effects caused by movement of the structures.

Over the years, attempts have been made to correct for PVE by using several data acquisition strategies.[14,15] Partial volume correction (PVC) is a necessity and should not be ignored in the clinical setting. Studies of patients with lung lesions have shown that PVC leads to an increase the accuracy of SUV estimates from 55% to 89% in lesions smaller than 2 cm.[16]

GLOBAL DISEASE BURDEN: ASSESSING GLOBAL METABOLIC ACTIVITY

The concept of global metabolic activity assessment was introduced in 1993 for quantifying overall metabolic activity in patients with Alzheimer disease compared with age-matched controls.[17] This innovative approach revealed substantial differences between the 2 populations and led to a new beginning in PET quantification. This idea was based on combining volumetric and metabolic data into a single parameter, named global disease burden. In the late 1990s, the concept of total lesion glycolysis (TLG) was introduced to measure the overall metabolic response of the lesion to cancer treatment.[18]

Studies show that this approach correlates with other PET response parameters and is reproducible. Thus, global disease measurement gives information that is complementary to that of conventional SUV and its variants and further enhances the role of PET.

With the advances made in medical image segmentation of various structures, global disease assessment has become more powerful. Commercial image analysis software now provides schemes for the generation of highly reproducible and accurate data with excellent agreement with manual measurements.

Recent publications indicate the feasibility of the global assessment methods for assessing malignant mesothelioma,[19] lymphoma,[20] sarcoidosis,[19] Crohn disease,[21] radiation pneumonitis,[22,23] brain disorders,[24,25] and atherosclerosis.[26–28] By adopting commercially available software, 18F-fluorodeoxyglucose (FDG)–avid abnormalities can be segmented to generate the metabolically active volume (MAV) and the partial volume corrected SUV_{mean} ($pvcSUV_{mean}$). These values permit the calculation of the partial volume corrected metabolic volume product (pvcMVP), which leads to $pvcMVP_{mean} = MAV \times pvcSUV_{mean}$. In addition, global disease activity score can be obtained by summing pvcMVPs in all FDG-avid lesions in the body. One review of metabolic tumor volume and total glycolysis in solid tumors concluded that "both metabolic tumor volume and TLG have the potential to become valuable as prognostic biomarkers for survival outcome, clinical staging, and response to both neoadjuvant and concurrent therapies."[29] Therefore, the authors anticipate the development of more sophisticated and automated software schemes that will permit the generation of these quantitative parameters for assessing disease activity. Such measurements may provide clinicians with a single number summing up the overall disease activity throughout the body for monitoring and evaluating treatment response which can be potentially used in pediatric imaging.[30]

SUMMARY

The introduction of hybrid PET/CT has allowed clinicians to combine structural and molecular data at the same setting, and this has brought about a paradigm shift in diagnostic imaging. At present, molecular imaging with PET is at the forefront of patient management in many disciplines, including pediatrics. This powerful combined modality can be used in the initial diagnosis and later phases of the disease, and following various interventions. Adopting PET/CT spares patients from futile and costly therapies as well as considerable risks. The application of novel quantitative methods described in this article will enhance the impact of modern imaging modalities in variety of clinical settings. This modality will further improve the outcome from many serious diseases and disorders and will also result in reducing health care costs.

ACKNOWLEDGMENTS

The content of this article was adapted from a previous publication on the same topic by the same authors.[9]

REFERENCES

1. Zaidi H, Alavi A, Naqa IE. Novel quantitative PET techniques for clinical decision support in oncology. Semin Nucl Med 2018;48(6):548–64.

2. Raynor WY, Zadeh MZ, Kothekar E, et al. Evolving role of PET-based novel quantitative techniques in the management of hematological malignancies. PET Clin 2019;14(3):331–40.

3. Seraj SM, Ayubcha C, Zadeh MZ, et al. The evolving role of PET-based novel quantitative techniques in the interventional radiology procedures of the liver. PET Clin 2019;14(4):419–25.

4. Br J Radiol. 2019 Feb;92(1094):20180584. DOI:10.1259/BJR.20180584. (PMID: 30383441).

5. PET Clin. 2019 Jan;14(1):145-174. doi:10.1016/j.cpet.2018.08.008. (PMID: 30420216).

6. Zaidi H, editor. Quantitative analysis in nuclear medicine imaging. Boston: Springer; 2006.

7. Kole AC, Nieweg OE, Pruim J, et al. Standardized uptake value and quantification of metabolism for breast cancer imaging with FDG and L-[1-11C]tyrosine PET. J Nucl Med 1997;38(5):692–6.

8. Minn H, Leskinen-Kallio S, Lindholm P, et al. [18F]fluorodeoxyglucose uptake in tumors: kinetic vs. steady-state methods with reference to plasma insulin. J Comput Assist Tomogr 1993;17(1):115–23.

9. Houshmand S, Salavati A, Hess S, et al. An update on novel quantitative techniques in the context of evolving whole-body PET imaging. PET Clin 2015; 10(1):45–58.

10. Keyes JW Jr. SUV: standard uptake or silly useless value? J Nucl Med 1995;36(10):1836–9.

11. Boellaard R. Standards for PET image acquisition and quantitative data analysis. J Nucl Med 2009; 50(Suppl 1):11S–20S.

12. Bundschuh RA, Martinez-Möller A, Ziegler SI, et al. Misalignment in PET/CT: relevance for SUV and therapy management. Nuklearmedizin 2008;47(2): N14–5.

13. Salavati A, Borofsky S, Boon-Keng TK, et al. Application of partial volume effect correction and 4D PET in the quantification of FDG avid lung lesions. Mol Imaging Biol 2015;17(1):140–8.

14. Rousset O, Rahmim A, Alavi A, et al. Partial volume correction strategies in PET. PET Clin 2007;2(2): 235–49.

15. Alavi A, Werner TJ, Høilund-Carlsen PF, et al. Correction for partial volume effect is a must, not a luxury, to fully exploit the potential of quantitative PET imaging in clinical oncology. Mol Imaging Biol 2018;20(1):1–3.

16. Hickeson M, Yun M, Matthies A, et al. Use of a corrected standardized uptake value based on the lesion size on CT permits accurate characterization of lung nodules on FDG-PET. Eur J Nucl Med Mol Imaging 2002;29(12):1639–47.

17. Alavi A, Newberg AB, Souder E, et al. Quantitative analysis of PET and MRI data in normal aging and Alzheimer's disease: atrophy weighted total brain metabolism and absolute whole brain metabolism as reliable discriminators. J Nucl Med 1993;34(10): 1681–7.

18. Larson SM, Erdi Y, Akhurst T, et al. Tumor treatment response based on visual and quantitative changes in global tumor glycolysis using PET-FDG imaging. The visual response score and the change in total lesion glycolysis. Clin Positron Imaging 1999;2(3): 159–71.

19. Basu S, Saboury B, Werner T, et al. Clinical utility of FDG-PET and PET/CT in non-malignant thoracic disorders. Mol Imaging Biol 2011;13(6):1051–60.

20. Berkowitz A, Basu S, Srinivas S, et al. Determination of whole-body metabolic burden as a quantitative measure of disease activity in lymphoma: a novel approach with fluorodeoxyglucose-PET. Nucl Med Commun 2008;29(6):521–6.

21. Saboury B, Salavati A, Brothers A, et al. FDG PET/CT in Crohn's disease: correlation of quantitative FDG PET/CT parameters with clinical and endoscopic surrogate markers of disease activity. Eur J Nucl Med Mol Imaging 2014;41(4):605–14.

22. Abdulla S, Salavati A, Saboury B, et al. Quantitative assessment of global lung inflammation following radiation therapy using FDG PET/CT: a pilot study. Eur J Nucl Med Mol Imaging 2014;41(2): 350–6.

23. Jahangiri P, Pournazari K, Torigian DA, et al. A prospective study of the feasibility of FDG-PET/CT imaging to quantify radiation-induced lung inflammation in locally advanced non-small cell lung cancer patients receiving proton or photon radiotherapy. Eur J Nucl Med Mol Imaging 2019; 46(1):206–16.

24. Peter J, Houshmand S, Werner TJ, et al. Novel assessment of global metabolism by 18F-FDG-PET

for localizing affected lobe in temporal lobe epilepsy. Nucl Med Commun 2016;37(8):882–7.

25. Khosravi M, Peter J, Wintering NA, et al. 18F-FDG is a superior indicator of cognitive performance compared to 18F-Florbetapir in Alzheimer's disease and mild cognitive impairment evaluation: a global quantitative analysis. J Alzheimers Dis 2019;70(4): 1197–207.

26. Bural GG, Torigian DA, Chamroonrat W, et al. Quantitative assessment of the atherosclerotic burden of the aorta by combined FDG-PET and CT image analysis: a new concept. Nucl Med Biol 2006;33(8): 1037–43.

27. Beheshti M, Saboury B, Mehta NN, et al. Detection and global quantification of cardiovascular molecular calcification by fluoro18-fluoride positron

emission tomography/computed tomography–a novel concept. Hell J Nucl Med 2011;14(2):114–20.

28. Mehta NN, Torigian DA, Gelfand JM, et al. Quantification of atherosclerotic plaque activity and vascular inflammation using [18-F] fluorodeoxyglucose positron emission tomography/computed tomography (FDG-PET/CT). J Vis Exp 2012;(63): e3777.

29. Van de Wiele C, Kruse V, Smeets P, et al. Predictive and prognostic value of metabolic tumour volume and total lesion glycolysis in solid tumours. Eur J Nucl Med Mol Imaging 2013;40(2):290–301.

30. Høilund-Carlsen PF, Edenbrandt L, Alavi A. Global disease score (GDS) is the name of the game! Eur J Nucl Med Mol Imaging 2019;46(9):1768–72.

Preparation and Logistic Considerations in Performing PET and PET/Computed Tomography in Pediatric Patients

Kevin W. Edwards, BSRT (N)(R), CNMT (RS,PET)*

KEYWORDS

• PET • Pediatrics • Screening

KEY POINTS

- Children's cerebral development is different; their emotional maturity is different, and their social interactions can differ greatly one from another and from 1 age group to another. Even their physiologic makeup differs from that of an adult. These differences factor into how performing PET imaging is approached on pediatric patients.
- As with any medical procedure, one must make sure the patient is prepared properly and has an understanding of the procedure they are about to undergo.
- With the advance in technology, PET/computed tomography can now be acquired in minimal time.

When I interviewed for a position as a pediatric nuclear medicine technologist, the interviewer asked me if I liked children. My honest reply was that "I like some children and dislike others in the same manner that I do adults but I am a very good nuclear medicine technologist and I am sure I will continue to be a very good nuclear medicine technologist even while working with children." The interviewer seemed to have a slight smile at my response, and I was hired. That was 19 years ago. I still am continuing to prove myself a very good nuclear medicine technologist except I now "proudly" identify as a pediatric nuclear medicine technologist. Pediatric nuclear medicine and pediatric PET imaging can be very challenging at times. Pediatric molecular imaging is often even more challenging than adult imaging for several reasons. The PET Center at The Children's Hospital of Philadelphia has performed not only numerous regular fludeoxyglucose (FDG)-PET/computed tomographic (CT) studies in the evaluation of pediatric malignancies[1–9] but also infectious/inflammatory disease[10,11] and myocardial viability studies. In addition, we have done ^{68}Ga-DOTATATE PET/CT[12,13] and ^{18}F-DOPA PET/CT studies[14–16] as well as PET/MR imaging studies. It is obvious that different types of studies in different children require different methods of preparation. This difference extends to the patients themselves, and we must be aware of the differences between adult and pediatric imaging and perform our tasks accordingly.

Despite our observing that children often look very similar to their parents and the frequent pronouncement of people that "oh, your son or daughter (fill in their name) looks just like you," …children are not smaller exact duplicates of their parents. This statement can be further extended by saying "children are not small adults."[17] Their cerebral development is different; their emotional maturity is different, and their social interactions can differ greatly one from another and from 1 age group to another. Even their physiologic

* The Children's Hospital of Philadelphia, Nuclear Medicine, 3NW80 Philadelphia, PA 19104, USA
E-mail address: edwardsk@email.chop.edu

PET Clin 15 (2020) 285–292
https://doi.org/10.1016/j.cpet.2020.03.001

makeup differs from that of an adult. These differences factor into how we approach performing PET imaging on pediatric patients. On the FDG-PET/CT images, some normal variants can only be observed in pediatric patients.[18] The pediatric PET/CT technologist should be aware of these variants. I have been using the term PET imaging but am to limiting this article to PET and primarily PET/CT imaging. I am not discussing PET/MR imaging in this article, although PET/MR imaging presents with many of the same challenges as PET and PET/CT imaging plus the added challenges of performing PET studies in the MR environment. My primary focus is on the current practice of pediatric PET/CT imaging.

As with any medical procedure, we must make sure the patient is prepared properly and has an understanding of the procedure they are about to undergo. Of the many considerations made when performing pediatric PET imaging, patient cooperation is one of the most important. The study, including the examination preparation, must be explained to each patient and their parents, and at their level of understanding. There should be no standard spiel. The vocabulary used must be tailored to the age group and indeed to the specific patient. The technologist should assess the patients by engaging them in conversation, about siblings, friends, pets, and favorite things to do. This conversation will allow the technologist to gain an understanding of the child's vocabulary, their social interactions, and comfort level; this, in turn, informs the technologist of how to explain the PET scan experience to the patient. Most patients less than 3 to 4 years old will be sedated or anesthetized. In these instances, the primary explanation of the procedure will be given to the parents. Patients 4 years and older may or may not be given some form of sedation or anesthesia. With the advance in PET imaging technology, many examinations can be completed in 10 to 20 minutes, and a fair number of patients in this population can complete the study without any sedation or anesthesia. At our institution, those patients who do require sedation or anesthesia are assessed by a sedation nurse practitioner to determine if sedation can be performed or if anesthesia is required. Because of the inability of voluntary voiding by sedated patients, urinary catheters will sometimes need to be placed especially when potential lesions in the pelvic region are being evaluated. The placement of urinary catheters must be performed by properly trained personnel. There is an increased possibility of urinary tract infection with each placement. At our institution, the nuclear medicine technologists are trained to place urinary catheters, and they typically place

catheters for this indication. Because of the risks of sedating or anesthetizing children, strict guidelines should be established for those sites that use sedation/anesthesia in their process.[19] Any reduction in the use of sedation/anesthesia reduces the risk of the patient suffering harm from sedation or anesthesia during the procedure.

With the advance in technology, PET/CT can now be acquired in minimal time. Pediatric PET/CT receives an even bigger bonus from this technological advancement because patients are often smaller, so scans are going to be shorter from the get-go, thus allowing much shorter scan times. Halftime imaging is a technique that takes advantage of some of the technology that was put into place for dose reduction. What the manufacturers of PET equipment had hoped to do was to achieve the same quality scan from using a smaller dose because of increased sensitivity of the PET detectors. What a savvy technologist can do to take advantage of this is to give the patient the same dose (which is rather small to start with) and then increase the speed of the scan by 2. This process can allow for a similar quality scan in half of the time, which should reduce the need for sedation/anesthesia. With the discussion in recent years over radiation exposure, we inevitably must consider whether PET radiation exposure from the injection can be reduced. The answer is...Yes! With the increased sensitivity of PET/CT systems, we are able to achieve high-quality imaging with less activity. It is quite possible to inject the patient with half of the FDG dose and scan at the normal time and achieve high-quality pictures along with a reduction in patient dose from the radiopharmaceutical injection.[20] Now, of course, for standard uptake value (SUV) tracking, whatever technique that was used on the initial scan should continue to be used on future scans of the patient, especially if you are tracking malignancy. However, you can take advantage of this technology to either reduce the patient's dose or perform the scan in a shorter period of time. Thereby, you may be able to avoid sedation or anesthesia in some patients, reducing the chance that there could be a reaction to the sedation medicines.

The patient preparation to FDG-PET/CT scans is very similar to adult preparation. Fasting, of course, is needed. Several sources have recommended fasting for a period of time from a minimum of 4 hours[21] to perhaps a minimum of 6 hours.[21] AT our institution, the recommendation is a 4-hour minimum oral time with the exception of water. Patients should be well hydrated before the scan, and there is voiding that is done immediately before scanning. If the patient is receiving intravenous fluids, the fluids should not contain any dextrose or glucose, just normal saline. Normal glucose ranges at our institution range from 60 mg/dL to 150 mg/dL; any measurement higher than 150 but equal or lower than 200 mg/dL requires the nuclear medicine physician's consent to continue. If the blood sugar is higher than 200 mg/dL, the test is rescheduled. It is also important that the patient refrain from any physical exercise for at least 24 hours before the scan.[21] If they are a person who regularly exercises or does strenuous physical activity, they should refrain for 48 hours before the scan, and if possible, it should be longer because we have seen the intense muscle FDG activity 4 days after strenuous exercise in the pediatric patient.[22] Failure to do so may cause uptake of the FDG in the muscles and decreased distribution to the rest of the body, possibly resulting in a decrease in the sensitivity of the test.[23,24] The playing of video games and/or excessive texting using your thumbs and fingers also should be refrained for 24 hours before the scan. Often there is uptake seen in the muscles of the hands and the forearms (**Fig. 1**) that was hard to explain until this phenomenon was looked into a bit more closely.[25]

There is a need to insure that the patient is warm enough to maintain body temperature and reduce the appearance of brown fat (brown adipose tissue); this is another common PET preparatory technique. Although brown fat activity is also seen in the adult population, it generally is more common and more extensive in distribution in the pediatric population and can appear in unusual locations (**Fig. 2**). Having the patient wear a sweater or jacket as they travel in for their PET scan is a good idea. Also, limiting the use of air conditioning in the car on the trip into the PET center may be beneficial. Warm blankets in the uptake room is another way to attempt to reduce the presence of brown fat on these scans.[21] Some sites may use medications to reduce the appearance of brown fat.[26] Our site does not do this typically but instead relies on physical and environmental controls to optimize imaging. Dimming the lights and having a low-stimulus environment during the uptake period also is a standard part of preparation.

Last menstrual cycle screening of female patients of child-bearing years is essential before injecting the patient for a PET scan. Screening typically begins at 10 years and up, although we routinely ask even 9-year-old female patients usually via their parents if they have begun their menstrual cycle. At our institution, if female patients have begun their menstrual cycle, then it is mandatory to perform a urine human chorionic gonadotropin pregnancy test. In instances when a urine test is unable to be obtained, then a serum pregnancy test may be performed in its stead. It is

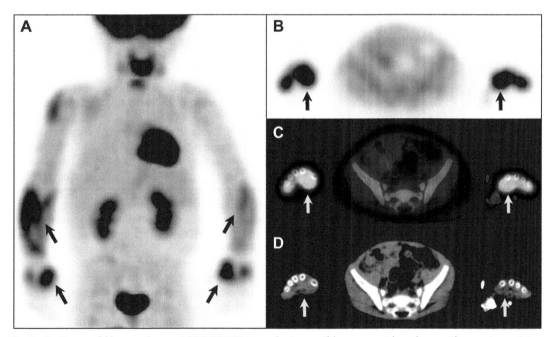

Fig. 1. An 8-year-old boy underwent FDG-PET/CT to evaluate possible recurrent lymphoma. The maximum intensity projection (MIP) images (*A*) revealed no evidence of lymphoma. However, there was diffuse activity in bilateral distal upper extremities (*arrows*). The axial images of the hand (*B*: PET; *C*: PET/CT fusion; *D*: CT) confirmed the intense activity (*arrows*) in the muscle. On the prescan questionnaire, the parents indicated that he had been playing a game on an Ipad for 3 hours before FDG injection.

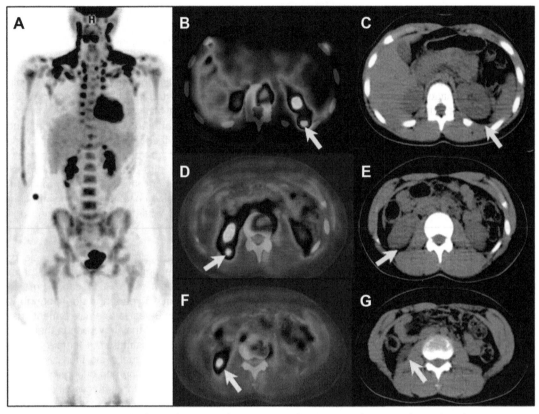

Fig. 2. A 15-year-old girl had lymphoma in the upper mediastinum and retroperitoneal region, status post chemotherapy. FDG-PET/CT was acquired to evaluate residual disease. The MIP images (*A*) revealed no evidence of upper mediastinum or retroperitoneal regions. However, there were numerous foci of intense activity in the neck, supraclavicular region, and paraspinal region. The axial images of the upper abdomen (B: PETCT fusion; C: CT; E: CT; D: PETCT fusion; E: CT; F: PETCT fusion) showed the perirenal activity (*arrows*) was located in the adipose tissue.

also important to know if certain medications were taken by the patient before their PET scan. Medications, including filgrastim and pegfilgrastim, which are used after chemotherapy to reduce the effects on the white blood cells and decrease the risk of infection may also affect the distribution of FDG in the bone marrow and spleen[27] (**Fig. 3**). It is paramount not to immediately perform FDG-PET/CT scan after using these hematopoietic factors when bone marrow malignant involvement is being evaluated.[28]

Screenings for PET scan should include a question concerning the use of these medications. As technologists, it is not in our scope of practice to dictate or determine the results of the scans, but we do have an obligation to make our interpreting doctors aware of all things that could affect the biodistribution of the radiopharmaceutical and the image quality of the scan. Proactive screening and review of medications allow us to best meet this obligation. Diabetic patients also require

awareness of this condition, so that optimal imaging techniques and patient preparation can occur.[21] Diabetic medications, such as metformin, may increase the uptake of FDG in the bowel.[29] Metformin may be stopped 24 to 48 hours before the study to reduce the risk of this effect. Metformin may also be prescribed for reasons other than diabetes, so a general screening question regarding the use of metformin should be standard protocol for FDG-PET scans.

PET/CT imaging in pediatric patients is performed for several reasons. For Oncology imaging, these reasons may be the following: initial diagnosis, staging, and response to therapy; disease progression; and in some cases, radiation therapy planning. Infectious imaging, neurology imaging, and cardiac imaging are also reasons that a PET/CT may be ordered. The indications or reasons for the PET scan should be known by the technologist because they can often cue the reading physician as to whether adequate patient

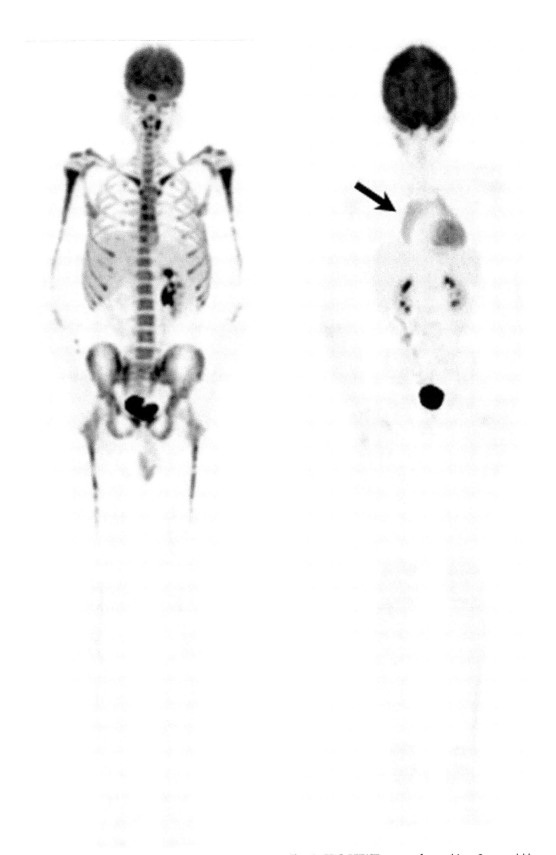

Fig. 3. An 11-year-old patient underwent FDG-PET/CT for restaging disease after chemotherapy. The patient received granulocyte colony-stimulating factor until 2 days before the scan. The image showed diffuse bone marrow uptake.

Fig. 4. FDG-PET/CT was performed in a 6-year-old boy without history of chemotherapy to determine whether he had active Rosai-Dorfman disease.[31–33] No abnormal activity typical of Rosai-Dorfman disease was noted. However, lambda-shaped activity in the region of the thymus (*arrow*) was noted, commonly seen in a pediatric patient.

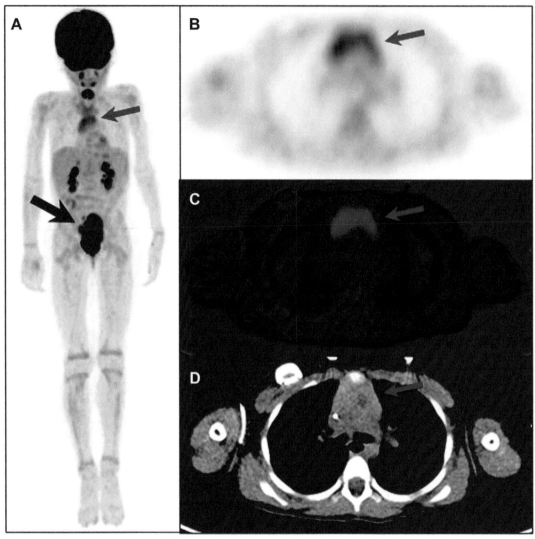

Fig. 5. A 4-year-old girl has newly diagnosed rhabdomyosarcoma in the pelvis. FDG-PET/CT was acquired for staging. The MIP image (*A*) showed not only large heterogeneous activity in the pelvis (*large black arrow*) but also increased activity in the midline upper chest (*red arrow*). On the axial images (*B*: PET; *C*: fusion; *D*: CT) of the upper chest, the activity (*red arrows*) was located in a prominent thymus.

preparations were followed, and the patient can be rescheduled as needed. One of the technologist's primary concerns is insuring optimal imaging is being achieved in addition to patient preparation and cooperation for the examination. Correct performance of the scanner, dose calibrator, and other equipment is necessary to achieve this. Quality control standards are put into place by the manufacturer, and adherence to all required testing procedures and intervals should be maintained. Operators of hybrid PET/CT scanners should make sure that all required testing on the CT components be performed as well. Local or state regulations may also require that certain testing be done on these units. Certification of your unit through the Intersocietal Commission for the Accreditation of Nuclear Medicine Laboratories[30] or American College of Radiology can help to insure that your scanner and related equipment are being maintained and operated under safe conditions and guidelines. Synchronizing the time between your scanner and your dose calibrator clock helps to insure the accuracy of SUV measurements and should be checked regularly. The responsibility of interpreting a PET or PET/CT scan is squarely on the shoulders of the reading nuclear medicine provider and falls outside the scope of a nuclear medicine technologist. However, there are normal variants that may appear on scans that the technologists should be aware of, such as the uptake of FDG into brown fat or adipose tissue we have discussed previously in this article. Another variant is the appearance of the thymus in pediatric patients, which is much more commonly seen than in the adult population. Especially, it can occur in many pediatric patients who had never received chemotherapy, especially in those preschool ages (**Figs. 4** and **5**), which is different from adult patients.

It is good for the nuclear medicine technologist to be aware of the normal variants and the appearance of a good-quality scan. The primary responsibility as a nuclear medicine technologist is to provide an optimal quality scan that maximizes the reading physician's ability to correctly interpret while using current radiation safety practices as the best possible experience is created for patients and families. Combining the radiation safety aspects (nuclear) with how care is provided (medicine) and the use of the most recent equipment (technology) is what defines a nuclear medicine technologist.

DISCLOSURE

The author has nothing to disclose.

REFERENCES

1. Cheng G, Servaes S, Zhuang H. Value of (18)F-fluoro-2-deoxy-D-glucose positron emission tomography/computed tomography scan versus diagnostic contrast computed tomography in initial staging of pediatric patients with lymphoma. Leuk Lymphoma 2013;54:737–42.
2. Codreanu I, Zhuang H. Disparities in uptake pattern of (123)I-MIBG, (18)F-FDG, and (99m)Tc-MDP within the same primary neuroblastoma. Clin Nucl Med 2014;39:e184–6.
3. Wen Z, Zhuang H. Burkitt's lymphoma involving multiple hormone-producing organs on FDG PET/CT. Clin Nucl Med 2019;44:995–7.
4. Wu C, Zhuang H. Congenital penile rhabdomyosarcoma on FDG PET/CT. Clin Nucl Med 2018;43:852–3.
5. Zadeh MZ, Wen Z, States LJ, et al. An isolated osseous Rosai-Dorfman disease shown on FDG PET/CT. Clin Nucl Med 2019;44:485–8.
6. Xie P, Zhuang H. FDG PET/CT findings of primary hepatic leiomyosarcoma in an immunocompetent pediatric patient. Clin Nucl Med 2017;42:323–4.
7. Wen Z, Zhuang H. Acral involvement of lymphoblastic lymphoma revealed on FDG PET/CT. Clin Nucl Med 2019;44:334–6.
8. Tolboom N, Servaes SE, Zhuang H. Neuroblastoma presenting as non-MIBG-avid widespread soft tissue metastases without bone involvement revealed by FDG PET/CT imaging. Clin Nucl Med 2017;42:643–4.
9. Zhang W, Zhuang H, Servaes S. Abnormal FDG and MIBG activity in the bones in a patient with neuroblastoma without detectable primary tumor. Clin Nucl Med 2016;41:632–3.
10. Yang J, Zhuang H, Servaes S. Fever of unknown origin: the roles of FDG PET or PET/CT. PET Clin 2012;7:181–9.
11. Codreanu I, Zhuang H. Isolated cholangiolitis revealed by 18F-FDG-PET/CT in a patient with fever of unknown origin. Hell J Nucl Med 2011;14:60–1.
12. Wen Z, Edwards KW, States LJ, et al. Heat-damaged red blood cell scintigraphy in helping interpretation of 68Ga-DOTATATE PET/CT. Clin Nucl Med 2019;44:927–8.
13. Wen Z, Zhang L, Batra V, et al. Elevated Ga68 DOTATATE activity in fibrous cortical defect. Clin Nucl Med 2020. https://doi.org/10.1097/RLU.0000000000002984.
14. Hardy OT, Hernandez-Pampaloni M, Saffer JR, et al. Accuracy of [18F]fluorodopa positron emission tomography for diagnosing and localizing focal congenital hyperinsulinism. J Clin Endocrinol Metab 2007;92:4706–11.
15. Hardy OT, Hernandez-Pampaloni M, Saffer JR, et al. Diagnosis and localization of focal congenital hyperinsulinism by 18F-fluorodopa PET scan. J Pediatr 2007;150:140–5.
16. Laje P, States LJ, Zhuang H, et al. Accuracy of PET/CT scan in the diagnosis of the focal form of congenital hyperinsulinism. J Pediatr Surg 2013;48:388–93.
17. Bachrach LK. Bare-bones fact–children are not small adults. N Engl J Med 2004;351:924–6.
18. Chen YJ, Tolboom N, States LJ, et al. Elevated FDG activity in the nonpneumatized sphenoid bone in an infant. Clin Nucl Med 2017;42:798–800.
19. Cote CJ, Wilson S. Guidelines for monitoring and management of pediatric patients before, during, and after sedation for diagnostic and therapeutic procedures. Pediatr Dent 2019;41:26E–52E.
20. Fahey FH, Ziniel SI, Manion D, et al. Administered activities in pediatric nuclear medicine and the impact of the 2010 North American Consensus guidelines on general hospitals in the United States. J Nucl Med 2016;57:1478–85.
21. Surasi DS, Bhambhvani P, Baldwin JA, et al. (1)(8)F-FDG PET and PET/CT patient preparation: a review of the literature. J Nucl Med Technol 2014;42:5–13.
22. Bai X, Wang X, Zhuang H. Long-lasting FDG uptake in the muscles after strenuous exercise. Clin Nucl Med 2015;40:975–6.
23. Vriens D, Visser EP, de Geus-Oei LF, et al. Methodological considerations in quantification of oncological FDG PET studies. Eur J Nucl Med Mol Imaging 2010;37:1408–25.
24. Nakatani K, Nakamoto Y, Togashi K. Risk factors for extensive skeletal muscle uptake in oncologic FDG-

PET/CT for patients undergoing a 4-h fast. Nucl Med Commun 2012;33:648–55.

25. Bai X, Wang X, Zhuang H. Relationship between the elevated muscle FDG uptake in the distal upper extremities on PET/CT scan and prescan utilization of mobile devices in young patients. Clin Nucl Med 2018;43:168–73.

26. Gelfand MJ, O'Hara SM, Curtwright LA, et al. Premedication to block [(18)F]FDG uptake in the brown adipose tissue of pediatric and adolescent patients. Pediatr Radiol 2005;35:984–90.

27. Jacene HA, Ishimori T, Engles JM, et al. Effects of pegfilgrastim on normal biodistribution of 18F-FDG: preclinical and clinical studies. J Nucl Med 2006; 47:950–6.

28. Badr S, Kotb M, Elahmadawy MA, et al. Predictive value of FDG PET/CT versus bone marrow biopsy in pediatric lymphoma. Clin Nucl Med 2018;43: e428–38.

29. Ozulker T, Ozulker F, Mert M, et al. Clearance of the high intestinal (18)F-FDG uptake associated with metformin after stopping the drug. Eur J Nucl Med Mol Imaging 2010;37:1011–7.

30. Katanick SL, Intersocietal Commission for the Accreditation of Nuclear Medicine Laboratories. Fundamentals of ICANL accreditation. J Nucl Med Technol 2005;33:19–23.

31. Pucar D, Laskin WB, Saperstein L. Isolated multinodular soft-tissue Rosai-Dorfman disease on FDG PET/CT. Clin Nucl Med 2018;43:e53–5.

32. Whipple NS, Marion LL, Dansie DM, et al. [(18)F] FDG-PET for evaluating pediatric Rosai-Dorfman disease. Pediatr Hematol Oncol 2018;35:177–80.

33. Kong Z, Wang Y, Ma W, et al. FDG PET/CT image for a Rosai-Dorfman disease with pituitary and bone involvement in a pediatric patient. Clin Nucl Med 2019;44:873–5.

Radiation Safety Concerns Related to PET/Computed Tomography Imaging for Assessing Pediatric Diseases and Disorders

Dennise Magill, MS[a],*, Abass Alavi, MD, MD (Hon), PhD (Hon), DSc (Hon)[b]

KEYWORDS

- PET/CT • Radiation dose • Pediatric

KEY POINTS

- PET/computed tomography (CT) is a common hybrid imaging modality utilized in a variety of diagnostic applications for both adult and pediatric patients.
- When considering radiation safety, the combination of PET and Computed Tomography (CT) as a dual-modality imaging system presents not only concerns associated with each modality independently but also with those that would apply to the combined modalities as a single imaging tool.
- When focusing on patient radiation safety in the context of PET/CT imaging, the main focus is radiation dose reduction, which translates to a reduction in the potential cancer risk.

INTRODUCTION: RADIATION RISK AND CONTROVERSY IN DIAGNOSTIC IMAGING

PET/computed tomography (CT) is a common hybrid imaging modality utilized in a variety of diagnostic applications for both adult and pediatric patients. The Society of Nuclear Medicine and Molecular Imaging (SNMMI) has published multiple procedure protocol standards for the use of PET/CT in 5 diagnostic categories, including oncology, cardiology, and neurology, and new procedures are in development.[1] When considering radiation safety, the combination of PET and Computed Tomography (CT) as a dual-modality imaging system presents concerns associated not only with each modality independently but also with those that would apply to the combined modalities as a single imaging tool.

When focusing on patient radiation safety in the context of PET/CT imaging, the main focus is radiation dose reduction, which translates to a reduction in potential cancer risk. In PET/CT, radiation risk refers primarily to an assumed increased potential for the induction of a cancerous process later in life.[2] Although many of the radiation reduction techniques in PET/CT are applicable in both adult and pediatric imaging populations, they are especially important in pediatrics due to the increased radiosensitivity of this population. This increased radiosensitivity in children is due in part to their actively developing organs at the time of exposure and their longer postexposure life expectancy. Specifically, children have shown a higher relative risk of leukemia, brain, breast, skin, and thyroid cancers compared with adults exposed to radiation postadolescence.[3,4] Much of the data examined in children and adults are derived from the Life Span Study as well as other occupational radiation exposure accidents and medical radiation treatments.[3,5] Essentially, the creditable human dose-response data are

[a] Environmental & Radiation Safety, University of Pennsylvania, 3160 Chestnut Street, Suite 400, Philadelphia, PA 19104, USA; [b] 168 John Morgan West, Division of Nuclear Medicine, Department of Radiology, Perelman School of Medicine, Hospital of the University of Pennsylvania, 3400 Spruce Street, Philadelphia, PA 19104, USA
* Corresponding author.
E-mail address: magilld@upenn.edu

PET Clin 15 (2020) 293–298
https://doi.org/10.1016/j.cpet.2020.03.012

compiled from cohorts receiving doses on the order of 1 Sv, which is an order of magnitude more than doses received during diagnostic imaging, specifically with PET/CT.[6]

The 2006 National Academy of Sciences Biological Effects of Ionizing Radiation (BEIR) VII report has been frequently cited in discussions of potential cancer risk to adult and pediatric populations in medical imaging.[5] The committee issuing this report focused on low-dose, low-energy transfer radiation for the purpose of developing potential risk estimates for human subjects. For solid cancers, the report is predicated predominantly on the linear no-threshold (LNT) model, which simplistically maintains that any radiation exposure carries a potential risk of inducing cancer. For select malignant processes, such as leukemia, the committee decided to use a linear-quadratic model, and in some cases linear threshold models have been applied.[5]

The validity of using the LNT derived from high-dose and high-dose rate data to model low-dose, low low-energy transfer radiation like that used in PET/CT imaging has been controversial. In recent years, several investigators have called for a reassessment of the data.[6–8] Even the BEIR VII report acknowledges that at dose levels of 0 mSv to 100 mSv, the data are intrinsically limited for defining a radiation risk-response curve. Nevertheless, several national and international committees continue to use the LNT model, and, therefore, regulatory agencies like the Nuclear Regulatory Commission continue to promulgate regulations based on this simplistic risk model.[9] In response, organizations like the American Association of Physicists in Medicine (AAPM) and the International Organization for Medical Physics have previously released position statements about the speculative nature of applying an LNT model to cohort data to draw conclusions at the low-dose levels used in patient imaging.[10,11] The Society for Pediatric Radiology also released a statement specific to pediatric CT to quell public fears about data extrapolated for cancer risk and applied to CT imaging.[12] The ongoing controversy and debate over the legitimate use of the LNT model and extrapolated data to low-dose radiation underline the prudence for clinicians to strive to reduce unnecessary patient radiation dose in PET/CT imaging while balancing the clinical necessity for diagnostically beneficial scanning technique.

PET/COMPUTED TOMOGRAPHY HYBRID IMAGING OPTIMIZATION

Optimization of the utilization of PET/CT is a significant means of reducing unnecessary patient radiation dose in adults and pediatrics. To this end, appropriate use criteria (AUC) have been proposed in the scientific literature and evidence-based guidelines have been developed by various organizations.[13,14] **Table 1** lists a few prominent organizations disseminating AUC guidelines for PET/CT imaging. For example, in the scientific literature, Jadvar and colleagues[13] published an AUC for fluorodeoxyglucose (^{18}F-FDG)PET/CT with representation from 6 major national and international organizations. They reviewed a total of 2665 published studies and determined that 45 studies meet their inclusion criteria. They chose 7 cancerous processes that ^{18}F-FDG PET/CT could be indicated for as initial staging, assessment of therapy response, or restaging when new or recurrent malignancy was expected. The group reviewed the existing scientific data and assigned appropriateness criteria for imaging of various scenarios within each cancer type. For ease of use, these AUC are listed in table format and assigned both a numeric value on a scale of 1 to 9 and a label of "appropriate," "may be appropriate," or "rarely appropriate," with a higher numeric score tending toward "appropriate" and the lower numeric score indicating "rarely appropriate."[13] Resources for determining if a patient's clinical indication meets the AUC are available and should be consulted prior to ordering imaging.

Moreover, it is judicious to use PET/CT AUC to consider if other nonionizing imaging modalities

Table 1
Resources for appropriate use criteria and clinical guidelines

Organization	Document	Resource
American College of Radiology	Appropriateness Criteria	https://www.acr.org/Clinical-Resources/ACR-Appropriateness-Criteria
SNMMI	Clinical Guidelines	http://www.snmmi.org/ClinicalPractice/content.aspx?ItemNumber=10817&navItemNumber=10786
EANM	Guidelines	https://www.eanm.org/publications/guidelines/

may be of greater value or could be substituted in place of PET/CT depending on a patient's clinical indication. When applicable, imaging modalities, such as ultrasound and MR imaging, can provide diagnostically relevant information without any additional ionizing radiation risk.[14]

Another key component in the reduction of patient radiation dose is related to the optimization of the clinical PET/CT imaging equipment. Proper quality assurance (QA) programs set in accordance with national guidelines and accreditation bodies help ensure that the imaging equipment is functioning optimally.[15–17] Poorly functioning or inefficient equipment can lead to image degradation and translate to an inability to maintain lower patient radiation doses while still achieving acceptable diagnostic quality images. Physicist resources related to establishing and implementing a QA program can be found in the AAPM Task Group Report No. 126 for PET/CT for acceptance testing on new installations and routine QA thereafter.[18] These evaluations generally are performed by technologists and physicists at various specified frequencies. Examples of routine QA include daily manufacturer's recommended QA; quarterly PET normalization, calibration, and PET/CT image registration testing; and annual spatial resolution, PET sensitivity, and count rate performance measurements, to name a few.

PET RADIATION SAFETY FOR PEDIATRICS

The factor directly effecting patient radiation dose for PET imaging is the amount of radiopharmaceutical activity administered for the examination. Specifically, for pediatric patients, a variety of formulas have been proposed to scale an adult reference activity. These have included scaling the adult administration activity by a child's weight normalized to a standard adult weight of 70 kg, normalizing a child's body surface area to that of a standard adult of 1.73 m^2, Webster's formula, and the European Association of Nuclear Medicine (EANM) pediatric dosing card.[19–21]

Since 2008, when the initial survey of 13 North American pediatric hospitals showed wide variation in administration activities used in nuclear medicine studies, efforts were made to provide recommendations to standardize and reduce radiopharmaceutical activities.[22] The North American Consensus Guidelines for Pediatric Administered Radiopharmaceutical Activities were released in 2010 and updated in 2016. These guidelines included recommendations for ^{18}F-FDG for brain and body as well as ^{18}F-sodium fluoride for skeletal PET imaging.[19,23] Although the administered activity per kilogram

recommendations did not change between 2010 and the 2016 updates, the minimum administration activity decreased for brain, body and skeletal pediatric PET imaging. For ^{18}F-FDG imaging of the body and brain, the minimum administration activity decreased from 37 MBq (1.0 mCi) for both to 26 MBq (0.7 mCi) and 14 MBq (0.37 mCi), respectively.[19,23] For a 1-year old patient, this is an effective dose reduction of 1.05 mSv in body imaging and 2.19 mSv for brain imaging.[24] Similarly, the recommended administration activity per kilogram for ^{18}F-sodium fluoride did not change between 2010 and 2016. The minimum administered activity dropped, however, from 18.5 MBq (0.5 mCi) to 14 MBq (0.38 mCi), yielding a 0.5-mSv effective dose savings for a 1-year-old patient.[19,23,24] Additionally, both the 2016 North American Guidelines and EANM dose card provide recommendations for ^{68}Ga-labeled peptides in pediatric PET.[21,23]

Advances in PET technology also will assist in driving radiopharmaceutical activities and radiation doses to new optimized levels. With the successful launch of time-of-flight technology in 2005, the field of PET imaging has seen substantial increases in temporal resolution.[25] PET also has benefited from hardware improvements, resulting in evolving reconstruction algorithms.[26,27] Additionally the use of LSO and LYSO scintillators and silicon photomultiplier detectors are decreasing temporal resolution times further.[28,29] The PennPET Explorer[29–31] took a novel approach to the PET imaging evolution by developing an extended axial field-of-view whole-body PET/CT imaging system, which would have the ability to scan up to 2 m in axial length simultaneously when scaled. Also, the introduction of PET/MR imaging instruments to pediatric studies will reduce radiation dose from this approach further.[32] Continued research in these areas undoubtedly will introduce a need to continually evaluate radiopharmaceutical guidelines for adults and pediatrics.

CT RADIATION SAFETY FOR PEDIATRICS

The CT modality provides attenuation correction (AC) data for compensation of the gamma ray attenuation experienced during PET imaging, anatomic mapping for colocalization with the PET, and in some cases a diagnostic quality scan that can be interpreted independently of the PET.[25,33] Clinicians should determine what purpose the CT scan will serve prior to imaging. If CT data only are needed for AC, then a relatively small signal-to-noise ratio is adequate, allowing for a significant decrease in radiation dose. If a diagnostic CT is needed in addition to the PET/

CT, however, then combining a diagnostic quality CT image at the time of the PET/CT can reduce the amount of sedation time for the child and potentially reduce the radiation dose by acquiring a single set of CT data versus 2 independent repetitive sets.[34]

It is important to understand that the CT dose index (CTDI) and dose-length product (DLP) reported by a CT system are not patient-specific. The reported CTDI corresponds to a volumetric radiation dose in either a polymethyl methacrylate 16-cm head or 32-cm body phantom. For example, if the whole-body CT scan is performed on a 1-year-old patient with a 15.1-cm anteroposterior diameter, the scanner-reported CTDI would under-report the dose by 89% because the reported CTDI is assuming an effective diameter of 32 cm.[35,36] The AAPM Report No. 204 provides the basis for scaling the reported CTDI based on size-specific dose estimates in both the head and body.[35] Because the DLP is predicated on the CTDI multiplied by the scan length, it inherently suffers from the same issue, and care should be taken when comparing these values across multiple scanners or institutions. Further caution is needed when reviewing the indicated CTDI values for pediatric abdomen scans. CT scanners report pediatric abdomen CTDI and DLP values in either a 16-cm or 32-cm phantom, depending on the CT manufacturer. The phantom size used by a particular scanner when evaluating the CTDI and DLP values must be taken into account.

A survey of 19 North American pediatric PET/CT clinics was conducted by Fahey and colleagues[33] in 2017. Their survey incorporated data from 14 dedicated pediatric hospitals and 5 academic hospitals with large pediatric imaging populations. Their findings showed considerable variations in imaging parameters, notably in the quality reference milliampere-seconds (mAs) for the Siemens Medical Solutions (Erlangen, Germany) systems and noise index values for the GE Healthcare (Chicago, Illinois ,USA) systems. Although most sites were using automated tube current modulation (ATCM) for both nondiagnostic CT and diagnostic CT, the ATCM parameters varied significantly. This same study suggested there is yet another option for CT using an integrated multiscan method to combine a diagnostic CT scan over the area of interest, with 1 or more CT AC scans taken over the areas not covered by diagnostic CT.[26] All acquired CT image data from this multiscan acquisition then were used to meet the needs for the PET, thus producing a PET/CT scan and a diagnostic CT with minor overlap and reduced radiation exposure to the patient. Clinicians also can consider CT dose optimizations by minimizing Z-axis coverage when longer scans are not warranted; using tube voltage (kilovolts) modulation and/or ATCM when appropriate; increasing pitch; and utilizing advanced reconstruction algorithms to reduce the radiation needed to produce adequate image data.[14]

Alternatively, whole-body MR imaging techniques may help reduce the overall cumulative patient radiation dose by eliminating the CT dose detriment in favor of nonionizing image data for AC and anatomic mapping.[14] Whole-body MR imaging techniques using conventional T1-weighted, T2-weighted, and diffusion-weighted sequences, in combination with nanoparticle contrast agents, such as iron oxide, have all been reported in the literature.[37–39] MR imaging is not without its own set of patient risks. These may include physical injuries related to displacement of or malfunctioning implant devices, skin burns, and potential for projectiles. Schmidt and colleagues[40] concluded that between 1995 and 2005 the Food and Drug Administration Manufacturer and User Facility Device Experience database showed 389 reported accidents with a majority related to patient burns. The risk of MR imaging–induced DNA double-strand breaks (DSBs) also has been a recent topic for debate.[41] Some studies have shown increased evidence of DSB post–MR imaging whereas others have shown no correlation, and others have argued that the resulting DSB may not be as damaging as the complex DSBs resulting from exposure to ionizing radiation.[42–45]

SUMMARY

The Image Gently Nuclear Medicine Working Group published a 10-year update in 2019.[46] The ongoing goals listed by this working group include continuing to harmonize the North American guidelines with the EANM pediatric dosing guidelines, and continuing to promote incorporation of these guidelines in North American pediatric PET imaging facilities. The update also acknowledged the need for standardization of CT parameters in hybrid imaging and also will seek to tackle this issue as one of its future goals.[46] Between efforts by these working groups, nuclear medicine researchers, and evolutions in PET technology, the future of PET/CT radiation safety for adult and pediatric imaging is looking bright.

ACKNOWLEDGMENTS

The authors would like to acknowledge and thank Marc Felice and Natalie Beckmann for their support of this literature review.

DISCLOSURE

The authors have nothing to disclose.

REFERENCES

1. SNMMI Procedure Standards. Society of nuclear medicine and molecular imaging website. Available at: http://www.snmmi.org/ClinicalPractice/content.aspx?ItemNumber=6414&navItemNumber=10790. Accessed January 23, 2020.

2. Fahey FH, Treves ST, Adelstein SJ. Minimizing and communicating radiation risk in pediatric nuclear medicine. J Nucl Med 2011;52:1240–51.

3. Kutanzi KR, Lumen A, Koturbash I, et al. Pediatric exposures to ionizing radiation: carcinogenic considerations. Int J Environ Res Public Health 2016; 13:1056–7.

4. United Nations Scientific Committee on the Effects of Atomic Radiation (UNSCEAR). Sources, effects, and risks of ionizing radiation: United States scientific committee on the effects of atomic radiation: UNSCEAR 2013 report to the general assembly with scientific annexes. Vienna (Austria): UNSCEAR; 2013.

5. National Research Council of the National Academies. Health risks from exposure to low levels of ionizing radiation: BEIR VII phase 2. Washington, DC: The National Academies Press; 2006. p. 245.

6. Siegel J, Greenspan BS, Maurer AH, et al. The BEIR VII estimates of low-dose radiation health risks are based on faulty assumptions and data analyses: a call for reassessment. J Nucl Med 2018;59:1017–9.

7. Hansen CL, Hingorani R. LNT RIP: it is time to bury the linear no threshold hypothesis. J Nucl Cardiol 2019;26:1358–60.

8. Weber W, Zanzonico P. The controversial linear no-threshold model. J Nucl Med 2017;58:7–8.

9. Cardarelli JJ, Ulsh BA. It is time to move beyond the linear no-threshold theory for low-dose radiation protection. Dose Response 2018;16. 1559325818779651.

10. American Association of Physicists in Medicine. AAPM website. AAPM position statement on radiation risks from medical imaging procedures 2018. Available at: https://www.aapm.org/org/policies/details.asp?id=318&type=PP&current=true. Accessed January 27, 2020.

11. Pradhan AS. On the risk to low doses (< 100 mSv) of ionizing radiation during medical imaging procedures- IOMP policy statement. J Med Phys 2013;38:57–8.

12. Society of Pediatric Radiology. Risks and benefits in pediatric CT. Pediatr Radiol 2001;31:387.

13. Jadvar H, Colletti PM, Delgado-Bolton R, et al. Appropriate use criteria for FDG PET/CT in restaging and treatment response assessment of malignant disease. J Nucl Med 2017;58:2026–37.

14. Akin EA, Torigian DA, Colletti PM, et al. Optimizing oncologic FDG-PET/CT scans to decrease radiation exposure. Image Wisely website. 2017. Available at: https://www.imagewisely.org/Imaging-Modalities/Nuclear-Medicine/Optimizing-Oncologic-FDG-PETCT-Scans. Accessed January 23, 2020.

15. American College of Radiology. ACR accreditation support website. Quality control: PET 2019. Available at: https://accreditationsupport.acr.org/support/solutions/articles/11000062295-quality-control-pet. Accessed January 28, 2020.

16. Intersocietal Accreditation Commission. The IAC standards and guidelines for nuclear/PET accreditation. IAC 2016; 35-37. Available at: https://accreditationsupport.acr.org/support/solutions/articles/11000062295-quality-control-pet. Accessed January 28, 2020.

17. The Joint Commission. Revised requirements for diagnostic imaging services: Environment of Care (EC) 02.04.03. The Joint Commission: Oakbrook Terrace, Illinois;2015; Issued January 2015.

18. American Association of Physicists in Medicine. AAPM report No 126: PET/CT acceptance testing and quality assurance. Alexandria, Virginia: AAPM; 2019. Available at: https://www.aapm.org/pubs/reports/RPT_126.pdf. Accessed January 27, 2020.

19. Gelfand MJ, Parisi MT, Treves ST. Pediatric radiopharmaceutical administered doses: 2010 North American consensus guidelines. J Nucl Med 2011; 52:318–22.

20. Accorsi R, Karp JS, Surti S. Improved dose regimen in pediatric PET. J Nucl Med 2010;51:293–300.

21. Jacobs F, Thierens H, Piepsz A, et al. Optimized tracer-dependent dosage cards to obtain weight-independent effective doses. Eur J Nucl Med Mol Imaging 2005;32:581–8.

22. Treves ST, Davis RT, Fahey FH. Administered radiopharmaceutical doses in children: a survey of 13 pediatric hospitals in North America. J Nucl Med 2008; 49:1024–7.

23. Treves ST, Gelfand MJ, Fahey FH, et al. 2016 update of the North American consensus guidelines for pediatric administered radiopharmaceutical activities. J Nucl Med 2016;57:15N–8N.

24. Mattsson S, Johansson L, Leide Svegborn S, et al. ICRP publication 128: radiation dose to patients from radiopharmaceuticals: a compendium of current information related to frequently used substances. Ann ICRP 2015;44(2_suppl):7–321.

25. Walrand S, Hesse M, Jamar F. Update on novel trends in PET/CT technology and its clinical applications. Br J Radiol 2018;89:20160534.

26. Surti S, Karp JS. Advances in time-of-flight PET. Phys Med 2016;32:12–22.

27. Vandenberghe S, Mikhaylova E, D'Hoe E, et al. Recent developments in time-of-flight PET. EJNMMI Phys 2016;3:3.

28. Gundacker S, Auffray E, Pauwels K, et al. Measurement of intrinsic rise times for various L(Y)SO and LuAG scintillators with a general study of prompt photons to achieve 10 os in TOF_PET. Phys Med Biol 2016;61:2802–37.

29. Karp JS, Viswnath V, Geagan MJ, et al. PennPET explorer: design and preliminary performance of a whole-body imager. J Nucl Med 2020;61:136–43.

30. Pantel AR, Viswanath V, Daube-Witherspoon ME, et al. PennPET explorer: human imaging on a whole-body imager. J Nucl Med 2020;61:144–51.

31. Badawi RD, Shi H, Hu P, et al. First human imaging studies with the EXPLORER total-body PET scanner. J Nucl Med 2019;60:299–303.

32. Pichler BJ, Kolb A, Nägele T, et al. PET/MRI: paving the way for the next generation of clinical multimodality imaging applications. J Nucl Med 2010;51:333–6.

33. Fahey FH, Goodkind A, MacDougall RD, et al. Operational and dosimetric aspects of pediatric PET/CT. J Nucl Med 2017;58:1360–6.

34. Alessio AM, Kinahan PE. CT protocol selection in PET-CT imaging. Image Wisely website. 2012. Available at: https://www.imagewisely.org/~/media/ImageWisely-Files/NucMed/CT-Protocol-Selection-in-PETCT-Imaging.pdf. Accessed January 30, 2020.

35. American Association of Physicists in Medicine. AAPM report No 204: size-specific Dose Estimates (SSDE) in pediatric and adult body CT examinations. Alexandria, Virginia: AAPM; 2011. Available at: https://www.aapm.org/pubs/reports/RPT_204.pdf. Accessed January 30, 2020.

36. International Commission on Radiation Units and Measurement. ICRU report 74: patient dosimetry for X-rays used in medical imaging. J ICRU 2005; 5:89.

37. Kwee TC, van Ufford HM, Beek FJ, et al. Whole-body MRI, including diffusion-weighted imaging, for initial staging of malignant lymphoma: comparison to computed tomography. Invest Radiol 2009;44:683–90.

38. van Ufford HM, Kwee TC, Beek FJ, et al. Newly diagnosed lymphoma: initial results with whole-body T1-weighted, STIR, and Diffusion-weighted MRI compared with 18F-FDG PET/CT. AJR Am J Roentgenol 2011;196:662–9.

39. Klenk C, Gawande R, Uslu L, et al. Ionising radiation-free whole-body MRI versus ^{18}F-fluorodeoxyglucose PET/CT scans for children and young adults with cancer: a prospective, non-radomised, single-centre study. Lancet Oncol 2014;15:275–85.

40. Schmidt MH, Marshall J, Downie J, et al. Pediatric magnetic resonance research and the minimal-risk standard. IRB 2011;33(5):1–6.

41. Lassman M, Eberlein U, Yosi G, et al. Correspondence: 18F-FDG PET/CT scans for children and adolescents. Lancet Oncol 2014;15:e243.

42. Fiechter M, Stehli J, Fuchs TA, et al. Impact of cardiac magnetic resonance imaging on human lymphocyte DNA integrity. Eur Heart J 2013;34:2340–5.

43. Foster KR, Moulder JE, Budinger TF. Will an MRI examination damage your genes? Radiat Res 2017; 187:1–6.

44. Reddig A, Fatahi M, Roggenbuck D, et al. Impact of in vivo high-field-strength and ultra-high-field-strength MR imaging on DNA double-strand-break formation in human lymphocytes. Radiology 2017; 282:782–9.

45. Frankel J, Wilén J, Hansson Mild K. Assessing exposures to magnetic resonance imaging's complex mixture of magnetic fields for in vivo, in vitro, and epidemiologic studies of health effects for staff and patients. Front Public Health 2018;6:66.

46. Treves ST, Gelfand M, Parisi M, et al. Update: image gently and nuclear medicine at 10 years. J Nucl Med 2019;60:7N–9N.

PET in Pediatric Lymphoma

Jennifer Gillman, MD, MSCI[a], Lisa J. States, MD[b,c,d], Sabah Servaes, MD[b,c,d],*

KEYWORDS

• Tomography • Pediatrics • Lymphoma

KEY POINTS

• Pediatric lymphoma is the third most common childhood cancer, consisting of 15% of all pediatric malignancies.
• Hodgkin lymphoma often presents with dominant nodal disease in the chest and neck.
• Evaluation of the extent of disease is essential for appropriate risk stratification and treatment planning.

INTRODUCTION
Epidemiology

Pediatric lymphoma is the third most common childhood cancer, consisting of 15% of all pediatric malignancies. About 55% of new pediatric lymphoma diagnoses are Hodgkin lymphoma (HL), which occurs more frequently in older children and adolescents, classically involving contiguous nodal groups. According to the National Cancer Institute Surveillance, Epidemiology and End Results statistics, the most common subtypes of HL include nodular sclerosis (70%), mixed cellularity (16%), and lymphocytic predominant (7%).[1] The overall 5-year survival rate for pediatric HL is 91%, noting higher rates of survival are seen in children with lower stage disease.[2,3]

Pediatric non-Hodgkin lymphoma (NHL) is more common is children younger than 9 years old, and consists of four major subtypes of disease: (1) Burkitt lymphoma (40%), (2) diffuse large B-cell lymphoma (DLBCL) (20%), (3) lymphoblastic lymphoma (30%), and (4) anaplastic large cell lymphoma (10%).[4] The 5-year survival rate of pediatric NHL is 72%, which is overall better when compared with adults, but worse when compared with pediatric HL.[1]

Although HL is often curable in greater that 90% of children with chemotherapy or combination chemotherapy/radiation therapy, survivors are at risk for secondary cancers in or close to the field of radiation. This includes breast cancers in women, thyroid cancers, and sarcomas.[5,6] These patients are at a 14-fold increased cumulative risk of secondary life-limiting neoplasms with a 20- to 30-year latency period after radiotherapy.[7] The use of radiation therapy can be limited or avoided in children demonstrating an early response to chemotherapy on fluorodeoxyglucose (FDG) PET/computed tomography (CT) (defined as a complete metabolic response on FDG PET/CT after two treatment cycles).[8]

Presentation

HL often presents with dominant nodal disease in the chest and neck. Approximately one-third of patients present with "B" symptoms, including fever, night sweats, and weight loss; these symptoms are the result of cytokine release. which is associated with biologic aggressiveness and worse prognosis.[9] Imaging is valuable early in the diagnostic work-up of lymphoma, with enlarged palpable lymphadenopathy usually first evaluated with ultrasound, often followed by CT imaging. Based on the location of the patient's disease, CT or ultrasound-guided biopsies are performed to avoid more invasive surgical excisional biopsies. For most subtypes of lymphoma, FDG

^a Department of Radiology, Hospital of the University of Pennsylvania, 3400 Spruce St, Philadelphia, PA 19104, USA; ^b Department of Radiology, The Children's Hospital of Philadelphia, 3401 Civic Center Blvd, Philadelphia, PA 19104, USA; ^c Perelman School of Medicine, University of Pennsylvania, 3400 Civic Center Blvd, Philadelphia, PA 19104, USA; ^d Section of Oncologic Imaging, Department of Radiology, The Children's Hospital of Philadelphia, 3401 Civic Center Boulevard, Philadelphia, PA 19104, USA
* Corresponding author.
E-mail address: servaes@email.chop.edu

PET Clin 15 (2020) 299–307
https://doi.org/10.1016/j.cpet.2020.03.007

PET/CT is the technique of choice for staging and treatment response evaluation.

FLUORODEOXYGLUCOSE PET/COMPUTED TOMOGRAPHY FOR STAGING

Evaluation of the extent of disease is essential for appropriate risk stratification and treatment planning. More specifically, the stage of disease at presentation helps define the patient's chemotherapy regimen and the potential extent of the field for radiation therapy. Currently, the standard whole-body staging assessment is FDG PET/CT.[10,11] The Lugano classification, a modification of the Ann Arbor classification, formally incorporates the use of FDG PET/CT for staging and treatment response. Low-risk disease is defined as nonbulky disease stage IA or IIA. Intermediate-risk disease is defined as bulky stage IA or IIA, or stage IB, IIB, IIAE, IIIA, or IVA disease regardless of bulk. High-risk disease is defined as stage IIIB or IVB. Examples of stage IIB disease, stage IIIA disease, and stage IV disease are seen in **Figs. 1–3**, respectively.

Before the standardization of FDG PET/CT in staging for lymphoma, conventional staging methods included history; physical examination; laboratory screening; chest radiography; ultrasound of peripheral lymph nodes and abdomen; CT of the chest, abdomen, and pelvis; echocardiography; bone scintigraphy; and bone marrow examination, with optional MR imaging. In a prospective blinded study by Kabickova and colleagues,[12] pretreatment FDG-PET alone accurately staged 80.3% of children with pediatric lymphoma, and altered staging in 28% of patients when compared with conventional staging methods. FDG-PET demonstrated greater specificity and accuracy compared with conventional staging methods, with 100% versus 60%, and 96.7% versus 85.2%, respectively.[12]

Dual-modality fusion imaging with FDG PET/CT more accurately detects malignant lesions in children with lymphoma. London and colleagues[13] studied 209 patients with 5014 regional lymph nodes and found greater specificity and fewer false-positive results with FDG PET/CT when compared with conventional imaging. Furthermore, FDG-PET/CT more accurately predicts lesion response to therapy, which contributes to patient risk-stratification and treatment regimens.

FDG PET/CT provides added value to pretherapy testing by influencing disease staging and defining the extent of the field involved in radiation therapy, if necessary. In a smaller study involving 30 children with HL, Robertson and colleagues found that FDG-PET/CT changed the clinical stage in 50% of patients, resulting in upstaging in eight patients (27%) and downstaging in seven patients (23%). The overall volume of the radiation field was adjusted in 21 patients (70%) based on the PET imaging; a total of 47 radiation sites were adjusted, and 15 (31.9%) were excluded from the radiation field as a result of the PET imaging.[14]

Staging FDG-PET has also demonstrated high sensitivity and specificity for detecting skeletal lymphomatous involvement, which obviates more invasive evaluation with bone marrow biopsy.[15–17] According to the new Lugano criteria, bone marrow biopsy is no longer indicated for routine staging of HL.[10] Skeletal involvement of lymphoma is often focal/multifocal and the utility of posterior iliac crest bone marrow sampling is limited. However, bone marrow biopsy is still recommended in staging of NHL, specifically DLBCL; the National Comprehensive Cancer Network International Prognostic Index for DLBCL uses bone marrow sampling for risk stratification and does not incorporate image-based bone marrow involvement.[18,19]

FDG PET/CT protocol for staging extends from skull base to mid-thigh. The use of whole-body (WB) FDG PET/CT from skull vertex to toes does not impact clinical staging of pediatric lymphoma or treatment course.[20] Advantages of the more limited field of view include reduced radiation exposure, decreased table time, and potentially decreased anesthesia time. WB FDG-PET/CT may be of use in rare cases of pediatric cutaneous T-cell lymphoma to document all sites of cutaneous involvement.

INTERIM TREATMENT FLUORODEOXYGLUCOSE PET/COMPUTED TOMOGRAPHY

In practice, post-treatment response by FDG PET/CT is determined using the five-point Deauville score criteria (**Table 1**). Early response to chemotherapy is assessed by FDG PET/CT performed after two cycles of chemotherapy; complete metabolic response is defined by a score of one, two, or three, whereas a score of four or five indicates the presence of hypermetabolic disease related to lymphoma. After the completion of chemotherapy, a complete metabolic response is defined by Deauville score of one or two. The Deauville score is more specific than subjective visual PET interpretations with a positive predictive value of 72.7% compared with 44.4%, respectively, and with similar negative predictive values of 95.6% and 95.1%.[21]

Patients with low-risk lymphoma who are early responders to chemotherapy can safely avoid

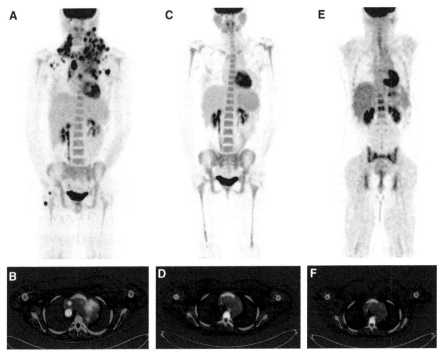

Fig. 1. A 19-year-old man with Hodgkin lymphoma stage IIB. (A) FDG PET maximum intensity projection (MIP) shows multiple hypermetabolic foci in the neck and chest and no disease below the diaphragm. (B) Axial fused PET/CT shows hypermetabolic mediastinal lymphadenopathy. (C) FDG-PET MIP after two cycles of chemotherapy with complete metabolic response. Diffuse marrow activity in the axial skeleton and long bones caused by granulocyte colony–stimulating factor therapy. (D) Axial fused PET/CT image shows residual activity in the mediastinum greater than aortic blood pool (Deauville 3). (E) FDG-PET coronal image at the end of therapy shows residual activity in the mediastinum. The coronal image allows more accurate visual comparison with the liver. (F) Axial fused PET/CT image shows residual activity in mediastinal tissue (Deauville 3).

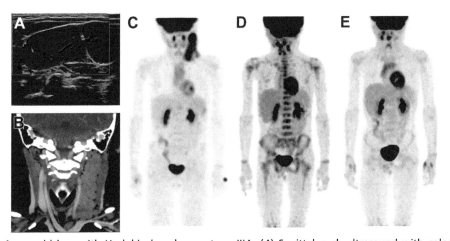

Fig. 2. A 4-year-old boy with Hodgkin lymphoma stage IIIA. (A) Sagittal neck ultrasound with color Doppler shows lymphadenopathy with loss of normal architecture and areas of peripheral blood flow suggestive of malignancy. (B) Coronal contrast-enhanced CT image shows left neck bulk lymphadenopathy measuring 8.0 cm in dimension. (C) FDG-PET MIP at diagnosis shows hypermetabolic left neck lymphadenopathy and a small focus in the spleen. Physiologic uptake is seen in the adenoids, thymus, and terminal ileum. (D) FDG-PET MIP after two cycles of chemotherapy shows complete metabolic response and diffuse marrow uptake caused by granulocyte colony–stimulating factor therapy. (E) FDG-PET MIP at the end of therapy shows complete metabolic response. Mild FDG uptake in a mildly enlarged thymus is consistent with thymic rebound. Note uptake in hand muscles caused by device use.

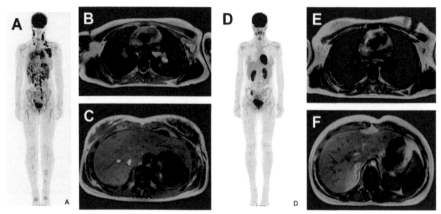

Fig. 3. A 14-year-old girl with nodular lymphocyte-predominant Hodgkin lymphoma stage IV, FDG PET/MR imaging. (*A*) Coronal MIP shows hypermetabolic lymph nodes above and below the diaphragm and lungs, liver, and spleen. (*B, C*) Axial fused PET/T1-weighted images shows FDG avid hilar lymph nodes, nodular pulmonary infiltrates, liver, and spleen. (*D–F*) FDG PET MIP and fused PET/T1 images after three cycles of chemotherapy show a complete metabolic response.

additional aggressive radiation therapy regimens. This has been demonstrated by the international trial GPOH-HD95, a prospective trial in which low-risk patients demonstrated an overall high progression-free survival with or without the use of targeted radiation therapy.[22]

Early interim treatment FDG PET/CT is also of value in children diagnosed with intermediate-risk lymphoma. An early response to chemotherapy in intermediate-risk children is defined as greater than or equal to 60% reduction in disease volume after two cycles of chemotherapy. In the Children's Oncology Group AHOD 0031 trial, there was no significant difference in event-free survival (EFS) with the omission of in-field radiation in intermediate-risk children with early rapid responses to chemotherapy (EFS, 86.8% vs 83.8%; P = .29).[23] Similarly, intermediate-risk rapid responders also demonstrated an equivalent 3-year progression-free survival whether or not they received in-field radiation therapy.[24] Therefore, with the use of interim treatment FDG PET/

CT, additional radiation therapy may be avoided in rapid-responding intermediate-risk children.

SURVEILLANCE FLUORODEOXYGLUCOSE PET/COMPUTED TOMOGRAPHY

Low-risk children who are early rapid responders have a better prognosis, and additional routine surveillance PET-CT in asymptomatic children after the completion of therapy does not impact overall survival.[25–27] Voss and colleagues[25] as part of the Children's Oncology Group study demonstrated that routine surveillance of 216 asymptomatic children identified relapse in only four patients (1.9%). The most important predictor of survival was mean time to relapse with the worst outcomes in those who relapse within the first year, independent of the mode of detection.[25] Therefore, patients who achieve a complete response require no additional surveillance imaging. Because these patients are at a low risk of relapse, positive findings of surveillance PET imaging should be scrutinized for potential false positives.

In particular, patients initially diagnosed with low-risk HL respond well to therapy, often only requiring chemotherapy alone; these patients could avoid aggressive or frequent post-treatment surveillance with FDG-PET. Schwartz and colleagues[28] validated the Childhood Hodgkin International Prognostic Score (CHIPS), which can predict rapid early responders/complete response to therapy, with CHIPS zero to one versus two to three having a 4-year EFS of 90.6% versus 75.9%, respectively. In comparison, patients with

Table 1
Deauville score criteria

1	No FDG uptake
2	FDG uptake less than or equal to mediastinal blood pool
3	FDG uptake greater than mediastinal blood pool but less than or equal to liver
4	FDG uptake moderately greater than liver
5	FDG uptake markedly greater than liver and/or new sites of disease

evidence of response by CT/PET-CT had an EFS of 85% to 88%.[28]

Therefore, the role of post-treatment imaging is indicated for those with residual disease or who develop new symptoms. Imaging is targeted to the site of concern, noting that most recurrent disease is detected by history and physical examination.[29]

FLUORODEOXYGLUCOSE PET PITFALLS

FDG PET/CT has limited use in the setting of surveillance after the completion of therapy because of its high sensitivity (95%), but low positive predictive value (53%).[30] Avid findings on PET imaging are found in malignancy, and are other hypermetabolic processes including infection, inflammation, or increased physiologic activity in the setting of thymic rebound or brown adipose tissue.

Thymus and Lymphoid Tissue

Normal thymic metabolic activity is seen from childhood into early adulthood, characterized in 28% of pediatric patients. Diminutive in size and activity during times of systemic illness and physiologic stress, the thymus can undergo physiologic hyperplasia after chemotherapy. This results in "thymic rebound," which demonstrated relative hypermetabolism on post-treatment FDG-PET (see **Fig. 2**E). Although anterior mediastinal involvement of lymphoma is common, when other sites of disease improve post-treatment, an increase in thymic uptake may be seen. Furthermore, thymic avidity should be homogeneous, and a suspicion for thymic lymphomatous involvement is suggested if thymic uptake is focal or multifocal.[31] In addition, Brink and colleagues[32] evaluated FDG uptake in the thymus of 168 patients and characterized the uptake with respect to age and treatment.

Similarly, increased FDG-uptake is seen within the tonsils or within hypertrophic reactive parapharyngeal lymphoid tissues on the completion of chemotherapy.[33]

Brown Fat

Brown adipose tissue becomes metabolically active in response to cold temperatures and sympathetic nervous system activation; marked brown adipose activity can interfere with FDG-PET imaging interpretations. Sites of brown fat often localize to sites that commonly demonstrate lymphomatous involvement, including the neck, supraclavicular regions, and axillae, and less often within the perivascular mediastinum (**Fig. 4**).[25,34] FDG

activity within brown fat may result in false-positive interpretations; however, if CT imaging is also acquired the avidity is better localized within adipose tissue. Solutions to decreasing the likelihood of brown fat activation include raising the temperature in patient areas or providing warm blankets. Alternative pharmacologic solutions to suppress brown fat activity include the administration of nonselective β-blockers, such as propranolol,[35] or the use of benzodiazepines.[36] Note that pharmacologic brown adipose tissue suppression is off-labeled use for these medications.[37]

Lung Involvement

Although primary pulmonary lymphoma is rare in children, secondary lung involvement occurs in up to 10% of children with HL.[38] CT is more sensitive for the evaluation of pulmonary involvement of lymphoma, because lung nodules less than 5 mm in size are lower than the spatial resolution of FDG-PET. This limitation is in part because of inherent respiratory motion and the resolution of PET scanners.[12] Therefore, the definition of pulmonary

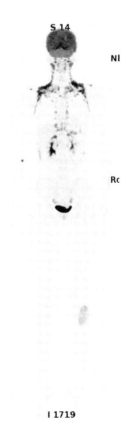

Fig. 4. Whole-body MIP image demonstrating extensive FDG uptake within brown fat of the neck, trapezius musculature, and thoracic paravertebral musculature.

lymphoma involvement is based on dedicated breath-held chest CT imaging. According to the EuroNEt-PHL-C2 trial, lung lymphoma involvement is defined by having at least three foci greater than or equal to 2 mm in size or at least one lesion greater than or equal to 10 mm on CT.[37]

PET/MR IMAGING

To reduce radiation exposure "as low as reasonably achievable" and to follow the principles of "image gently," there has been increased interest in the use of MR imaging in children with lymphoma.[39] Combined imaging with PET/MR imaging reduces exposure from diagnostic radiation by approximately 65% to 73% compared with PET/CT.[40,41] In addition, when using time of flight PET/MR imaging, there is potential for maintaining diagnostic image quality at half the FDG dose.[42] The use of MR imaging also has greater soft tissue contrast compared with CT.

The PET/MR imaging WB MR imaging sequences vary depending on the institutional protocols. At our institution the protocol for lymphoma includes axial T1-weighted two-point Dixon (three-dimensional) sequence and axial diffusion-weighted imaging (DWI) with b values of 50, 400, and 800 performed simultaneously during a 3-minute PET acquisition. Patients with a known diagnosis of Hodgkin disease are scanned from skull base to thighs and patients with NHL are scanned from vertex to toes. Additional axial T2 fast spin echo with fat saturation through the chest, abdomen, and pelvis is performed with a smaller field of view to improve resolution. DWI has largely replaced the need for contrast-enhanced MR imaging for lymph node assessment. Postcontrast imaging is not used, which reduces the risk of contrast-related side effects, such as allergic reactions in children, and the unknown effects of gadolinium deposition in the brain, which is currently under investigation.[43] Alternative intravenous contrast agents, such as ferumoxytol, are being evaluated.[44] PET/MR imaging scan time is approximately 75 minutes.[45]

PET/MR Imaging Versus Whole-Body MR Imaging

WB MR imaging has also been used at some institutions as an additional form of imaging in pediatric lymphoma. Kirchner and colleagues[40] evaluated WB MR imaging with DWI compared with three different PET/MR imaging protocols (unenhanced PET/MR imaging, contrast-enhanced PET/MR imaging, and contrast-enhanced PET/MR imaging with DWI) for staging or monitoring pediatric lymphoma. Although WB

MR imaging demonstrated good specificity and positive predictive value, all PET/MR imaging protocols demonstrated significantly greater sensitivity, negative predictive value, and diagnostic accuracy compared with WB MR imaging (sensitivity, specificity, positive predictive value, negative predictive value, and diagnostic accuracy were 96%, 96.5%, 97%, 95%, and 96% for unenhanced PET/MR imaging; 97%, 96.5%, 97%, 96.5%, and 97% for contrast-enhanced PET/MR imaging; 97%, 96.5%, 97%, 96.5%, and 97% for contrast-enhanced PET/MR imaging with DWI PET/MR imaging; and 77%, 96%, 96%, 78.5%, and 86% for MR imaging-DWI). There was also no significant difference between the different PET/MR imaging protocols.[40]

PET/Computed Tomography and PET/MR Imaging

There are a limited number of studies comparing the use of FDG PET/CT and FDG PET/MR imaging in the pediatric population. In the adult literature, similar diagnostic accuracy has been shown between these two modalities.[46,47] Among children with a variety of different cancers, Schäfer and colleagues[41] found equivalent cancer detection rates and significantly reduced radiation exposure.

Within the pediatric lymphoma literature, few studies comparing PET/CT and PET/MR imaging have been performed. Sher and colleagues[48] performed 40 prospective sequential PET/CT and PET/MR imaging with children with known diagnoses of lymphoma (PET/MR imaging was performed first in 31 of these patients). Between these two modalities, there was no statistically significant difference in lesion detection or diagnostic accuracy, and no differences in Ann Arbor clinical staging.[48]

Similarly, Ponisio and colleagues[49] performed sequential FDG-PET/CT and FDG-PET/MR imaging examinations in patients with pediatric lymphoma to evaluate the feasibility and diagnostic performance. The evaluation of nine PET/MR images in eight patients and found comparable lesion detection and 100% concordance in examination interpretation.[49]

Even when sequentially performed, SUV for PET/CT and PET/MR imaging were strongly correlated, but PET/MR imaging underestimated lesion SUV when it was the first of the two studies performed.[48,49] The reason for this is unclear, but may in part be caused by the amount of time between FDG dose injection and PET image acquisition between PET/CT and PET/MR imaging examinations. For example, in the study performed by Sher and colleagues,[48] the average time between PET image acquisition when PET/CT was performed first was 34 minutes, versus 61 minutes when PET/MR imaging was performed first; this may result in higher SUV values in the PET/CT performed at the later time point. Nonetheless, the diagnostic quality of these examinations was not statistically different.[48]

Potential PET/MR Imaging Disadvantages

Although FDG-PET/MR imaging is a promising new modality, there is not yet enough data to support its routine use for staging or surveillance of children with lymphoma. PET/MR imaging protocols are still under development, and its availability globally is limited.

In addition to the cost of performing PET/MR imaging fused imaging, PET/MR imaging can take 60 to 90 minutes or longer to acquire compared with approximately less than 30 minutes with FDG-PET/CT. In children, this additional time may also require extended periods of anesthesia to limit motion degradation.[50]

Furthermore, the use of MR imaging for attenuation correction and anatomic correlation is a potential limitation of PET/MR imaging. There are inherent difficulties in using MR imaging for attenuation correction of the lungs. For example, Schäfer and colleagues[41] noted a case of lung metastases missed on PET/MR imaging. However, given the limitations of FDG-PET for resolving small lung lesions, dedicated chest CT imaging might be necessary when staging children at risk for lung metastases. Regarding the use of MR imaging for anatomic correlation, although Sher and colleagues[48] noted no difference in diagnostic accuracy between PET/MR imaging and PET/CT, one discordant finding/false-positive finding on PET/MR imaging was physiologic FDG uptake within bowel mistaken as mesenteric lymphadenopathy. Potential variability in MR imaging for anatomic correlation may change with altered PET/MR imaging protocols.

Although there is reduced diagnostic radiation exposure with PET/MR imaging, therapeutic radiation doses have a stronger contribution to the risk of secondary neoplasms in patients with pediatric lymphoma.[51] Therefore, the cost-benefit of using PET/MR imaging has not yet been established, especially because annual post-treatment surveillance imaging with FDG-PET is not necessary in most patients with lymphoma. Further research into the use of PET/MR imaging in pediatric oncology patients is needed with continued collaborations among institutions.

DISCLOSURE

The authors have nothing to disclose.

ACKNOWLEDGMENTS

The authors thank Dr. David Mankoff for his help and mentorship as an advisor on this paper.

REFERENCES

1. Percy CL, Smith MA, Linet M, et al. Lymphomas and reticuloendothelial neoplasms. In: Ries LA, Smith MA, Gurney JG, et al, editors. Cancer incidence and survival among children and adolescents: United States SEER program 1975-1995. Bethesda, Maryland: National Cancer Institute; 1999. p. 1–170. Available at: http://www-seer.ims.nci.nih.gov.

2. Smith MA, Seibel NL, Altekruse SF, et al. Outcomes for children and adolescents with cancer: challenges for the twenty-first century. J Clin Oncol 2010;28(15):2625–34.

3. Freed J, Kelly KM. Current approaches to the management of pediatric Hodgkin lymphoma. Pediatr Drugs 2010;12(2):85–98.

4. Abramson SB, Jacob D, Rosenfeld M, et al. A 3-year M.D.: accelerating careers, diminishing debt. N Engl J Med 2013;369:1085–7.

5. Friedman DL, Chen L, Wolden S, et al. Dose-intensive response-based chemotherapy and radiation therapy for children and adolescents with newly diagnosed intermediate-risk Hodgkin lymphoma: a report from the Children's Oncology Group Study AHOD0031. J Clin Oncol 2014;32(32):3651–8.

6. Mauz-Körholz C, Metzger ML, Kelly KM, et al. Pediatric Hodgkin lymphoma. J Clin Oncol 2015;33(27):2975–85.

7. Holmqvist AS, Chen Y, Berano Teh J, et al. Risk of solid subsequent malignant neoplasms after childhood Hodgkin lymphoma: identification of high-risk populations to guide surveillance. A report from the Late Effects Study Group. Cancer 2019;125(8):1373–83.

8. Metzger ML, Weinstein HJ, Hudson MM, et al. Association between radiotherapy vs no radiotherapy based on early response to VAMP chemotherapy and survival among children with favorable-risk Hodgkin lymphoma. JAMA 2012;307(24):2609–16.

9. Kaplan HS. Hodgkin's disease. 2nd edition. Cambridge (MA): Harvard University Press;1980.

10. Cheson BD, Fisher RI, Barrington SF, et al. Recommendations for initial evaluation, staging, and response assessment of Hodgkin and non-Hodgkin lymphoma: the Lugano classification. J Clin Oncol 2014;32(27):3059–67.

11. Barrington SF, Mikhaeel NG, Kostakoglu L, et al. Role of imaging in the staging and response

assessment of lymphoma: consensus of the International Conference on Malignant Lymphomas Imaging Working Group. J Clin Oncol 2014;32(27):3048–58.

12. Kabickova E, Sumerauer D, Cumlivska E, et al. Comparison of 18F-FDG-PET and standard procedures for the pretreatment staging of children and adolescents with Hodgkin's disease. Eur J Nucl Med Mol Imaging 2006;33(9):1025–31.

13. London K, Cross S, Onikul E, et al. 18F-FDG PET/CT in paediatric lymphoma: comparison with conventional imaging. Eur J Nucl Med Mol Imaging 2011;38(2):274–84.

14. Robertson VL, Anderson CS, Keller FG, et al. Role of FDG-PET in the definition of involved-field radiation therapy and management for pediatric Hodgkin's lymphoma. Int J Radiat Oncol Biol Phys 2011;80(2):324–32.

15. Cheng G, Chen W, Chamroonrat W, et al. Biopsy versus FDG PET/CT in the initial evaluation of bone marrow involvement in pediatric lymphoma patients. Eur J Nucl Med Mol Imaging 2011;38(8):1469–76.

16. Yağci-Küpeli B, Koçyiğit-Deveci E, Adamhasan F, et al. The value of 18F-FDG PET/CT in detecting bone marrow involvement in childhood cancers. J Pediatr Hematol Oncol 2019;41(6):438–41.

17. Badr S, Kotb M, Elahmadawy MA, et al. Predictive value of FDG PET/CT versus bone marrow biopsy in pediatric lymphoma. Clin Nucl Med 2018;43(12):e428–38.

18. Adams HJA, Kwee TC. Do not abandon the bone marrow biopsy yet in diffuse large B-cell lymphoma. J Clin Oncol 2015;33(10):1217.

19. Zhou Z, Sehn LH, Rademaker AW, et al. An enhanced International Prognostic Index (NCCN-IPI) for patients with diffuse large B-cell lymphoma treated in the rituximab era. Blood 2014;123(6):837–42.

20. Cerci JJ, Etchebehere EC, Nadel H, et al. Is true whole-body 18 F-FDG PET/CT required in pediatric lymphoma? An IAEA multicenter prospective study. J Nucl Med 2019;60(8):1087–93.

21. Sedig LK, Bailey JJ, Wong KK, et al. Do Deauville scores improve the clinical utility of end-of-therapy FDG PET scans for pediatric Hodgkin lymphoma? Am J Roentgenol 2019;212(2):456–60.

22. Dörffel W, Rühl U, Lüders H, et al. Treatment of children and adolescents with Hodgkin lymphoma without radiotherapy for patients in complete remission after chemotherapy: final results of the multinational trial GPOH-HD95. J Clin Oncol 2013;31(12):1562–8.

23. Charpentier AM, Friedman DL, Wolden S, et al. Predictive factor analysis of response-adapted radiation therapy for chemotherapy-sensitive pediatric Hodgkin lymphoma: analysis of the Children's

Oncology Group AHOD 0031 Trial. Int J Radiat Oncol Biol Phys 2016;96(5):943–50.

24. Friedman D, Wolden S, Constine L, et al. AHOD0031: a phase III study of dose-intensive therapy for intermediate risk Hodgkin lymphoma: a report from the Children's Oncology Group. Blood 2010;116(21):766.

25. Voss SD, Chen L, Constine LS, et al. Surveillance computed tomography imaging and detection of relapse in intermediate- and advanced-stage pediatric Hodgkin's lymphoma: a report from the Children's Oncology Group. J Clin Oncol 2012;30(21):2635–40.

26. Gallamini A, Hutchings M, Rigacci L, et al. Early interim 2-[18F]fluoro-2-deoxy-D-glucose positron emission tomography is prognostically superior to international prognostic score in advanced-stage Hodgkin's lymphoma: a report from a joint Italian-Danish study. J Clin Oncol 2007;25(24):3746–52.

27. Hutchings M, Loft A, Hansen M, et al. FDG-PET after two cycles of chemotherapy predicts treatment failure and progression-free survival in Hodgkin lymphoma. Blood 2006;107(1):52–9.

28. Schwartz CL, Chen L, McCarten K, et al. Childhood Hodgkin international prognostic score (CHIPS) predicts event-free survival in Hodgkin lymphoma: a report from the Children's Oncology Group. Pediatr Blood Cancer 2017;64(4).

29. Friedmann AM, Wolfson JA, Hudson MM, et al. Relapse after treatment of pediatric Hodgkin lymphoma: outcome and role of surveillance after end of therapy. Pediatr Blood Cancer 2013;60(9):1458–63.

30. Rhodes MM, Delbeke D, Whitlock JA, et al. Utility of FDG-PET/CT in follow-up of children treated for Hodgkin and non-Hodgkin lymphoma. J Pediatr Hematol Oncol 2006;28(5):300–6.

31. Jerushalmi J, Frenkel A, Bar-Shalom R. Physiologic thymic uptake of 18F-FDG in children and young adults: a PET/CT evaluation of incidence, patterns, and relationship to treatment. J Nucl Med 2009;50(6):849–53.

32. Brink I, Reinhardt MJ, Hoegerle S, et al. Increased metabolic activity in the thymus gland studied with 18F-FDG PET: age dependency and frequency after chemotherapy. J Nucl Med 2001;42(4):591–5. Available at: http://www.ncbi.nlm.nih.gov/pubmed/11337547.

33. Okuyama C, Matsushima S, Nishimura M, et al. Increased 18 F-FDG accumulation in the tonsils after chemotherapy for pediatric lymphoma: a common physiological phenomenon. Ann Nucl Med 2019;33(5):368–73.

34. Kaste SC, Howard SC, McCarville EB, et al. 18F-FDG-avid sites mimicking active disease in pediatric Hodgkin's. Pediatr Radiol 2005;35(2):141–54.

35. George A, Sinha P, Conrad G, et al. Pilot study of propranolol premedication to reduce FDG uptake in brown adipose tissue on PET scans of adolescent and young adult oncology patients. Pediatr Hematol Oncol 2017;34(3):149–56.

36. Cousins J, Czachowski M, Muthukrishnan A, et al. Pediatric brown adipose tissue on 18F-FDG PET: diazepam intervention. J Nucl Med Technol 2017; 45(2):82–6.

37. Kluge R, Kurch L, Georgi T, et al. Current role of FDG-PET in pediatric Hodgkin's lymphoma. Semin Nucl Med 2017. https://doi.org/10.1053/j.semnuclmed.2017.01.001.

38. Urasinski T, Kamienska E, Gawlikowska-Sroka A, et al. Pediatric pulmonary Hodgkin lymphoma: analysis of 10 years data from a single center. Eur J Med Res 2010;15(2):206–10.

39. Treves ST, Gelfand M, Parisi M, et al. Update: image gently and nuclear medicine at 10 years. J Nucl Med 2019;60(4):7N–9N. Available at:http://www.ncbi.nlm.nih.gov/pubmed/30936261.

40. Kirchner J, Deuschl C, Schweiger B, et al. Imaging children suffering from lymphoma: an evaluation of different 18F-FDG PET/MRI protocols compared to whole-body DW-MRI. Eur J Nucl Med Mol Imaging 2017;44(10):1742–50.

41. Schäfer JF, Gatidis S, Schmidt H, et al. Simultaneous whole-body PET/MR imaging in comparison to PET/CT in pediatric oncology: initial results. Radiology 2014;273(1):220–31.

42. Schmall J, Nevo E, Edwards K, et al. Investigating low-dose image quality in pediatric TOF-PET/MRI. J Nucl Med 2018;59(supplement 1):304.

43. Mayerhoefer ME, Archibald SJ, Messiou C, et al. MRI and PET/MRI in hematologic malignancies. J Magn Reson Imaging 2019. https://doi.org/10.1002/jmri.26848.

44. Toth GB, Varallyay CG, Horvath A, et al. Current and potential imaging applications of ferumoxytol for magnetic resonance imaging. Kidney Int 2017; 92(1):47–66.

45. Klenk C, Gawande R, Uslu L, et al. Ionising radiation-free whole-body MRI versus (18)F-fluorodeoxyglucose PET/CT scans for children and young adults with cancer: a prospective, non-randomised, single-centre study. Lancet Oncol 2014;15(3): 275–85.

46. Drzezga A, Souvatzoglou M, Eiber M, et al. First clinical experience with integrated whole-body PET/MR: comparison to PET/CT in patients with oncologic diagnoses. J Nucl Med 2012;53(6):845–55.

47. Heusch P, Nensa F, Schaarschmidt B, et al. Diagnostic accuracy of whole-body PET/MRI and whole-body PET/CT for TNM staging in oncology. Eur J Nucl Med Mol Imaging 2015;42(1):42–8.

48. Sher AC, Seghers V, Paldino MJ, et al. Assessment of sequential PET/MRI in comparison with PET/CT of pediatric lymphoma: a prospective study. Am J Roentgenol 2016;206(3):623–31.

49. Ponisio MR, McConathy J, Laforest R, et al. Evaluation of diagnostic performance of whole-body simultaneous PET/MRI in pediatric lymphoma. Pediatr Radiol 2016;46(9):1258–68.

50. Ehman EC, Johnson GB, Villanueva-Meyer JE, et al. PET/MRI: where might it replace PET/CT? J Magn Reson Imaging 2017;46(5):1247–62.

51. Nievelstein RAJ, Van Ufford HMEQ, Kwee TC, et al. Radiation exposure and mortality risk from CT and PET imaging of patients with malignant lymphoma. Eur Radiol 2012;22(9):1946–54.

Roles of F-18-Fluoro-2-Deoxy-Glucose PET/Computed Tomography Scans in the Management of Post-Transplant Lymphoproliferative Disease in Pediatric Patient

Yan-Feng Xu, MD, PhD, Ji-Gang Yang, MD, PhD*

KEYWORDS

- PTLD • Pediatrics • PET/CT

KEY POINTS

- PET/computed tomography scanning plays a pivotal role in the early diagnosis of the lesions, in guiding biopsy, and in the surveillance of treatment response in patients with post-transplant lymphoproliferative disease.
- Although PET/computed tomography scanning has been shown to be potentially useful in post-transplant lymphoproliferative disease of adults, the evidence in children is insufficient.
- PET/computed tomography scanning is supposed to be a useful tool for staging and follow-up of pediatric patients with post-transplant lymphoproliferative disease and can detect occult lesions not visualized on other imaging modalities.

INTRODUCTION

Post-transplant lymphoproliferative disease (PTLD) is a relatively new disease entity that is now widely recognized. It is a serious complication after solid organ and hematopoietic stem cell transplantation, decreasing both patient and organ survival.[1] PTLD may develop at any time with a first peak incidence within 1 year after transplantation and a second peak after 4 to 5 years.[2] It is the second most common malignancy in adult transplant recipients and the most common post-transplant malignancy in children. The incidence of PTLD may vary from 1% to 20%,[3] and risk factors for the development of PTLD include a high level of immunosuppression, Epstein-Barr virus (EBV) infection, human leukocyte antigen mismatching, and T-cell depletion.

CLINICAL FEATURES AND TREATMENT OF POST-TRANSPLANT LYMPHOPROLIFERATIVE DISORDER

PTLD are specific types of lymphoma. The vast majority of PTLD cases (approximately 85%) are of B-cell origin and out of these, 80% are associated with EBV infection.[1] The incidence of EBV-associated PTLD has been reported to be 1.2% in adults and up to 8.4% in children,[4] which is most likely owing to the transmission of the

Nuclear Medicine Department, Beijing Friendship Hospital, Capital Medical University, 95 Yong An Road, Xi Cheng District, Beijing 100050, China
* Corresponding author.
E-mail address: 13681221974@163.com

PET Clin 15 (2020) 309–319
https://doi.org/10.1016/j.cpet.2020.03.006
1556-8598/20/© 2020 Elsevier Inc. All rights reserved.

infection from an organ from an EBV-seropositive donor to a seronegative recipient (D+/R−).[5] Despite the strong association between EBV and PTLD, disease biology has not been well-understood.[6]

As a serious complication after transplantation, PTLD has a heterogeneous clinical presentation, which may resemble allograft dysfunction or developing lymphadenopathy or other mass lesions, but may also be limited to nonspecific symptoms including weight loss, fever, or malaise. At diagnosis, the clinical spectrum ranges from solitary asymptomatic process to fulminant systemic disease.[7] The diagnosis of PTLD is based on histopathologic confirmation after clinical suspicion. However, unusual or unexpected presentations can hinder early diagnosis.[8–14] PTLD is defined by the presence of specific histopathologic changes that include benign plasmacytic hyperplasia and malignant lymphoma. According to the World Health Organization 2008 classification, PTLD has 4 main pathologic categories: (a) hyperplastic (or early) lesions, (b) polymorphic lesions, (c) monomorphic (ie, lymphomatous, invariably monoclonal) lesions, which are further subcategorized along recognized lines of B-cell, T-cell, or natural killer cell neoplasia, and (d) other lymphoproliferative disorders, including Hodgkin lymphoma.[15]

Because of the similarities in pathology, treatment of PTLD is largely based on insights in lymphomagenesis in immunocompetent patients. Decreasing immunosuppression and targeting B-cell proliferation with rituximab alone or in combination with chemotherapy drugs are commonly used strategies in PTLD treatment. Data show that the addition of rituximab to the standard CHOP (cyclophosphamide, adriamycin, vincristine, and prednisone) regimen as first-line treatment for late PTLD should be strongly considered. Some researchers believe that rituximab consolidation is superior to regimens without consolidation for patients in complete remission after rituximab induction therapy.[16] In case of EBV-positive PTLD, preemptive treatment with rituximab is often initiated based on EBV DNA levels. However, a considerable limitation of this approach is the lack of standardized cut-off values, monitoring time points, and sampling source.[17] The role of antiviral prophylaxis for the prevention of PTLD remains controversial, and a systematic review showed that antiviral prophylaxis had no influence on the incidence of PTLD, regardless of the antiviral agent, the duration of antiviral prophylaxis, or the age of the recipient.[18] Many other drugs are being tested for PTLD, including immunomodulatory agents (such as leflunomide and its active metabolite teriflunomide), the checkpoint inhibitor blockade (specially the programmed death 1/programmed death ligand 1 pathway) and anti-CD30 monoclonal antibody (brentuximab vedotin).

CLINICAL FEATURES OF POST-TRANSPLANT LYMPHOPROLIFERATIVE DISORDER IN PEDIATRIC PATIENTS

PTLD is the most common malignancy affecting children after transplantation.[19] The risk of PTLD is higher in children than in adults, probably because of the greater incidence of pretransplant EBV infection in children.[20] A research from Australia compared overall and site-specific incidences of cancer after kidney transplantation in childhood recipients by using standardized incidence ratios. This study showed that the standardized incidence ratio for non-skin cancer was 8.23 (95% confidence interval, 6.92–9.73), with the highest risk for PTLD (standardized incidence ratio, 45.80; 95% confidence interval, 32.71–62.44).[21] However, although the overall mortality rate is relatively high, the prognosis is likely to be better in children than in adults.[22]

THE VALUE OF F-18-FLUORO-2-DEOXY-GLUCOSE PET/COMPUTED TOMOGRAPHY SCANS IN ADULT POST-TRANSPLANT LYMPHOPROLIFERATIVE DISORDER

In recent years, F-18-fluoro-2-deoxy-glucose (FDG) PET/computed tomography (CT) scanning has gained clinical importance in the evaluation of PTLD, which is special type of lymphoma. FDG PET/CT scanning plays pivotal roles in the early detection of the lesions, in guiding biopsy, and in the surveillance of treatment response in patients with various other types of lymphomas in different clinical settings.[23–45] A research showed that FDG PET scans detected more lesions in smaller lymph nodes and bone/bone marrow, whereas CT scanning was superior in detecting lesions in the bowel and stomach.[46] Although FDG PET/CT scanning has proven as an indispensable an imaging modality in the staging, restaging, and evaluation of treatment response in many other types of lymphomas,[47,48] there is no universally accepted standardized imaging approach to assess PTLD, either at staging or for response evaluation to therapy at this moment.

A published single-institution series including 150 patients with suspected PTLD showed that

FDG PET scanning had high specificity (89%) in differentiating PTLD from benign etiologies,[49] which suggest that PET scanning is useful in directing the most appropriate site for biopsy to confirm the diagnosis. FDG PET/CT scan is useful in resolving equivocal findings on CT scans. In a case series, PET/CT scans upstaged 2 of 5 patients with biopsy-proven PTLD after renal transplantation.[50] In another case series, PET/CT scans detected occult lesions not identified on other imaging modalities in 57% of patients.[51] Panagiotidis et al[52] investigated the roles of FDG PET/CT scans in the evaluation of PTLD in 40 patients and demonstrated that PET/CT scans had a sensitivity of 88.2% and a specificity of 91.3%, while the diagnostic performance of CT scans had a sensitivity of 87.5% and a specificity of 88.8%.[52] A small study involving 5 cases showed that FDG PET/CT scans revealed more lesions than CT scans, upstaged the disease, and detected 3 extranodal findings that were not visualized in conventional imaging.[52] Noraini et al[53] reported PET/CT scans showed comparable sensitivity (75% vs 83%), similar specificity (100% in both modalities), and comparable accuracy (77% vs 85%) compared with conventional imaging during staging at diagnosis. Pooled data from 7 studies showed that PET/CT scans identified additional lesions in 27.8% (95% confidence interval, 17.0%–42.0%) not detected by morphologic imaging (CT scans or MR imaging).[54] A recent meta-analysis showed that the pooled sensitivity and specificity of FDG PET/CT scans in the evaluation of adult PTLD are 89.7% and 90.9%, respectively.[55]

It is known that FDG uptake in classically indolent or low-grade lymphomas is relatively low, although patients with non-Hodgkin lymphoma and a standardized uptake value of (SUV) of greater than 10 have a high likelihood for aggressive disease.[56] Takehana et al[51] retrospectively reviewed the records of 30 patients who underwent FDG PET/CT scanning for the evaluation of PTLD and demonstrated that the more aggressive PTLD histologic subtypes had higher a maximum SUV (SUV_{max}) compared with the less aggressive subtypes (10.9 ± 7.5 vs 4.5 ± 3.0), which indicated that FDG PET/CT scans might predict the PTLD subtype, because the lesions with higher pathologic grade presenting with significantly higher SUV_{max} compared with the less aggressive forms.

FDG PET/CT is not only an accurate diagnostic tool for staging, but also helpful for the treatment assessment and follow-up of patients with PTLD.[57] In comparison with anatomic imaging, PET/CT scanning was found to be superior to conventional imaging modalities at follow-up, with greater sensitivity (100% vs 81%), and comparable specificity (80% vs 100%), and accuracy (97% vs 83%).[53] To evaluate the role of PET/CT in response assessment by the end of treatment, Zimmermann et al[58] performed a retrospective, multicenter study of 37 patients with CD20-positive PTLD after solid organ transplantation treated with uniform, up-to-date, first-line protocols. This study demonstrated that the positive predictive value of end-of-treatment PET/CT scans for PTLD relapse was 38%, and the negative predictive value was 92%. Time to progression and progression-free survival were significantly longer in the PET negative group ($P = .019$ and $P = .013$). End-of-treatment PET scans in PTLD identified patients at low risk of relapse and offered clinically relevant information, particularly in patients in a partial remission by CT results.[58] Another report found that FDG PET/CT scanning turned out to be an excellent predictor of progression-free survival in patients with PTLD. Five patients reached complete remission confirmed by both CT and FDG PET/CT scans and remained progression free with a median follow-up of 37 months (range, 3–46 months).[59] The investigation involving the largest patient population was from Montes de Jesus et al[60] with 91 consecutive patients. In this retrospective study, the authors noted that FDG PET/CT scanning has a sensitivity of 85% and a specificity of 90% with good interobserver agreement. Interestingly, the sensitivity of FDG PET/CT seems related to the patients' lactate dehydrogenase levels.[60]

Bone marrow biopsy (BMB) remains the standard to detect bone marrow involvement, but is prone to sampling error. Gheysens et al[61] retrospectively investigated whether PET/CT scans could identify bone marrow involvement in patients with PTLD with sufficient accuracy in comparison with staging BMB. Twenty-five patients diagnosed with PTLD who underwent PET/CT scans and BMB within 1 month were evaluated, and 6 patients (24%) were considered positive for bone marrow involvement on PET/CT scans compared with 1 by BMB. Although they could not completely exclude false-positive results on the PET/CT scans, data demonstrated a significantly higher sensitivity of PET/CT scanning compared with BMB (100% vs 17%), but a similar specificity. These data confirmed the high diagnostic performance of 18-F-FDG-PET/CT scans for detecting bone marrow involvement, but prospective studies are still needed to determine whether 18-F-FDG-PET/CT scans could indeed replace BMB in PTLD.[61]

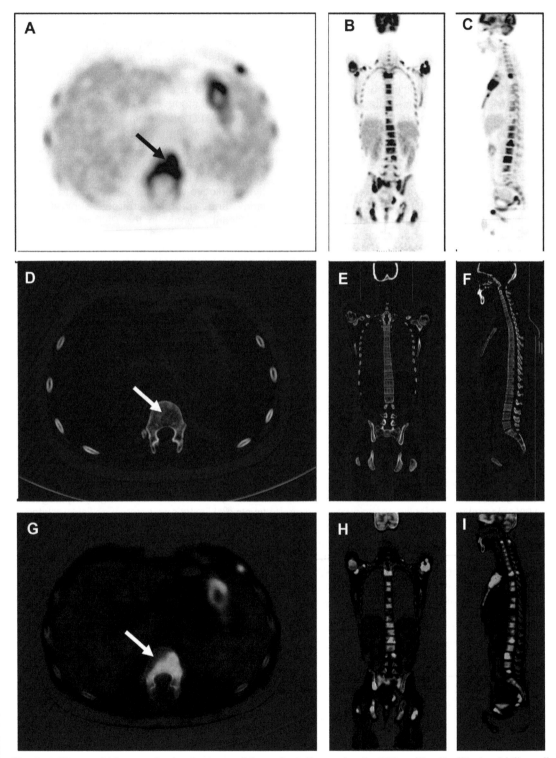

Fig. 1. A 17-year-old boy received auto stem cell transplantation owing to EBV-positive T-cell/natural killer cell lymphoproliferative disease and developed PTLD. PET images show multiple bone lesions with intense FDG up-take (*A*, axial; *B*, coronal; *C*, sagittal). CT images did not show obvious abnormalities of bone (*D*, axial; *E*, coronal; *F*, sagittal). Fused PET/CT images show multiple bone lesions with intense FDG uptake (*G*, axial; *H*, coronal; *I*, sagittal). Arrows in Fig. 1. A, D, G showed one of the bone lesions in the patient.

THE VALUE OF PET/COMPUTED TOMOGRAPHY SCANS IN POST-TRANSPLANT LYMPHOPROLIFERATIVE DISORDER OF PEDIATRIC PATIENTS

F-18-Fluoro-2-Deoxy-Glucose PET/Computed Tomography Scans in the Initial Evaluation of Pediatric Post-Transplant Lymphoproliferative Disorder

The current literature showed that FDG PET/CT scanning has additional value in the initial evaluation of pediatric patients with PTLD. A cohort study involving 34 pediatric patients showed that FDG PET scans can provide more information compared with conventional CT scans in the initial staging of PTLD in pediatric patients (**Fig. 1**).[46] FDG PET scans detected more lesions than conventional CT scans and upstaged 20.5% of patients.[46] However, because PET scans lack anatomic details, correlative CT scans are essential to clearly localize the lesions on PET scanning and to minimize false-positive results. This finding is particularly important in patients with PTLD, because many patients have extranodal sites of involvement. At the same time, CT scans also can detect some lesions not detected by 18-F-FDG PET scans. 18-F-FDG PET and CT scans are complementary at initial staging of pediatric PTLD, and extranodal involvement in patients with PTLD were observed in 70% patients.[51] FDG PET/CT scans represented a good alternative imaging method to avoid contrast-related nephrotoxicity in patients who developed impaired renal function secondary to chronic immunosuppressive therapy.

FDG PET/CT scans may be used to guide biopsy in pediatric patients suspected of having PTLD, because combining the detailed anatomic information from CT scans with the metabolic information from PET scans can enable the precise localization of high FDG uptake (**Fig. 2**). Adding FDG PET to CT scans can improve the diagnostic accuracy of CT scans and guide biopsies by indicating areas of high metabolic activity, rather than

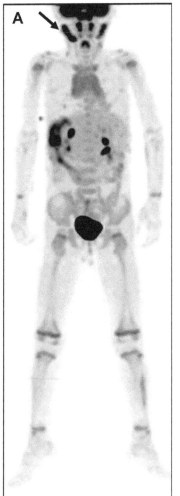

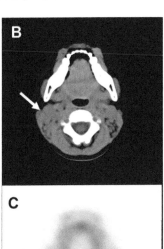

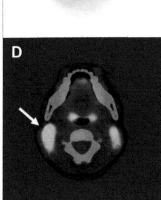

Fig. 2. A 3-year-old patient with PTLD after liver transplantation owing to bird amino acid carbamoyltransferase deficiency. Laboratory tests showed a positive result in EBV load. PET/CT scanning showed multiple enlarged lymph nodes on the bilateral cervix, stomach, spleen, abdominal aorta, and mesentery. The largest located in the right neck II area about 2.3 × 1.4 cm with an SUV_{max}/mean of 7.8/4.8. Excision biopsy of right lateral cervical lymph node confirmed early lesions of PTLD after transplantation. (*A*) Maximum image projection. (*B*) CT scam. (*C*) PET scan. (*D*) Fusion imaging. Arrows in Fig. 2 showed the enlarged lymph node on the right cervix.

necrosis and fibrosis, within a mass. In patients with multiple lesions, FDG PET/CT scans can show the most prominent and active lesions, which may guide the interventionists to biopsy areas of highest 18-F-FDG uptake, potentially leading to early histologic diagnosis and fewer false-negative results.[62] Accurate biopsy at the correct site will decrease the need for repeating biopsy, as well as the potential risk of reseeding tumors by multiple sampling.[62]

Vali et al[46] retrospectively evaluated the value of PET/CT scans in 34 consecutive pediatric patients with PTLD. On lesion-based analysis, 18-F-FDG PET scans showed more lesions than conventional CT scans (168 vs 134), but CT scans revealed 22 lesions negative on PET. These findings indicated that FDG PET and CT scans were complementary at the initial staging of pediatric PTLD.[46] Based on 3 studies, FDG PET/CT scan findings upstaged patients compared with CT scans alone in 15.3%.[56] FDG PET/CT scanning was used to clarify dubious lesions seen on morphologic imaging in 29.1%.[46,51,52] However, one of the most recent investigations involving 28 pediatric patients with PTLD suggests that FDG PET/CT scanning has excellent specificity and positive predicative value, but that the sensitivity and negative predicative value are less ideal.[63] This is because FDG PET/CT scans can fail to detect histologically confirmed PTLD in the regions where there was high physiologic background FDG uptake, including the brain, kidneys, or heart.[49,52]

F-18-Fluoro-2-Deoxy-Glucose PET/Computed Tomography Scans in the Diagnosis of Pathologic Types of Pediatric Post-Transplant Lymphoproliferative Disorder

FDG PET/CT scanning has been tried in the differential diagnosis of pathologic types of pediatric PTLD. One report showed that the SUV_{max} determined by FDG PET/CT scanning was significantly higher in monomorphic/Hodgkin subtypes than in polymorphic subtypes of PTLD (10.9 ± 7.5 vs 4.5 ± 3.0).[52] Another investigation reported that less FDG uptake in patients with early and polymorphic PTLD, with an SUV_{max} of 4.8 ± 2.3 and 5.1 ± 2.8, respectively, comparing the SUV_{max} in the monomorphic PTLD, which was 8.9±6.3.[46] Highly malignant subtypes showed a higher SUV_{max} than early and polymorphic subtypes (**Fig. 3**). However, the difference was not statistically significant ($P = .11$). These results suggest that the monomorphic types of PTLD in children is more aggressive. However, it should be emphasized that 18-F-FDG PET/CT scans could not definitely differentiate or diagnose the different types of PTLD in pediatric patients.

F-18-Fluoro-2-Deoxy-Glucose PET/Computed Tomography Scans in the Evaluation of the Therapy Response of Pediatric Post-Transplant Lymphoproliferative Disorder

FDG PET/CT scanning is a useful imaging modality in the staging and evaluation of therapy response in both adult and pediatric lymphoma, and increased

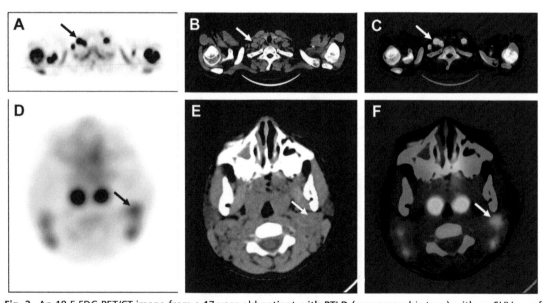

Fig. 3. An 18-F-FDG PET/CT image from a 17-year-old patient with PTLD (monomorphic type) with an SUV_{max} of 22.3 (A) PET scan. (B) CT scan. (C) Fusion imaging. The 18-F-FDG PET/CT images of a 2-year-old patient with PTLD (early lesions) with an SUV_{max} of 3.1. (D) PET scan. (E) CT scan. (F) Fusion imaging. Arrows in Fig.3 A-C showed the enlarged lymph node on the right supraclavicular of the patient with monomorphic type. Arrows in Fig.3 D-F showed the enlarged lymph node on the left cervix of the patient with early lesions.

the sensitivity and specificity of disease assessment over conventional imaging method in detecting additional lesions, with modification of clinical stage in 15% to 20% of adult patients, and 50% in pediatric patients.[64] Besides, FDG PET/CT scanning is also more accurate than CT scanning alone in evaluating response after the completion of therapy or determining recurrence because of its advantage in distinguishing between viable tumor and necrosis or fibrosis in residual masses.[65]

The potential roles of PET/CT scanning in adult PTLD has been well-recognized. However, there is its use in pediatric PTLD is less reported. PET/CT scanning may have an important role in the staging and follow-up of pediatric patients with PTLD[66] (**Fig. 4**). In a small cohort of 9 pediatric

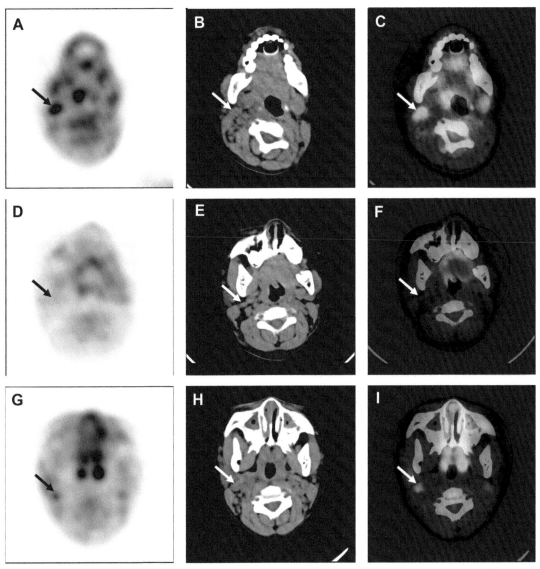

Fig. 4. A 3-year-old child underwent liver transplantation owing to cryptogenic cirrhosis 1 year ago. After transplantation, the patient regularly received antirejection treatment. PET/CT scans showed multiple enlarged lymph nodes in the bilateral cervix, and some of them showed abnormal FDG uptake with an SUV$_{max}$/mean of 2.6/1.6 (PET/CT scan on October 25, 2017). (A) PET scan. (B) CT scan. (C) Fusion imaging. A left cervical lymph node biopsy demonstrated early pathologic changes of PTLD. One year after treatment with decreasing antirejection dose and rituximab, a PET/CT scan demonstrated that cervical lymph nodes reduced significantly, without obvious FDG uptake (PET/CT on September 12, 2018). (D) PET scan. (E) CT scan. (F) Fusion imaging. Two years after treatment, a PET/CT scan showed the enlargement of cervical lymph nodes again, with increased FDG uptake and an SUV$_{max}$/mean of 1.9/1.3. (G–I) PET/CT scan on January 23, 2019. (G) PET scan. (H) CT scan. (I) Fusion imaging, which suggested disease progress. Arrows in Fig.4 showed the enlarged lymph node on the right cervix of the patient.

patients, it was found that PET/CT results helped to stop treatment in a significant proportion of patients (6 of 9), including 3 cases where CT results on their own might have mandated continuation of treatment, and the use of PET/CT scanning guided or altered clinical management in 8 patients (89% of cases).[67] Von Falck and colleagues[68] studied a pediatric population of 7 patients with PTLD both at staging and during treatment. In this cohort, initial staging PET/CT scans correlated with cross-sectional imaging in all cases. PET/CT scans helped to clarify equivocal findings in 3 of 7 cases and it was able to demonstrate remission earlier than conventional cross-sectional imaging in 3 patients. Patients with complete metabolic response in PET/CT had no evidence of recurrent disease for at least 9 months.[68] These studies concluded that a single whole-body PET/CT examination had comparable performance to conventional imaging in initial staging of pediatric PTLD and was more accurate in the evaluation of the therapeutic efficacy than conventional imaging.

Available studies reported promising results in detection, staging, and therapy evaluation, but suffered from methodologic shortcomings. Because inflammatory and infectious lesions can accumulate FDG and lead to false-positive findings on PET/CT scans, concerns remain with regard to occurrence of false negatives owing to physiologic high background activity and early PTLD lesions as well as false positives owing to inflammatory conditions. A higher SUV_{max} in the monomorphic subtype of PTLD and its association with serum lactate dehydrogenase level suggest that SUV_{max} may be considered an indicator of tumor aggressiveness in pediatric PTLD. SUV_{max} was significantly correlated with serum concentration of lactate dehydrogenase (correlation = 0.55; $P = .03$), a marker of PTLD activity that has been associated with unfavorable prognosis.[69] Further investigations are required to evaluate the prognostic value of SUV_{max} in pediatric PTLD.

SUMMARY

The data from most investigation supported a view that FDG PET/CT is a relatively accurate diagnostic tool for staging and for the follow-up of pediatric patients with PTLD. It has the ability to help resolve equivocal imaging findings and can detect occult lesions not visualized by other imaging modalities. Together with established clinical, laboratory, and radiological markers, FDG PET/CT scans can support the decision whether to stop or reduce treatment when there is complete metabolic response, therefore reducing the burden of treatment in this vulnerable population. In conclusion, FDG PET/CT scanning could play important roles in the diagnosis and management of PTLD in pediatric patients.

DISCLOSURE

Jigang YANG was partially supported by National Natural Science Foundation of China (No: 81771860, 81971642), Beijing Natural Science Foundation (No:7192041), National Key Research and Development Plan (No: 2017YFC0114003).

REFERENCES

1. Parker A, Bowles K, Bradley JA, et al. Diagnosis of post-transplant lymphoproliferative disorder in solid organ transplant recipients - BCSH and BTS guidelines. Br J Haematol 2010;149:675–92.
2. Camacho JC, Moreno CC, Harri PA, et al. Posttransplantation lymphoproliferative disease: proposed imaging classification. Radiographics 2014;34:2025–38.
3. Cockfield SM. Identifying the patient at risk for post-transplant lymphoproliferative disorder. Transpl Infect Dis 2001;3:70–8.
4. Caillard S, Lelong C, Pessione F, et al. Post-transplant lymphoproliferative disorders occurring after renal transplantation in adults: report of 230 cases from the French Registry. Am J Transplant 2006;6:2735–42.
5. Green M. Management of Epstein-Barr virus-induced post-transplant lymphoproliferative disease in recipients of solid organ transplantation. Am J Transplant 2001;1:103–8.
6. Dharnidharka VR, Webster AC, Martinez OM, et al. Post-transplant lymphoproliferative disorders. Nat Rev Dis Primers 2016;2:15088.
7. Al-Mansour Z, Nelson BP, Evens AM. Post-transplant lymphoproliferative disease (PTLD): risk factors, diagnosis, and current treatment strategies. Curr Hematol Malig Rep 2013;8:173–83.
8. Bai X, Yang H, Zhuang H. FDG PET/CT findings of the recurrent posttransplantation lymphoproliferative disorder in a pediatric liver transplant recipient with right leg pain as the only complaint. Clin Nucl Med 2015;40:832–4.
9. Bahmanyar M, Shakibazad N, Imanieh MH, et al. Soft palate ulcer: an unusual presentation of a post-transplant lymphoproliferative disorder. J Pediatr Hematol Oncol 2017;39:e97–9.
10. Bawane P, Jain M, Balkrishnan M, et al. A rare cause of gastrointestinal bleeding in the post-transplant setting. Clin Exp Hepatol 2017;3:215–7.
11. Keshtkari A, Dehghani SM, Haghighat M, et al. Croup as unusual presentation of post-transplantation lymphoproliferative disorder after liver transplantation in an 18-month-old child. Int J Organ Transplant Med 2016;7:57–60.

12. Samolitis NJ, Bharadwaj JS, Weis JR, et al. Post-transplant lymphoproliferative disorder limited to the skin. J Cutan Pathol 2004;31:453–7.

13. Derlin T, Braubach P, Kreipe HH, et al. 18F-FDG PET for detection of primary Tracheobronchial T-/natural killer-cell-derived posttransplant lymphoproliferative disorder after lung transplantation. Clin Nucl Med 2017;42:988–9.

14. Yadav P, Kumar N, Prasad N, et al. Late posttransplant lymphoproliferative disease: report of a rare case and role of positron emission tomography-computed tomography. Indian J Nephrol 2018;28:393–6.

15. Sabattini E, Bacci F, Sagramoso C, et al. WHO classification of tumours of haematopoietic and lymphoid tissues in 2008: an overview. Pathologica 2010;102:83–7.

16. Trappe RU, Dierickx D, Zimmermann H, et al. Response to rituximab induction is a predictive marker in B-cell post-transplant lymphoproliferative disorder and allows successful stratification into rituximab or R-CHOP consolidation in an international, prospective, multicenter phase II trial. J Clin Oncol 2017;35:536–43.

17. Bakker NA, van Imhoff GW, Verschuuren EA, et al. Presentation and early detection of post-transplant lymphoproliferative disorder after solid organ transplantation. Transpl Int 2007;20:207–18.

18. AlDabbagh MA, Gitman MR, Kumar D, et al. The role of antiviral prophylaxis for the prevention of Epstein-Barr virus-associated posttransplant lymphoproliferative disease in solid organ transplant recipients: a systematic review. Am J Transplant 2017;17:770–81.

19. Feng S, Buell JF, Chari RS, et al. Tumors and transplantation: the 2003 Third Annual ASTS State-of-the-Art Winter Symposium. Am J Transplant 2003;3:1481–7.

20. Dharnidharka VR, Tejani AH, Ho PL, et al. Post-transplant lymphoproliferative disorder in the United States: young Caucasian males are at highest risk. Am J Transplant 2002;2:993–8.

21. Francis A, Johnson DW, Craig JC, et al. Incidence and predictors of cancer following kidney transplantation in childhood. Am J Transplant 2017;17:2650–8.

22. Gallego S, Llort A, Gros L, et al. Post-transplant lymphoproliferative disorders in children: the role of chemotherapy in the era of rituximab. Pediatr Transplant 2010;14:61–6.

23. Minamimoto R, Fayad L, Advani R, et al. Diffuse large B-cell lymphoma: prospective multicenter comparison of early interim FLT PET/CT versus FDG PET/CT with IHP, EORTC, deauville, and PERCIST criteria for early therapeutic monitoring. Radiology 2016;280:220–9.

24. Bund C, Heimburger C, Trensz P, et al. FDG PET to diagnose neurolymphomatosis in a case of triple-hit B-cell lymphoma. Clin Nucl Med 2017;42:458–60.

25. Liu E, Wang S, Lai P, et al. "Hepatic Superscan" in a patient with hepatosplenic alphabeta T-cell lymphoma: 18F-FDG PET/CT findings. Clin Nucl Med 2018;43:595–8.

26. Press OW, Li H, Schoder H, et al. US intergroup trial of response-adapted therapy for stage III to IV Hodgkin lymphoma using early interim fluorodeoxyglucose-positron emission tomography imaging: Southwest Oncology Group S0816. J Clin Oncol 2016;34:2020–7.

27. Moon SH, Cho SK, Kim WS, et al. The role of 18F-FDG PET/CT for initial staging of nasal type natural killer/T-cell lymphoma: a comparison with conventional staging methods. J Nucl Med 2013;54:1039–44.

28. Gonzalez-Barca E, Canales M, Cortes M, et al. Predictive value of interim (1)(8)F-FDG-PET/CT for event-free survival in patients with diffuse large B-cell lymphoma homogenously treated in a phase II trial with six cycles of R-CHOP-14 plus pegfilgrastim as first-line treatment. Nucl Med Commun 2013;34:946–52.

29. Lopci E, Meignan M. Current evidence on PET response assessment to immunotherapy in lymphomas. PET Clin 2020;15:23–34.

30. Cottereau AS, Nioche C, Dirand AS, et al. (18)F-FDG PET dissemination features in diffuse large B-cell lymphoma are predictive of outcome. J Nucl Med 2020;61:40–5.

31. Wen Z, Zhuang H. Burkitt's lymphoma involving multiple hormone-producing organs on FDG PET/CT. Clin Nucl Med 2019;44:995–7.

32. Pan Q, Luo Y, Cao X, et al. Spontaneous regression of clinically indolent lymphomas revealed by 18F-FDG PET/CT. Clin Nucl Med 2019;44:321–3.

33. Albano D, Bosio G, Pagani C, et al. Prognostic role of baseline 18F-FDG PET/CT metabolic parameters in Burkitt lymphoma. Eur J Nucl Med Mol Imaging 2019;46:87–96.

34. Ganeshalingam R, Roach P, Schembri GP. Diffuse large B-cell lymphoma recurring as neurolymphomatosis on FDG PET/CT. Clin Nucl Med 2019;44:145–7.

35. Liu Z, Yang X, Liu J, et al. FDG PET/CT demonstrated precursor B-cell lymphoblastic lymphoma in a pediatric patient with hemophilia B. Clin Nucl Med 2019;44:683–5.

36. Hod N, Levin D, Anconina R, et al. 18F-FDG PET/CT in intramuscular mantle cell lymphoma with elongated lymphomatous neurovascular extension. Clin Nucl Med 2019;44:e298–300.

37. Brady JL, Binkley MS, Hajj C, et al. Definitive radiotherapy for localized follicular lymphoma staged by (18)F-FDG PET-CT: a collaborative study by ILROG. Blood 2019;133:237–45.

38. Wen Z, Zhuang H. Acral involvement of lymphoblastic lymphoma revealed on FDG PET/CT. Clin Nucl Med 2019;44:334–6.

39. Kostakoglu L, Nowakowski GS. End-of-treatment PET/computed tomography response in diffuse large B-cell lymphoma. PET Clin 2019;14:307–15.

40. Baba S, Abe K, Isoda T, et al. Impact of FDG-PET/CT in the management of lymphoma. Ann Nucl Med 2011;25:701–16.

41. Cheng G, Chen W, Chamroonrat W, et al. Biopsy versus FDG PET/CT in the initial evaluation of bone marrow involvement in pediatric lymphoma patients. Eur J Nucl Med Mol Imaging 2011;38:1469–76.

42. Zhang M, Yang X, Wang W, et al. Anaplastic large cell lymphoma involving 7 different organs in a pediatric patient demonstrated by FDG PET/CT. Clin Nucl Med 2020;45:255–7.

43. Donald JS, Barnthouse N, Chen DL. Rare variant of intravascular large B-cell lymphoma with hemophagocytic syndrome. Clin Nucl Med 2018;43: e125–6.

44. Kan Y, Wang Y, Wang W, et al. Unexpected corpus callosum involvement of diffuse large B-cell lymphoma on FDG PET/CT. Clin Nucl Med 2018;43: 933–5.

45. Hotta M, Minamimoto R. Orbital adult T-cell leukemia/lymphoma with skin involvement demonstrated on FDG PET/CT. Clin Nucl Med 2019;44:993–4.

46. Vali R, Punnett A, Bajno L, et al. The value of 18F-FDG PET in pediatric patients with post-transplant lymphoproliferative disorder at initial diagnosis. Pediatr Transpl 2015;19:932–9.

47. Cheson BD. Staging and response assessment in lymphomas: the new Lugano classification. Chin Clin Oncol 2015;4:5.

48. Cheson BD. Role of functional imaging in the management of lymphoma. J Clin Oncol 2011;29: 1844–54.

49. Dierickx D, Tousseyn T, Requile A, et al. The accuracy of positron emission tomography in the detection of posttransplant lymphoproliferative disorder. Haematologica 2013;98:771–5.

50. O'Conner AR, Franc BL. FDG PET imaging in the evaluation of post-transplant lymphoproliferative disorder following renal transplantation. Nucl Med Commun 2005;26:1107–11.

51. Takehana CS, Twist CJ, Mosci C, et al. (18)F-FDG PET/CT in the management of patients with post-transplant lymphoproliferative disorder. Nucl Med Commun 2014;35:276–81.

52. Panagiotidis E, Quigley AM, Pencharz D, et al. (18) F-fluorodeoxyglucose positron emission tomography/computed tomography in diagnosis of post-transplant lymphoproliferative disorder. Leuk Lymphoma 2014;55:515–9.

53. Noraini AR, Gay E, Ferrara C, et al. PET-CT as an effective imaging modality in the staging and follow-up of post-transplant lymphoproliferative disorder following solid organ transplantation. Singapore Med J 2009;50:1189–95.

54. Montes de Jesus FM, Kwee TC, Nijland M, et al. Performance of advanced imaging modalities at diagnosis and treatment response evaluation of patients with post-transplant lymphoproliferative disorder: a systematic review and meta-analysis. Crit Rev Oncol Hematol 2018;132:27–38.

55. Ballova V, Muoio B, Albano D, et al. Diagnostic performance of (18)F-FDG PET or PET/CT for detection of post-transplant lymphoproliferative disorder: a systematic review and a bivariate meta-analysis. Diagnostics (Basel) 2020;10(2).

56. Schoder H, Noy A, Gonen M, et al. Intensity of 18fluorodeoxyglucose uptake in positron emission tomography distinguishes between indolent and aggressive non-Hodgkin's lymphoma. J Clin Oncol 2005;23:4643–51.

57. Chowdhury FU, Sheerin F, Bradley KM, et al. PET/CT staging and response evaluation of post-transplantation lymphoproliferative disease (PTLD). Clin Nucl Med 2009;34:386–7.

58. Zimmermann H, Denecke T, Dreyling MH, et al. End-of-treatment positron emission tomography after uniform first-line therapy of B-cell posttransplant lymphoproliferative disorder identifies patients at low risk of relapse in the prospective German PTLD registry. Transplantation 2018;102:868–75.

59. Bakker NA, Pruim J, de Graaf W, et al. PTLD visualization by FDG-PET: improved detection of extranodal localizations. Am J Transplant 2006;6:1984–5.

60. Montes de Jesus FM, Kwee TC, Kahle XU, et al. Diagnostic performance of FDG-PET/CT of post-transplant lymphoproliferative disorder and factors affecting diagnostic yield. Eur J Nucl Med Mol Imaging 2020;47:529–36.

61. Gheysens O, Thielemans S, Morscio J, et al. Detection of bone marrow involvement in newly diagnosed post-transplant lymphoproliferative disorder: (18)F-fluorodeoxyglucose positron emission tomography/computed tomography versus bone marrow biopsy. Leuk Lymphoma 2016;57:2382–8.

62. Rakheja R, Makis W, Skamene S, et al. Correlating metabolic activity on 18F-FDG PET/CT with histopathologic characteristics of osseous and soft-tissue sarcomas: a retrospective review of 136 patients. AJR Am J Roentgenol 2012;198:1409–16.

63. Montes de Jesus F, Glaudemans A, Tissing W, et al. (18)F-FDG PET/CT in the diagnostic and treatment evaluation of pediatric post-transplant lymphoproliferative disorders. J Nucl Med 2020. https://doi.org/10.2967/jnumed.119.239624.

64. Montravers F, McNamara D, Landman-Parker J, et al. [(18)F]FDG in childhood lymphoma: clinical utility and impact on management. Eur J Nucl Med Mol Imaging 2002;29:1155–65.

65. Seam P, Juweid ME, Cheson BD. The role of FDG-PET scans in patients with lymphoma. Blood 2007; 110:3507–16.

66. Makis W, Lisbona R, Derbekyan V. Hodgkin lymphoma post-transplant lymphoproliferative disorder following pediatric renal transplant: serial imaging with F-18 FDG PET/CT. Clin Nucl Med 2010;35:704–5.

67. Guerra-Garcia P, Hirsch S, Levine DS, et al. Preliminary experience on the use of PET/CT in the management of pediatric post-transplant lymphoproliferative disorder. Pediatr Blood Cancer 2017;64(12). https://doi.org/10.1002/pbc.26685. Epub 2017 Jun 14.

68. von Falck C, Maecker B, Schirg E, et al. Post transplant lymphoproliferative disease in pediatric solid organ transplant patients: a possible role for [18F]-FDG-PET(/CT) in initial staging and therapy monitoring. Eur J Radiol 2007;63:427–35.

69. Choquet S, Leblond V, Herbrecht R, et al. Efficacy and safety of rituximab in B-cell post-transplantation lymphoproliferative disorders: results of a prospective multicenter phase 2 study. Blood 2006;107:3053–7.

Roles of PET/Computed Tomography in the Evaluation of Neuroblastoma

Zhe Wen, MD, PhD[a], Lin Zhang, MD[b], Hongming Zhuang, MD, PhD[c],*

KEYWORDS

- Neuroblastoma • PET/CT • ^{18}F FDG • ^{18}F DOPA • ^{68}Ga DOTATATE • ^{18}F MFBG

KEY POINTS

- ^{123}I Metaiodobenzylguanidine (MIBG) scan with single-photon emission computed tomography/computed tomography remains a major molecular imaging modality in patients with neuroblastoma.
- ^{18}F Fluorodeoxyglucose PET/computed tomography plays an important role in the evaluation of neuroblastoma, especially in non-MIBG-avid lesions.
- Other PET tracers, including ^{18}F DOPA, ^{68}Ga DOTATATE, and ^{18}F MFBG, have shown potential in the assessment of neuroblastoma.

Neuroblastoma, the most common extracranial pediatric solid tumor, accounts for about 7% of all pediatric neoplasms. Neuroblastoma arises from primitive neuroblasts of the embryonic neural crest and can grow anywhere along the sympathetic nervous system chain, but most primary neuroblastomas occur in the abdomen, especially in the adrenals, which account for approximately half of the total cases.[1] Metastases are present at the diagnosis in approximately half of the patients.

Imaging plays a crucial role in the management of patients with neuroblastoma. The International Neuroblastoma Risk Group Staging System emphasizes determining the disease stage before any therapy and depends on using 20 imaging-defined risk factors (IDRFs) across multiple organ systems at the diagnosis. IDRFs are important in determining whether the primary tumor was resectable. The imaging modalities used to determine IDRF can include ultrasonography, magnetic resonance (MR) imaging, computed tomography (CT), and scintigraphy. Accurate determination of the extent of disease at the onset of the disease is crucial in formulating a proper treatment strategy. Surgical resection is the mainstay for primary tumor when no distant metastasis is identified, whereas more complicated combined therapy is required for metastatic disease.

GENERAL IMAGING IN NEUROBLASTOMA

Anatomically, the primary tumor, especially those tumors in the abdomen, can be assessed using ultrasound, CT, or MR imaging. MR imaging is preferred for the initial evaluation because it can better assess liver, bone marrow, and spinal canal involvement. Lesions from neuroblastoma generally showed hyperintense signal on T2-weighted images (Fig. 1). However, MR imaging is less ideal in the evaluation of therapy response. After therapy, residual tumors are less hyperintense or become hypointense on T2-weighted image, which renders evaluation difficult. In addition, the

a Department of Nuclear Medicine, Beijing Shijitan Hospital, Capital Medical University, No. 10 Tieyi Road, Haidian District, Beijing, 100038, PR China; b Department of Radiology, Xiamen Children's Hospital, Xiamen Branch Hospital, Children's Hospital, FUDAN University, #92 Yibin Road, Huli District, Xiamen, Fujian 361006, PR China; c Department of Radiology, The Children's Hospital of Philadelphia, Perelman School of Medicine, University of Pennsylvania, 34th and Civic Center Boulevard, Philadelphia, PA 19104, USA
* Corresponding author.
E-mail address: zhuang@email.chop.edu

PET Clin 15 (2020) 321–331
https://doi.org/10.1016/j.cpet.2020.03.003
1556-8598/20/© 2020 Elsevier Inc. All rights reserved.

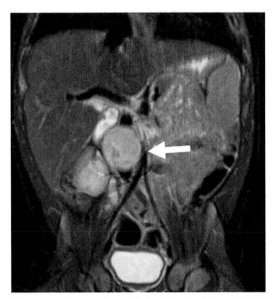

Fig. 1. MR image (T2-weighted) of a 2-month-old, which revealed a right retroperitoneal soft tissue mass about 2.7 × 2.1 × 3.1 cm in size (arrow). Postsurgical examination confirmed neuroblastoma.

bone marrow signal abnormalities after therapy are not necessarily due to lesions from neuroblastoma,[2,3] which leads to reduced positive predicative value. The findings by anatomic imaging are indispensable in surgical planning.

Many different nuclear medicine tracers, including [99]mTc methylene diphosphonate (MDP), [99]mTc Sestamibi, and ^{67}Ga, had been used before in the evaluation of neuroblastoma.[4–9] However, in recent years, all of these nuclear medicine imaging modalities have been largely replaced by metaiodobenzylguanidine (MIBG) scan or fluorodeoxyglucose (FDG)-PET/CT study.[10]

METAIODOBENZYLGUANIDINE IMAGING

In general, accurate staging neuroblastoma requires a combination of cross-sectional imaging and nuclear medicine functional imaging. At the present time, functional imaging with metaiodobenzylguanidine (MIBG) plays an indispensable role in the staging of neuroblastoma (**Fig. 2**). MIBG scan is the most commonly used imaging modality in patients with neuroblastoma and is regarded as standard of care. At present, ^{123}I MIBG study is the mainstay of imaging neuroblastoma in comparison to ^{131}I MIBG imaging because of its better imaging characteristics.[11] Inclusion of single-photon emission computed tomography (SPECT)/CT as part of the MIBG imaging is crucial in accurate determination of not only the anatomic

location of the abnormal activity but also the tumor burden.[12] Higher MIBG uptake correlates with unfavorable histopathology.[13] Many confusing or inconclusive findings on planar MIBG images can become better defined on SPECT/CT images.[14–24]

[123]I MIBG study is a 2-day study, which is not convenient to patients and their families. In addition, the image quality is less ideal, which could pose a challenge to inexperienced interpreters. Some investigators have attempted to use [124]I-MIBG,[25,26] which can acquire PET/CT images and which generally has much better image quality. However, at the current time, [124]I-MIBG scan has not become popular except for use in dosimetry study for radiation planning with ^{131}I-MIBG, mainly because of its about 10 times higher radiation compared with ^{123}I MIBG,[27,28] which is a very serious concern in the pediatric population.

[18]F FLUORODEOXYGLUCOSE PET/COMPUTED TOMOGRAPHY IN NEUROBLASTOMA

[18]F FDG-PET/CT has become one of the most important imaging modalities in the evaluation of most types of malignancies.[29–48] However, its use in the management of the patients with pediatric neuroblastoma is still less defined. Shulkin and colleagues[49,50] were among the earliest to note that most neuroblastoma lesions had elevated ^{18}F FDG accumulation. Their early work demonstrated that about 94% of neuroblastomas would have elevated ^{18}F FDG activity.[49] Interestingly, the FDG-avid but MIBG-negative and MIBG-avid but FDG-negative neuroblastoma can coexist in the same tumor.[51] Some investigators think that FDG-PET/CT is more sensitive than ^{123}I MIBG scan in the evaluation of neuroblastoma[52] (**Fig. 3**).

However, the more important use of ^{18}F FDG-PET/CT in patients with neuroblastoma is to evaluate the small portion of the neuroblastoma that does not have increased MIBG activity. Approximately 10% of neuroblastomas are not MIBG-avid,[53] for which ^{18}F FDG-PET/CT should be used. FDG-PET/CT plays an important role in the evaluation of non-MIBG-avid but ^{18}F FDG-positive[54,55] neuroblastoma (**Figs. 4** and **5**). The specificity, overall accuracy, and positive predictive values of ^{18}F FDG-PET/CT are significantly higher than whole-body diffusion-weighted MR imaging with background body suppression.[56]

Parameters obtained from ^{18}F FDG-PET/CT have been proposed as prognostic factors in neuroblastoma. In a prospective study including 28 patients with high-risk neuroblastoma, Papathanasiou and colleagues[57] noted that 24 of them had lesions with elevated FDG accumulation. A pattern of more prominent FDG activity than [123]I

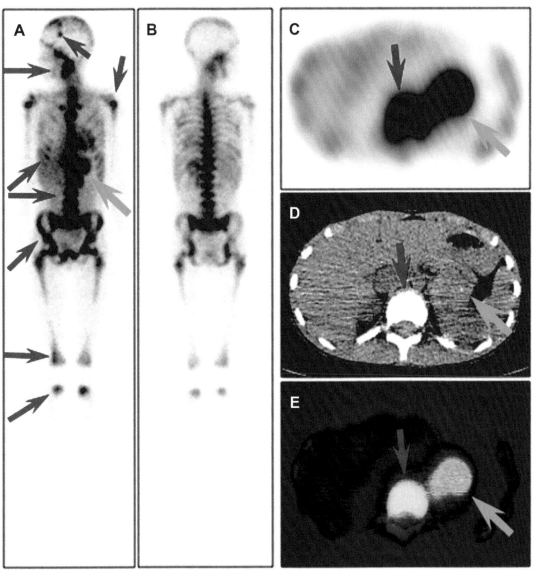

Fig. 2. A 10-year-old previously healthy girl presented with progressive fatigue, migratory bony and muscular pain for 4 weeks. Physical examination revealed no lymphadenopathy. Radiographic examination showed compression fractures in the L2 and L3 vertebral bodies without other prominent findings. Routine laboratory examination revealed worsening anemia and significantly increased lactate dehydrogenase. The overall findings are potentially concerning for an oncologic process, including leukemia. For this reason, bone marrow biopsy was performed, which demonstrated high-risk neuroblastoma. The patient subsequently underwent ^{123}I MIBG scan for staging. The whole-body planar images (A: anterior; B: posterior) showed widespread bony activity (*red arrows*) in the skull, spine, ribs, sternum, humeri, pelvic bones, femurs, and tibias, consistent with osseous metastases. In addition, large activity was noted in the left upper abdomen (*green arrow*). On the axial SPECT/CT images of the upper abdomen (C: SPECT; D: CT; E: fusion), activity in both the T12 vertebral body (*red arrows*) and the primary left adrenal soft tissue mass (*green arrow*) was confirmed.

MIBG corresponded to more aggressive disease and worse outcome.[57] In 25 patients with neuroblastoma, Liu and colleagues[58] found that nonsurvivors tended to have higher tracer uptake in primary tumors on pretherapy ^{18}F FDG-PET/CT scan. Based on 20 patients with MIBG-avid disease, Kang and colleagues[59] reported that the progression-free survival of the patients with neuroblastoma was negatively related to the primary tumor's maximum uptake value and tumor-to-background ratio on pretherapy ^{18}F FDG-PET/CT images. Lee and colleagues[60] analyzed 50

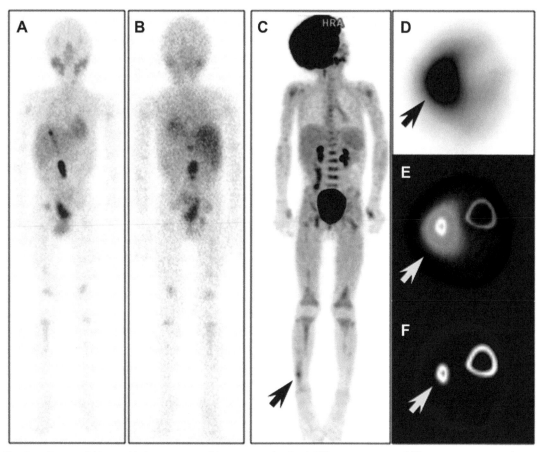

Fig. 3. A 5-year-old boy with known neuroblastoma under both ^{123}I MIBG scan and ^{18}F FDG-PET/CT scan for re-staging. The planar whole-body MIBG images (*A*: anterior; *B*: posterior) revealed abnormal activity in bilateral humeri, lower thoracic spine, bilateral pelvic bones, bilateral femurs, and bilateral tibias, whereas the activity in the middle abdomen and overlapping the liver was an injection artifact. All of these foci of abnormal activity shown on MIBG scan were also demonstrated on the maximum intensity projection image (*C*) of the FDG-PET/CT acquired 3 days later. Many of these lesions are more extensive on ^{18}F FDG-PET/CT images. In addition, there was a distinct focal activity in the right distal lower extremity (*arrow*) that was not seen on MIBG images. On the distal tibial level of the axial images of the PET/CT (*D*: PET; *E*: fusion; *F*: CT), this new activity was located in the distal right fibula (*arrows*), consistent with hypermetabolic malignant lesion not shown on MIBG images, which was confirmed by follow-up studies.

patients with pretherapy ^{18}F FDG-PET/CT and found that 2-year progression-free survival and overall survival were more than 80.0% in patients with low ^{18}F FDG uptake, but the patients with high FDG uptake had 2-year progression-free survival and overall survival progression-free survival of less than 30.0% and 55.0%, respectively. In addition, higher metabolic tumor volume, total lesion glycolysis, and abnormal activity in the bone marrow on FDG-PET/CT study are also regarded as poor prognostic factors.[61]

[18]F FDG-PET/CT might also be more accurate in the evaluation of therapy response in patients with neuroblastomas that are both MIBG and ^{18}F FDG avid. In an 8-year-old boy with stage 4

neuroblastoma, posttherapy imaging showed persistent abnormal accumulation on ^{123}I MIBG scintigraphy but normal ^{18}F FDG distribution. However, without further therapy, the patient was still in remission 3 years later, which indicated false positive posttherapy MIBG study.[62] Similarly, Garcia and colleagues[63] reported their observation that a 5-year-old stage IV neuroblastoma patient had persistent posttherapy residual abnormal MIBG activity but normal FDG distribution. The therapy was terminated, but the patient remained tumor free for 3 years.[63] The findings indicate that the treated neuroblastomas have matured to benign ganglioneuromas,[64–66] which remain MIBG-avid[67,68] but will not commonly have

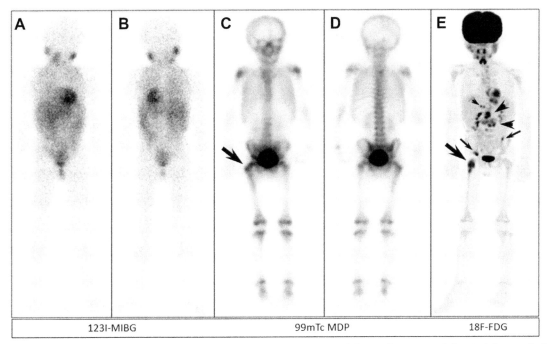

| 123I-MIBG | | 99mTc MDP | | 18F-FDG |

Fig. 4. A 3-year-old boy presented to the emergency room with acute abdominal pain. An abdominal CT revealed an upper abdominal soft tissue mass, which was proven pathologically as intermediate-risk neuroblastoma. The staging ^{123}I MIBG images (*A*: anterior; *B*: posterior) was normal without any abnormal activity. A ^{99m}Tc MDP bone scan (*C*: anterior; *D*: posterior) revealed only abnormal activity in the proximal right femur (*large arrow*). Nonetheless, the maximum intensity projection image of the ^{18}F FDG-PET/CT (*E*) acquired in the same week of ^{123}I MIBG study showed not only the abnormal activity in the right proximal femur (*large arrow*) but also the known primary tumor in the upper abdomen (*large arrowheads*) plus multiple sites of the bones (*smaller arrows*) and lymph nodes (*small arrowheads*).

elevated ^{18}F FDG activity. Interestingly, a comparison between MIBG and ^{18}F FDG-PET/CT involving 45 paired posttherapy follow-up study showed that ^{18}F FDG-PET/CT was negative in 9 MIBG-avid lesions.[69] Unfortunately, no further follow-up was provided by this investigation, and therefore, it is unclear whether these MIBG-avid but ^{18}F FDG–non-avid lesions should be interpreted as false positive posttherapy MIBG study or false negative ^{18}F FDG study in regarding residual neuroblastomas.

One of the major limitations of ^{18}F FDG-PET/CT in the evaluation of neuroblastomas is that FDG can also have elevated activity not only in many other types of malignancies, which are rarely concurrent with neuroblastoma but also in numerous other nonneoplastic causes especially infectious/inflammatory processes,[70–77] which are very common in pediatric patients suffering neuroblastoma. This non–neuroblastoma-related ^{18}F FDG activity can potentially make ^{18}F FDG-PET/CT, although sensitive, less specific. In addition, although most neuroblastoma lesions will have elevated ^{18}F FDG activity, some do not, which leads to

decreased detection rate. All of these factors render ^{18}F FDG-PET/CT less ideal in comparison to MIBG imaging in the evaluation of neuroblastoma.[49,57]

OTHER PET TRACERS

Many other tracers suitable for PET/CT imaging in the evaluation of neuroblastomas have been developed over the years. However, no conclusion could be definitely drawn at this moment whether these tracers can have additional value over conventional ^{123}I MIBG-SPECT/CT images. Much more investigation in a large patient population is necessary to validate the utility of these promising tracers.

^{18}F Fluorodeoxyphenylalanine (^{18}F DOPA) PET/CT is reported to have better accuracy than common anatomic imaging modality in the evaluation of neuroblastoma. Many reports have suggested that ^{18}F DOPA PET/CT has a better detection rate of neuroblastoma lesions. Among 18 neuroblastoma lesions evaluated by both ^{123}I MIBG and ^{18}F DOPA-PET/CT imaging, Lu and

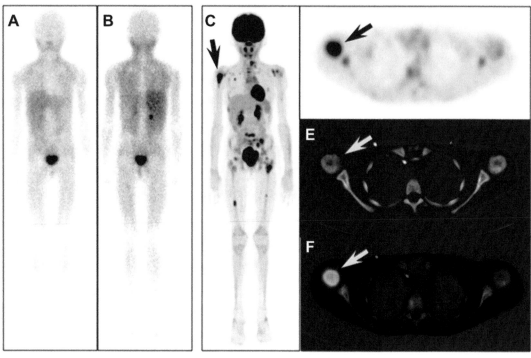

Fig. 5. A 10-year-old girl with a treated known neuroblastoma was transferred to the authors' hospital. A restaging ^{123}I MIBG scan (*A*: anterior; *B*: posterior) showed no abnormal activity except for foci of activity in the renal fossa caused by radioactive urine. However, maximal intensity projection image (*C*) of the ^{18}F FDG-PET/CT acquired 4 days later revealed multiple foci of abnormal activity throughout the body, consistent with hypermetabolic malignant processes. The most intense activity was in the proximal right proximal upper extremity (*arrow*), which was confirmed in the right proximal humerus (*arrows*) on the axial images (*D*: PET; *E*: CT; *F*: fusion). Biopsy result demonstrated recurrent neuroblastoma.

colleagues[78] found that 4 lesions with ^{123}I MIBG negative study had elevated ^{18}F DOPA activity. ^{18}F DOPA PET/CT can reveal lesions that were negative on pretherapy ^{123}I MIBG but only positive on post-^{131}I MIBG therapy scan.[79,80] With a series of investigation, Piccardo and colleagues[81–84] discovered that ^{18}F DOPA-PET/CT had significantly higher detection rate of neuroblastoma lesions than ^{123}I MIBG whole-body scan. One weakness is that SPECT/CT images were not acquired by all of these investigations, and therefore, at this moment, whether ^{18}F DOPA PET/CT is definitely better than ^{123}I MIBG-SPECT/CT, which is more accurate than whole-body images, is less certain. More studies are therefore necessary. Nonetheless, there is no doubt that ^{18}F DOPA PET/CT offers many advantages, in addition to much higher imaging quality, over ^{123}I MIBG-SPECT/CT imaging. First, the patient preparation for ^{18}F DOPA PET/CT is much simpler than the ^{123}I MIBG imaging. Second, the scanning time ^{18}F DOPA-PET/CT is much shorter than ^{123}I MIBG-SPECT/CT, which is very important in pediatric patients with neuroblastoma because many

procedures of sedation/anesthesia can be potentially avoided when scan time is much shorter. Third, ^{123}I MIBG-SPECT/CT is a 2-day procedure, whereas ^{18}F DOPA-PET/CT can be done in less than 2 hours from the time of injection. ^{18}F DOPA-PET/CT is not only able to save the patient and family 1 additional trip to the hospital/imaging facility but also enables early decision of the patient's management.[85] ^{18}F DOPA-PET/CT has an advantage over ^{18}F FDG-PET/CT in the evaluation of the possible intracranial lesion[86] because of its lack of normal brain activity.

^{18}F DOPA-PET/CT also had shown prognostic value in patients with neuroblastoma.[83,84] It appears that even with completely negative ^{123}I MIBG scan, positive ^{18}F DOPA-PET/CT scan indicates persistence or progression of the disease.[83] However, different from ^{18}F FDG-PET/CT studies described earlier, lower ^{18}F DOPA uptake seems related to poor prognosis,[58] which is currently poorly understood.

It is known that most patients' neuroblastoma cells express somatostatin receptors (SSTRs), especially SSTR2.[87] Interestingly, MIBG-avid neuroblastoma lesions have higher SSTR expression than those non-MIBG-avid neuroblastoma lesions.[87] PET tracers targeting SSTRs, including [68]Gallium-DOTA-(Tyr[3])-octreotate (^{68}Ga DOTA-TATE) and ^{68}Ga-DOTA-Nal3-Octreotide (^{68}Ga DOTANOC),[88] therefore, can be used in the evaluation of neuroblastoma. On the other hand, atypical distribution of ^{68}Ga DOTANOC can mimic neuroblastoma.[89] Some investigators think that ^{68}Ga DOTATATE-PET/CT is more sensitive compared with ^{123}I MIBG.[90,91] In an investigation with 5 patients with neuroblastoma, Kroiss and colleagues[90] showed that per lesion basis, ^{68}Ga DOTA-TOC-PET/CT was able to detect more lesions (97.2%) than ^{123}I MIBG (90.7%). Agrawal and colleagues[92] reported intense ^{68}Ga DOTA-TATE activity in the neck neuroblastoma soft tissue mass in a 12-year-old girl. Yurun[93] has shown DOTATATE-positive neuroblastoma lesions in bone marrow with negative ^{123}I MIBG activity. Similarly, Telli and colleagues[94] noted that in a 33-month-old girl, ^{68}Ga DOTATATE-PET/CT was able to detect early recurrent neuroblastoma lesions when ^{123}I MIBG was still negative. However, the significance of the positive ^{68}Ga DOTATATE activity at the sites of neuroblastoma at the current time is not to replace ^{123}I MIBG imaging. Instead, demonstration of such somatostatin-receptor-avidity enables ^{177}Lu DOTATATE therapy[95,96] in these patients.

[11]C Hydroxyephedrine (^{11}C HED) could also be a potentially useful PET tracer in the evaluation of neuroblastoma, which was first proposed by Shulkin and colleagues.[97] [11]C HED is a catecholamine analogue, and its uptake levels parallel the catecholamine levels.[98] In the initial investigation with 7 patients with neuroblastomas, Shulkin and colleagues[97] demonstrated that neuroblastomas had rapid ^{11}C HED accumulation in all 7 patients, and tumors became evident within a few minutes of tracer administration, which is an advantage over other MIBG scan and enables early decision of patient care. The major disadvantage of ^{11}C HED is the prominent activity in the liver and the urinary tract, which can limit evaluation of hepatic lesion or lesions adjacent to the urinary tract.[97] In a different study by Franzius and colleagues[99] in which ^{11}C HED and ^{123}I MIBG-SPECT/CT were compared, ^{11}C HED demonstrated slightly less sensitivity in detection of neuroblastic lesions than ^{123}I MIBG-SPET/CT. Because it is less sensitive and has very short half-time, ^{11}C HED is less likely to become popular than other potential tracers.

[18]F-labeled meta-fluorobenzylguanidine (^{18}F MFBG) was reported to have similar biodistribution with ^{123}I MIBG, but ^{18}F MFBG has much faster blood clearance.[100–102] In a pioneer study with 5 patients with recurrent neuroblastoma, Pandit-Taskar and colleagues[101] demonstrated that ^{18}F MFBG had significantly higher sensitivity than ^{123}I MIBG scan with a total of 122 lesions detected by ^{18}F MFBG PET/CT versus 68 lesions detected by ^{123}I MIBG. All lesions shown on the ^{123}I MIBG study were revealed by ^{18}F MFBG-PET/CT.[101] The sensitivity of the ^{18}F MFBG PET/CT images acquired at 3 to 4 hours after ^{18}F MFBG intravenous administration reached 100% with slightly reduced sensitivity if the interval between ^{18}F MFBG and image acquisition was shortened.[101] The reported overwhelmingly higher sensitivity of ^{18}F MFBG compared with ^{123}I MIBG warrants further investigation of this promising tracer.

SUMMARY

MIBG is still an indispensable imaging modality in the management of neuroblastoma. However, ^{18}F FDG-PET/CT can play a complementary role, especially in those non-MIBG-avid neuroblastomas. In addition, ^{18}F FDG-PET/CT might also be used in therapy response in those patients with persistent MIBG-avid lesions but in clinical remission. Other PET tracers, especially ^{18}F DOPA and ^{68}Ga DOTATATE, and ^{18}F MFBG, have shown promise. However, more investigations are warranted to validate their values in neuroblastoma patients.

DISCLOSURE

None.

REFERENCES

1. Irwin MS, Park JR. Neuroblastoma: paradigm for precision medicine. Pediatr Clin North Am 2015; 62:225–56.
2. Brisse HJ, McCarville MB, Granata C, et al. Guidelines for imaging and staging of neuroblastic tumors: consensus report from the International Neuroblastoma Risk Group Project. Radiology 2011;261:243–57.
3. Goo HW. Whole-body MRI of neuroblastoma. Eur J Radiol 2010;75:306–14.
4. Garty I, Koren A, Goshen Y, et al. The complementary role of sequential 99mTc-MDP and 67Ga-citrate scanning in the diagnosis and follow-up of neuroblastoma. Eur J Nucl Med 1985;11:224–9.
5. Connolly LP, Bloom DA, Kozakewich H, et al. Localization of Tc-99m MDP in neuroblastoma metastases to the liver and lung. Clin Nucl Med 1996;21: 629–33.

6. Macdonald WB, Stevens MM, Dalla Pozza L, et al. Gallium-67 and technetium-99m-methylene diphosphonate skeletal scintigraphy in determining prognosis for children with stage IV neuroblastoma. J Nucl Med 1993;34:1082–6.

7. Sty JR, Starshak RJ, Casper JT. Extraosseous accumulation of Tc-99m MDP. Metastatic intracranial neuroblastoma. Clin Nucl Med 1983;8:26–7.

8. Burak Z, Yuksel DA, Cetingul N, et al. The role of 99Tcm-sestamibi scintigraphy in the staging and prediction of the therapeutic response of stage IV neuroblastoma: comparison with 131I-MIBG and 99Tcm-MDP scintigraphy. Nucl Med Commun 1999;20:991–1000.

9. Berberoglu K, Unal SN, Kebudi R, et al. Role of 99mTc-hexakis-2-methoxyisobutylisonitrile for detecting marrow metastases in childhood solid tumours. Nucl Med Commun 2005;26:1075–80.

10. Orr KE, McHugh K. The new international neuroblastoma response criteria. Pediatr Radiol 2019; 49:1433–40.

11. Liu B, Zhuang H, Servaes S. Comparison of [123I] MIBG and [131I]MIBG for imaging of neuroblastoma and other neural crest tumors. Q J Nucl Med Mol Imaging 2013;57:21–8.

12. Liu B, Servaes S, Zhuang H. SPECT/CT MIBG imaging is crucial in the follow-up of the patients with high-risk neuroblastoma. Clin Nucl Med 2018;43:232–8.

13. Fendler WP, Melzer HI, Walz C, et al. High (1)(2)(3) I-MIBG uptake in neuroblastic tumours indicates unfavourable histopathology. Eur J Nucl Med Mol Imaging 2013;40:1701–10.

14. Zheng K, Zhuang H. Acrometastasis of neuroblastoma to the great toe revealed by MIBG scan. Clin Nucl Med 2017;42:397–400.

15. Zhao X, Zhuang H. Variable MIBG activity in the same renal cyst. Clin Nucl Med 2017;42:887–9.

16. Xie P, Shao F, Zhuang H. Primary neuroblastoma involving spinal canal. Clin Nucl Med 2016;41: 986–8.

17. Liu B, Yang H, Codreanu I, et al. Increased MIBG activity in the uterine cervix due to menstruation. Clin Nucl Med 2015;40:179–81.

18. Yang J, Codreanu I, Servaes S, et al. Persistent intense MIBG activity in the liver caused by prior radiation. Clin Nucl Med 2014;39:926–30.

19. Bai X, Zhuang H. Focally increased MIBG activity in the muscle: real lesion or LOVENOX injection artifact? Clin Nucl Med 2016;41:167–8.

20. Bai X, Zhuang H. MIBG activity in the gallbladder. Clin Nucl Med 2016;41:576–7.

21. Bai X, Wang X, Zhuang H. Increased gastric MIBG activity as a normal variant. Clin Nucl Med 2019;44: 761–3.

22. Liu B, Codreanu I, Yang J, et al. Diffuse elevated MIBG activity in the renal parenchyma caused by compromised renal blood flow. Clin Nucl Med 2014;39:1005–8.

23. Bai X, Yang H, Zhuang H. Asymmetric thoracic metaiodobenzylguanidine (MIBG) activity due to prior radiation therapy. Clin Nucl Med 2015;40: e338–40.

24. Bai X, Zhuang H. Persistent asymmetric brain MIBG activity related to a cerebrovascular infarct. Clin Nucl Med 2016;41:344–5.

25. Ott RJ, Tait D, Flower MA, et al. Treatment planning for 131I-mIBG radiotherapy of neural crest tumours using 124I-mIBG positron emission tomography. Br J Radiol 1992;65:787–91.

26. Cistaro A, Quartuccio N, Caobelli F, et al. 124I-MIBG: a new promising positron-emitting radiopharmaceutical for the evaluation of neuroblastoma. Nucl Med Rev Cent East Eur 2015;18:102–6.

27. Lee CL, Wahnishe H, Sayre GA, et al. Radiation dose estimation using preclinical imaging with 124I-metaiodobenzylguanidine (MIBG) PET. Med Phys 2010;37:4861–7.

28. Lopci E, Chiti A, Castellani MR, et al. Matched pairs dosimetry: 124I/131I metaiodobenzylguanidine and 124I/131I and 86Y/90Y antibodies. Eur J Nucl Med Mol Imaging 2011;38(Suppl 1):S28–40.

29. Hess S, Bjerring OS, Pfeiffer P, et al. Personalized clinical decision making in gastrointestinal malignancies: the role of PET. PET Clin 2016;11:273–83.

30. Yang Y, Wang W, Kan Y, et al. FDG PET/CT findings of polymorphic posttransplant lymphoproliferative disorders in a transplanted kidney. Clin Nucl Med 2018;43:441–4.

31. Parikh U, Marcus C, Sarangi R, et al. FDG PET/CT in pancreatic and hepatobiliary carcinomas: value to patient management and patient outcomes. PET Clin 2015;10:327–43.

32. Wu C, Zhuang H. Congenital penile rhabdomyosarcoma on FDG PET/CT. Clin Nucl Med 2018;43: 852–3.

33. Liu Y. Lung neoplasms with low F18-fluorodeoxyglucose avidity. PET Clin 2018;13:11–8.

34. Ng SH, Yen TC, Chang JT, et al. Prospective study of [18F]fluorodeoxyglucose positron emission tomography and computed tomography and magnetic resonance imaging in oral cavity squamous cell carcinoma with palpably negative neck. J Clin Oncol 2006;24:4371–6.

35. Burger IA, Casanova R, Steiger S, et al. 18F-FDG PET/CT of non-small cell lung carcinoma under neoadjuvant chemotherapy: background-based adaptive-volume metrics outperform TLG and MTV in predicting histopathologic response. J Nucl Med 2016;57:849–54.

36. Fonti R, Salvatore B, Quarantelli M, et al. 18F-FDG PET/CT, 99mTc-MIBI, and MRI in evaluation of patients with multiple myeloma. J Nucl Med 2008; 49:195–200.

37. Groheux D, Hindie E, Giacchetti S, et al. Triple-negative breast cancer: early assessment with 18F-FDG PET/CT during neoadjuvant chemotherapy identifies patients who are unlikely to achieve a pathologic complete response and are at a high risk of early relapse. J Nucl Med 2012; 53:249–54.

38. Houard C, Pinaquy JB, Mesguich C, et al. Role of (18)F-FDG PET/CT in posttreatment evaluation of anal carcinoma. J Nucl Med 2017;58:1414–20.

39. Robin P, Le Roux PY, Planquette B, et al. Limited screening with versus without (18)F-fluorodeoxyglucose PET/CT for occult malignancy in unprovoked venous thromboembolism: an open-label randomised controlled trial. Lancet Oncol 2016; 17:193–9.

40. Yang X, Wang W, Kan Y, et al. FDG PET/CT findings of a synovial sarcoma in a renal transplant. Clin Nucl Med 2019;44:259–61.

41. Wu X, Huang Y, Li Y, et al. A case of mediastinal leiomyosarcoma demonstrated on FDG PET/CT imaging. Clin Nucl Med 2019;44:e158–60.

42. Yeh CH, Chan SC, Lin CY, et al. Comparison of (18)F-FDG PET/MRI, MRI, and (18)F-FDG PET/CT for the detection of synchronous cancers and distant metastases in patients with oropharyngeal and hypopharyngeal squamous cell carcinoma. Eur J Nucl Med Mol Imaging 2020;47:94–104.

43. Yin H, Luo R, Xiu Y, et al. Thyroid metastasis from hepatocellular carcinoma visualized by 18F-FDG PET/CT imaging. Clin Nucl Med 2018;43:e455–7.

44. Laurens ST, Oyen WJ. Impact of fluorodeoxyglucose PET/computed tomography on the management of patients with colorectal cancer. PET Clin 2015;10:345–60.

45. Hicks RJ, Iravani A, Sandhu S. (18)F-fluorodeoxyglucose positron emission tomography/computed tomography for assessing tumor response to immunotherapy in solid tumors: melanoma and beyond. PET Clin 2020;15:11–22.

46. Vadi SK, Mittal BR, Gorla AKR, et al. 18F-FDG PET/CT in diagnostic and prognostic evaluation of patients with suspected recurrence of chondrosarcoma. Clin Nucl Med 2018;43:87–93.

47. Takahashi M, Soma T, Mukasa A, et al. Pattern of FDG and MET distribution in high- and low-grade gliomas on PET images. Clin Nucl Med 2019;44: 265–71.

48. Unterrainer M, Ruf V, Cyran CC, et al. Identification of distant metastases from recurrent gliosarcoma using whole-body 18F-FDG PET/CT. Clin Nucl Med 2019;44:923–4.

49. Shulkin BL, Hutchinson RJ, Castle VP, et al. Neuroblastoma: positron emission tomography with 2-[fluorine-18]-fluoro-2-deoxy-D-glucose compared with metaiodobenzylguanidine scintigraphy. Radiology 1996;199:743–50.

50. Shulkin BL, Mitchell DS, Ungar DR, et al. Neoplasms in a pediatric population: 2-[F-18]-fluoro-2-deoxy-D-glucose PET studies. Radiology 1995; 194:495–500.

51. Codreanu I, Zhuang H. Disparities in uptake pattern of (123)I-MIBG, (18)F-FDG, and (99m)Tc-MDP within the same primary neuroblastoma. Clin Nucl Med 2014;39:e184–6.

52. Melzer HI, Coppenrath E, Schmid I, et al. (1)(2)(3)I-MIBG scintigraphy/SPECT versus (1)(8)F-FDG PET in paediatric neuroblastoma. Eur J Nucl Med Mol Imaging 2011;38:1648–58.

53. Vik TA, Pfluger T, Kadota R, et al. (123)I-mIBG scintigraphy in patients with known or suspected neuroblastoma: results from a prospective multicenter trial. Pediatr Blood Cancer 2009;52: 784–90.

54. Tolboom N, Servaes SE, Zhuang H. Neuroblastoma presenting as non-MIBG-avid widespread soft tissue metastases without bone involvement revealed by FDG PET/CT imaging. Clin Nucl Med 2017;42: 643–4.

55. Colavolpe C, Guedj E, Cammilleri S, et al. Utility of FDG-PET/CT in the follow-up of neuroblastoma which became MIBG-negative. Pediatr Blood Cancer 2008;51:828–31.

56. Ishiguchi H, Ito S, Kato K, et al. Diagnostic performance of (18)F-FDG PET/CT and whole-body diffusion-weighted imaging with background body suppression (DWIBS) in detection of lymph node and bone metastases from pediatric neuroblastoma. Ann Nucl Med 2018;32:348–62.

57. Papathanasiou ND, Gaze MN, Sullivan K, et al. 18F-FDG PET/CT and 123I-metaiodobenzylguanidine imaging in high-risk neuroblastoma: diagnostic comparison and survival analysis. J Nucl Med 2011;52:519–25.

58. Liu CJ, Lu MY, Liu YL, et al. Risk stratification of pediatric patients with neuroblastoma using volumetric parameters of 18F-FDG and 18F-DOPA PET/CT. Clin Nucl Med 2017;42:e142–8.

59. Kang SY, Rahim MK, Kim YI, et al. Clinical significance of pretreatment FDG PET/CT in MIBG-avid pediatric neuroblastoma. Nucl Med Mol Imaging 2017;51:154–60.

60. Lee JW, Cho A, Yun M, et al. Prognostic value of pretreatment FDG PET in pediatric neuroblastoma. Eur J Radiol 2015;84:2633–9.

61. Li C, Zhang J, Chen S, et al. Prognostic value of metabolic indices and bone marrow uptake pattern on preoperative 18F-FDG PET/CT in pediatric patients with neuroblastoma. Eur J Nucl Med Mol Imaging 2018;45:306–15.

62. Sato Y, Kurosawa H, Sakamoto S, et al. Usefulness of 18F-fluorodeoxyglucose positron emission tomography for follow-up of 13-cis-retinoic acid treatment for residual neuroblastoma after

myeloablative chemotherapy. Medicine (Baltimore) 2015;94:e1290.

63. Garcia JR, Bassa P, Soler M, et al. Benign differentiation of treated neuroblastoma as a cause of false positive by (123)I-MIBG SPECT/CT. Usefulness of (18)F-FDG PET/CT. Rev Esp Med Nucl Imagen Mol 2019;38:389–90.

64. McLaughlin JE, Urich H. Maturing neuroblastoma and ganglioneuroblastoma: a study of four cases with long survival. J Pathol 1977;121:19–26.

65. Iwanaka T, Yamamoto K, Ogawa Y, et al. Maturation of mass-screened localized adrenal neuroblastoma. J Pediatr Surg 2001;36:1633–6.

66. Rozmus J, Langer M, Murphy JJ, et al. Multiple persistent ganglioneuromas likely arising from the spontaneous maturation of metastatic neuroblastoma. J Pediatr Hematol Oncol 2012;34:151–3.

67. van Hulsteijn LT, van der Hiel B, Smit JW, et al. Intraoperative detection of ganglioneuromas with 123I-MIBG. Clin Nucl Med 2012;37:768–71.

68. Geoerger B, Hero B, Harms D, et al. Metabolic activity and clinical features of primary ganglioneuromas. Cancer 2001;91:1905–13.

69. Gil TY, Lee DK, Lee JM, et al. Clinical experience with (18)F-fluorodeoxyglucose positron emission tomography and (123)I-metaiodobenzylguanine scintigraphy in pediatric neuroblastoma: complementary roles in follow-up of patients. Korean J Pediatr 2014;57:278–86.

70. Berrevoets MAH, Kouijzer IJE, Slieker K, et al. 18)F-FDG PET/CT-guided treatment duration in patients with high-risk staphylococcus aureus bacteremia: a proof of principle. J Nucl Med 2019;60:998–1002.

71. Kouijzer IJE, Kampschreur LM, Wever PC, et al. The value of (18)F-FDG PET/CT in diagnosis and during follow-up in 273 patients with chronic Q fever. J Nucl Med 2018;59:127–33.

72. Alavi A, Zhuang H. Finding infection–help from PET. Lancet 2001;358:1386.

73. Zhuang H, Alavi A. 18-fluorodeoxyglucose positron emission tomographic imaging in the detection and monitoring of infection and inflammation. Semin Nucl Med 2002;32:47–59.

74. Kaida H, Ishii K, Hanada S, et al. Incidental case of relapsing polychondritis detected by 18F-FDG PET/CT. Clin Nucl Med 2018;43:25–7.

75. Maffione AM, Rampin L, Rossella P, et al. False-positive 18F-FDG PET/CT due to filgrastim that induced extramedullary liver hematopoiesis in a Burkitt lymphoma. Clin Nucl Med 2018;43:e130–1.

76. Sanders V, Donald J, Siegel BA. Adrenal histoplasmosis. Clin Nucl Med 2018;43:502–3.

77. Incerti E, Tombetti E, Fallanca F, et al. (18)F-FDG PET reveals unique features of large vessel inflammation in patients with Takayasu's arteritis. Eur J Nucl Med Mol Imaging 2017;44:1109–18.

78. Lu MY, Liu YL, Chang HH, et al. Characterization of neuroblastic tumors using 18F-FDOPA PET. J Nucl Med 2013;54:42–9.

79. Piccardo A, Lopci E, Conte M, et al. Bone and lymph node metastases from neuroblastoma detected by 18F-DOPA-PET/CT and confirmed by posttherapy 131I-MIBG but negative on diagnostic 123I-MIBG scan. Clin Nucl Med 2014;39:e80–3.

80. Demirsoy U, Demir H, Corapcoglu F. Bone and lymph node metastases from neuroblastoma detected by (18)F-DOPA-PET/CT and confirmed by posttherapy (131)I-MIBG but negative on diagnostic (123)I-MIBG scan. Clin Nucl Med 2014;39:673.

81. Piccardo A, Lopci E, Conte M, et al. Comparison of 18F-DOPA PET/CT and 123I-MIBG scintigraphy in stage 3 and 4 neuroblastoma: a pilot study. Eur J Nucl Med Mol Imaging 2012;39:57–71.

82. Piccardo A, Lopci E, Foppiani L, et al. (18)F-DOPA PET/CT for assessment of response to induction chemotherapy in a child with high-risk neuroblastoma. Pediatr Radiol 2014;44:355–61.

83. Piccardo A, Morana G, Puntoni M, et al. Diagnosis, treatment response and prognosis. The role of (18)F-DOPA PET/CT in children affected by neuroblastoma in comparison with (123)I-mIBG scan. The first prospective study. J Nucl Med 2019;61(3):367–74.

84. Piccardo A, Puntoni M, Lopci E, et al. Prognostic value of (1)(8)F-DOPA PET/CT at the time of recurrence in patients affected by neuroblastoma. Eur J Nucl Med Mol Imaging 2014;41:1046–56.

85. Lopci E, Piccardo A, Nanni C, et al. 18F-DOPA PET/CT in neuroblastoma: comparison of conventional imaging with CT/MR. Clin Nucl Med 2012;37:e73–8.

86. Piccardo A, Morana G, Massollo M, et al. Brain metastasis from neuroblastoma depicted by (18)F-DOPA PET/CT. Nucl Med Mol Imaging 2015;49:241–2.

87. Alexander N, Marrano P, Thorner P, et al. Prevalence and clinical correlations of somatostatin receptor-2 (SSTR2) expression in neuroblastoma. J Pediatr Hematol Oncol 2019;41:222–7.

88. Malik D, Jois A, Singh H, et al. Metastatic neuroblastoma in adult patient, presenting as a super scan on 68Ga-DOTANOC PET/CT imaging. Clin Nucl Med 2017;42:697–9.

89. Vadi SK, Mittal BR, Parihar AS, et al. 68Ga-DOTANOC PET/CT in an atypical extraskeletal paravertebral hemangioma mimicking as neurogenic tumor in a known case of breast cancer. Clin Nucl Med 2019;44:e364–6.

90. Kroiss A, Putzer D, Uprimny C, et al. Functional imaging in phaeochromocytoma and neuroblastoma with 68Ga-DOTA-Tyr 3-octreotide positron

emission tomography and 123I-metaiodobenzyl-guanidine. Eur J Nucl Med Mol Imaging 2011;38: 865–73.

91. Alexander N, Vali R, Ahmadzadehfar H, et al. Review: the role of radiolabeled DOTA-conjugated peptides for imaging and treatment of childhood neuroblastoma. Curr Radiopharm 2018;11:14–21.

92. Agrawal K, Kumar R, Shukla J, et al. Ga-68 DOTA-TATE positron emission tomography/computer tomography in initial staging and therapy response evaluation in a rare case of primary neuroblastoma in neck. Indian J Nucl Med 2014;29:175–6.

93. Torun N. 68 Ga-DOTA-TATE in neuroblastoma with marrow involvement. Clin Nucl Med 2019;44: 467–8.

94. Telli C, Lay EE, Salancı BV, et al. The complementary role of Ga-68 DOTATATE PET/CT in neuroblastoma. Clin Nucl Med 2020;45:326–9.

95. Gains JE, Bomanji JB, Fersht NL, et al. 177Lu-DO-TATATE molecular radiotherapy for childhood neuroblastoma. J Nucl Med 2011;52:1041–7.

96. Kong G, Hofman MS, Murray WK, et al. Initial experience with gallium-68 DOTA-octreotate PET/CT and peptide receptor radionuclide therapy for pediatric patients with refractory metastatic neuroblastoma. J Pediatr Hematol Oncol 2016;38:87–96.

97. Shulkin BL, Wieland DM, Baro ME, et al. PET hydroxyephedrine imaging of neuroblastoma. J Nucl Med 1996;37:16–21.

98. Piccardo A, Lopci E, Conte M, et al. PET/CT imaging in neuroblastoma. Q J Nucl Med Mol Imaging 2013;57:29–39.

99. Franzius C, Riemann B, Vormoor J, et al. Metastatic neuroblastoma demonstrated by whole-body PET-CT using 11C-HED. Nuklearmedizin 2005;44:N4–5.

100. Garg PK, Garg S, Zalutsky MR. Synthesis and preliminary evaluation of para- and meta-[18F]fluorobenzylguanidine. Nucl Med Biol 1994;21:97–103.

101. Pandit-Taskar N, Zanzonico P, Staton KD, et al. Biodistribution and dosimetry of (18)F-meta-fluorobenzylguanidine: a first-in-human PET/CT imaging study of patients with neuroendocrine malignancies. J Nucl Med 2018;59:147–53.

102. Zhang H, Huang R, Cheung NK, et al. Imaging the norepinephrine transporter in neuroblastoma: a comparison of [18F]-MFBG and 123I-MIBG. Clin Cancer Res 2014;20:2182–91.

PET with ^{18}F-Fluorodeoxyglucose/ Computed Tomography in the Management of Pediatric Sarcoma

Douglas J. Harrison, MD, MS[a], Marguerite T. Parisi, MD, MS[b,c], Hedieh Khalatbari, MD, MBA[b], Barry L. Shulkin, MD, MBA[d],*

KEYWORDS

- Osteosarcoma • Ewing sarcoma • Rhabdomyosarcoma
- Non-rhabdomyosarcoma soft tissue sarcoma • ^{18}F- FDG PET/CT

KEY POINTS

- Sarcomas are an uncommon heterogeneous group of tumors that arise from connective tissue cells such as bone, muscle, nerves, and blood vessels. They are generally classified as bone or soft tissue tumors.
- The most frequent sarcomas in pediatric patients are osteosarcoma, rhabdomyosarcoma, and Ewing sarcoma.
- ^{18}F-FDG PET/CT is useful for the management of pediatric patients with sarcomas including at the time of staging, assessing response to therapy, and detection of recurrent disease.

INTRODUCTION

Although rare in adults, sarcomas represent a large proportion of pediatric malignancies. Although a broad range of subtypes exist, the most common sarcoma diagnoses in pediatrics remain osteosarcoma, rhabdomyosarcoma, and Ewing sarcoma. Other histologic subtypes are typically categorized under the classification of non-rhabdomyosarcoma soft tissue sarcomas (NRSTS). Sarcomas in pediatrics require a multimodal treatment approach that integrates systemic chemotherapy, surgical resection, and radiation therapy if indicated to achieve superior outcomes.

The most common sarcoma diagnosis in pediatrics is osteosarcoma, the most common primary malignant tumor of bone in both the adult and pediatric patient populations. Approximately 400 new cases of osteosarcoma are documented annually in the United States.[1] As with most pediatric sarcomas, curative therapy requires a multimodal approach, which in pediatric osteosarcoma, typically includes systemic chemotherapy in conjunction with full surgical resection of disease. Osteosarcoma is generally not considered to be a radiosensitive tumor, and as such, radiation therapy is not used in frontline therapy. Patients with localized disease treated with aggressive surgical resection and standard chemotherapy often do well with event-free survival (EFS) rates close to 70%.[2–4] Unfortunately, patients who present with metastatic and/or recurrent disease continue to have a poor

---

[a] Division of Pediatrics, MD Anderson Cancer Center, Unit 87, 1515 Holcombe Boulevard, Houston, TX 77030, USA; [b] Department of Radiology, Seattle Children's Hospital, M/S MA.7.220, 4850 Sand Point Way Northeast, Seattle, WA 98105, USA; [c] Department of Pediatrics, Seattle Children's Hospital, M/S MA.7.220, 4850 Sand Point Way Northeast, Seattle, WA 98105, USA; [d] Department of Radiology, Seattle Children's Hospital, M/S MA.7.220, 4800 Sand Point Way Northeast, Seattle, WA 98105, USA
* Corresponding author.
E-mail address: barry.shulkin@stjude.org

PET Clin 15 (2020) 333–347
https://doi.org/10.1016/j.cpet.2020.03.008

prognosis, with an overall survival between 10% and 40%.[5,6]

Rhabdomyosarcoma represents the most common soft tissue sarcoma in pediatrics and adolescents with 350 pediatric cases diagnosed annually in the United States.[7] An extensive risk classification system is used to delineate risk status that incorporates histologic subtype and cytogenetics, TMN stage, and the location of the primary tumor. A patient's individual risk status guides treatment as well as prognosis, with patients classified as low risk typically having an excellent prognosis with an EFS that approaches 90%.[8] Patients with intermediate-risk disease fare slightly worse, with an EFS of 65%, whereas high-risk patients, typically limited to patients who present with metastatic disease, and those with recurrent disease have a grim prognosis, with an EFS of less than 30%.[9–11] Patients with rhabdomyosarcoma similarly are treated with a combination of systemic chemotherapy, surgical resection (if feasible), and radiation therapy, as dictated by their risk stratification.

Ewing sarcoma is the second most common primary tumor of bone in pediatrics, although it can also arise in soft tissue. Approximately 200 children and adolescents are diagnosed annually in the United States, with treatment again incorporating high-intensity chemotherapy with surgical resection if negative margins can be obtained. Unlike osteosarcoma, Ewing sarcoma is significantly radiosensitive, and radiation therapy often will be included in local control measures. As with osteosarcoma and rhabdomyosarcoma, metastatic disease at presentation is a strong predictor of outcome, with patients who present with localized disease enjoying an EFS of approximately 75%, whereas patients who present with metastasis at diagnosis faring far worse with an EFS less than 30%.[12,13]

The remaining sarcoma diagnoses that arise in pediatric and adolescent patients are generally classified under the general category of NRSTS. Treatment again is multimodal, incorporating surgery, chemotherapy, and radiation therapy, and is governed by the specific histologic diagnosis and the risk status of the patient, which is typically delineated by histologic grade, the size of the primary tumor, and the presence or absence of metastatic disease.[14]

The most frequent sites of metastatic disease in pediatric sarcomas are the lungs followed by skeletal metastases. Staging at diagnosis generally includes imaging of the primary tumor via computed tomography (CT) scan or MR imaging, a noncontrast CT scan of the chest to screen for lung metastases, and historically [99m]Technetium methylene diphosphonate bone scintigraphy to evaluate for osseous metastatic disease. Of note, certain sarcomas, specifically Ewing sarcoma and rhabdomyosarcoma, will rarely metastasize to the bone marrow, and in these tumors, bilateral bone marrow aspirates and biopsies will be performed at diagnosis to screen for bone marrow infiltration.

The use of PET with fludeoxyglucose F 18 (^{18}F-FDG PET)/CT is becoming more widespread in the management of pediatric sarcomas. Current pediatric sarcoma protocols and treatment regimens are increasingly using this imaging modality to stage, prognosticate, and monitor response to therapy. Extensive research has been performed to improve the understanding of how best to incorporate this relatively novel tool into the management of pediatric sarcomas. This review examines the literature that has evaluated the role of ^{18}F-FDG PET/CT in pediatric sarcomas as a potential tool for screening for metastatic disease and as a biomarker that can be used to prognosticate and monitor treatment response with time.

THE USE OF PET WITH ^{18}F-FLUORODEOXYGLUCOSE/COMPUTED TOMOGRAPHY IN THE MANAGEMENT OF OSTEOSARCOMA
PET with ^{18}F-Fluorodeoxyglucose /Computed Tomography in Staging of Osteosarcoma

As mentioned previously, osteosarcoma is the most common malignant primary tumor of bone and the most common sarcoma seen in the pediatric patient population. Osteosarcoma most commonly presents in the metaphysis of long bones although can arise in any bone of the axial skeleton as well. As with all sarcomas, by far the most common location for osteosarcoma metastasis is the lungs, which will account for over 90% of all metastatic disease in osteosarcoma.[15] The remaining sites of metastasis in osteosarcoma include separate areas of bone, either in the same bone as the primary tumor which will typically be labeled as a skip lesion, or distant bones distinct from the location of the primary tumor. The initial staging of a patient with newly diagnosed osteosarcoma includes primary tumor imaging typically with plain radiographs as well as with CT or MR imaging, noncontrast CT of the chest to assess for pulmonary metastatic disease, and bone scintigraphy to screen for bone metastases. Recently, ^{18}F-FDG PET/CT has been identified as a potential powerful tool in the staging of osteosarcoma both at diagnosis and during surveillance. Indeed, several reports in the literature have suggested that ^{18}F-FDG PET/CT may more clearly identify pulmonary or bone metastatic lesions as compared with noncontrast chest CT and bone scintigraphy.[16]

The sensitivity of ^{18}F-FDG PET/CT in the identification of metastatic disease to bone in osteosarcoma is suggested to be greater than conventional bone scintigraphy according to several recent reports in the literature.[17,18] In a retrospective study of patients with osteosarcoma that directly compared the ability of each of these 2 imaging modalities to identify distant bone metastases, 18F-FDG PET/CT was found to have increased sensitivity, specificity, and diagnostic accuracy (95%, 98%, and 98%, respectively) over bone scintigraphy (76%, 97%, and 96%, respectively). Furthermore when both imaging modalities were used in combination, a 100% sensitivity rate was achieved in histologically confirmed bone metastases. In those patients whose metastatic lesions to bone were biopsied, 18F-FDG PET/CT alone had improved diagnostic sensitivity (93%) as compared with bone scintigraphy (73%) which led the authors to conclude that the diagnostic accuracy of 18F-FDG PET/CT was improved as compared with bone scintigraphy in identifying bone metastasis in osteosarcoma. The authors suggested that this could be a result of improved detection via 18F-FDG PET/CT of bone metastases which lay within the growth plate in pediatric patients as compared with bone scintigraphy.[17] A smaller retrospective study performed by the group at St. Jude Children's Research Hospital confirmed the findings of this relatively large series of patients. In the St Jude study, the imaging of 39 patients with osteosarcoma was retrospectively analyzed to compare 18F-FDG PET/CT to bone scintigraphy in the detection of bone metastases. The authors confirmed improved sensitivity of 18F-FDG PET/CT in the detection of distant bone metastases (79%) when compared with bone scintigraphy (32%).[18] The authors similarly found that the combination of 18F-FDG PET/CT and bone scintigraphy had improved sensitivity when compared with isolated bone scintigraphy. However, no statistical difference was identified in the sensitivity of isolated 18F-FDG PET/CT as compared with both imaging modalities in combination. These findings led the authors of this study to recommend that 18F-FDG PET/CT should replace bone scintigraphy in the staging of osteosarcoma due to its enhanced sensitivity in the identification of distant bone metastases.[18] These data have been confirmed in a recent study of the utility of 18F-FDG PET/CT in both osteosarcoma and Ewing sarcoma which similarly showed improved identification of bone metastases with superior sensitivity (100%) as compared with conventional imaging which included bone scintigraphy (20%).[19]

The data examining the role for 18F-FDG PET/CT in the identification of pulmonary metastatic disease are more limited, although a small study of patients with osteosarcoma found to have pulmonary nodules on noncontrast chest CT did confirm strong sensitivity (90.3%), specificity (87.5%), and positive and negative predictive values (87.5% and 90.3%, respectively) for 18F-FDG PET/CT in the screening of malignant versus benign pulmonary lesions which had been biopsy confirmed.[20] In this study, a maximum standardized uptake value (SUVmax) of greater than one was further established as a predictor of malignant versus benign histology in histologically evaluated pulmonary nodules.[20]

PET with 18F-Fluorodeoxyglucose/Computed Tomography in Long-Term Surveillance of Osteosarcoma

The literature is supportive of the use of 18F-FDG PET/CT as a tool to monitor for recurrent disease following completion of therapy for pediatric osteosarcoma. Specifically, a recent study evaluated the utility of 18F-FDG PET/CT in assessment of the site of the primary tumor after completion of therapy, determining that the imaging modality was able to effectively distinguish between local recurrence and postsurgical change. In this study, FDG uptake remained present at the primary site for more than 3 years after surgical resection. Lesions that continued to demonstrate a combination of elevated maximum standardized uptake value (SUVmax), as well as increase in SUVmax greater than 75%, were associated with high sensitivity, specificity, and accuracy in prediction of lesions that were at risk of future primary recurrence.[21] The potential utility of 18F-FDG PET/CT in identifying local recurrence in the primary site was confirmed in a recent small series of patients with osteosarcoma with documented local recurrence.[22] In this retrospective study of 8 patients with osteosarcoma with local recurrence, all were noted to have evidence of recurrence on 18F-FDG PET/CT. In the 5 patients who had a combination of 18F-FDG PET/CT and MR imaging, MR imaging was found to be nondiagnostic in 3, whereas in 4 recurrences of patients who had both 18F-FDG PET/CT imaging and bone scintigraphy, bone scintigraphy was negative in 3. These results, although in a retrospective study with a small sample size, led the investigators to conclude superiority of 18F-FDG PET/CT in diagnosis of local primary site osteosarcoma recurrence as compared with conventional imaging via MR imaging or bone scintigraphy.[22]

Further evidence supporting the use of 18F-FDG PET/CT in surveillance can be found in a combined study of patients with osteosarcoma and Ewing sarcoma in which 18F-FDG PET/CT was again shown to be effective in the identification of recurrent bone metastases following completion of therapy.[23] Although this study supported the use of the imaging modality in screening for bone metastases following completion of therapy, it was inconclusive regarding the utility of ^{18}F-FDG PET/CT in screening for recurrent pulmonary disease over conventional noncontrast chest CT. Certainly, pulmonary metastases were documented on ^{18}F-FDG PET/CT in patients enrolled in this study; however, the data showed inferior sensitivity along with an increased rate of false-negative results as compared with noncontrast chest CT.[23] Overall, there is definite data to support the use of ^{18}F-FDG PET/CT in osteosarcoma staging and surveillance, particularly in the identification of bone metastases; however, more data are needed to fully understand how best to use the modality in screening for and identification of pulmonary disease (**Fig. 1**).

PET with ^{18}F-Fluorodeoxyglucose/Computed Tomography as a Potential Biomarker in Osteosarcoma

As mentioned previously, the cornerstone of therapy for pediatric patients with osteosarcoma is systemic chemotherapy in conjunction with complete surgical resection with negative margins. Patients are treated typically with 2 cycles of neoadjuvant chemotherapy before surgery to provide for effective limb-sparing surgical resection, which is then followed by several cycles of adjuvant chemotherapy. Historically, the percentage of

necroses identified at the time of limb-sparing surgery following neoadjuvant chemotherapy has been used as a reliable predictor of overall outcome.[4,15]

Multiple studies in the literature have successfully correlated metabolic response via ^{18}F-FDG PET/CT evaluation with histologic response following neoadjuvant chemotherapy in pediatric osteosarcoma.[24–29] A recent study determined that the ratio of SUVmax at diagnosis to that following neoadjuvant chemotherapy was able to predict histologic response in patients with osteosarcoma.[24] Separate studies have shown that change in SUVmax can similarly predict histologic response following neoadjuvant chemotherapy. Specifically, a decrease in SUVmax by 62% was able to distinguish between patients classified as chemotherapy responders based on histologic response at limb-sparing surgery versus non-chemotherapy responders.[25] Further support for the utility of ^{18}F-FDG PET/CT in predicting histologic response can be found in a relatively large study of patients with osteosarcoma that attempted to evaluate and correlate several radiologic measures on both MR imaging and ^{18}F-FDG PET/CT with histologic response following neoadjuvant chemotherapy. Specifically, this study identified the combination of change in SUVmax in the primary tumor as assessed by ^{18}F-FDG PET/CT from the time of diagnosis to definitive surgery with change in the mean apparent diffusion coefficient on MR imaging of the primary tumor to have high sensitivity, specificity, and negative and positive predictive value in predicting

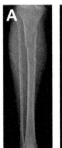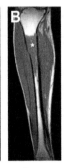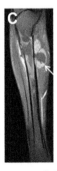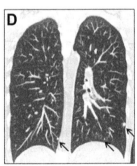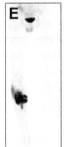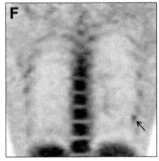

Fig. 1. Metastatic osteosarcoma. A 19-year-old man with history of chronic right leg pain presented with nontraumatic right tibial fracture. (*A*) Frontal radiograph of the right tibia demonstrated a pathologic fracture through a permeative, destructive lesion in the proximal tibial metadiaphysis. (*B, C*) Precontrast and postcontrast, coronal T1-weighted fat-saturated MR images demonstrated an osseous tumor (*asterisk*) and associated soft tissue mass (*arrow*). (*D*) Coronal image from a noncontrast CT chest obtained as part of staging workup demonstrated multiple pulmonary nodules (*arrows*). (*E*) Anterior ^{18}F-FDG PET maximum intensity projection (MIP) image of the lower extremities from a whole-body scan demonstrated marked FDG-avidity in the primary osseous lesion and adjacent soft tissue mass (SUVmax of 13.5). There were no osseous metastases. (*F*) Coronal image from the whole-body ^{18}F-FDG PET demonstrated increased FDG uptake only in the largest left lower lobe pulmonary nodule (*arrow*). Although ^{18}F-FDG PET/CT is an effective tool to delineate both the primary tumor and osseous metastases, noncontrast chest CT is the preferred modality for the detection of pulmonary metastases.

histologic response.[26] SUVmax on ^{18}F-FDG PET/CT following neoadjuvant chemotherapy on its own was similarly recently correlated to good histologic response in a small series of patients.[27] In a larger recent study, SUVmax on serial imaging at week 5 and week 10 of chemotherapy, as well as change in SUVmax from baseline to week 10, all predicted histologic response in osteosarcoma.[28] Finally, a meta-analysis of the current data confirmed both SUVmax as evaluated by ^{18}F-FDG PET/CT after neoadjuvant chemotherapy as well as the ratio of SUVmax at diagnosis and that following neoadjuvant chemotherapy as strong predictors of histologic response at the time of limb-sparing surgery in osteosarcoma.[29]

Because histologic response predicts overall outcome in osteosarcoma, it should follow that the previous ^{18}F-FDG PET/CT parameters would similarly predict outcome in the disease, and this has, indeed, been confirmed in several recent reports in the literature.[30–32] A recent study of patients with osteosarcoma performed at MD Anderson Cancer Center confirmed that an elevated SUVmax as measured at diagnosis as well as following neoadjuvant chemotherapy (>15 g/mL and 5 g/mL, respectively) were associated with an inferior progression-free survival (PFS). Similarly, in this study, an individually high SUVmax following neoadjuvant chemotherapy was associated with poor overall survival.[30] In an additional study of 40 patients with extremity osteosarcoma, a low SUVmax following neoadjuvant chemotherapy predicted an improved PFS.[31] A separate small study of patients with craniofacial bone sarcomas, of which 13 patients carried a diagnosis of osteosarcoma, identified change in SUVmax to be a more powerful predictor of disease-free survival than either successful surgical resection with negative margins or histologic response.[32] These data were confirmed in a recent prospective study of 34 patients performed at St. Jude's Children Research Hospital in collaboration with investigators at the University of Wisconsin. Enrolled patients had ^{18}F-FDG PET/CT performed at baseline, and at week 5 and 10 of chemotherapy. In this study, several measures on ^{18}F-FDG PET/CT were assessed, including both SUVmax and peak SUV (SUVp), as well as metabolic tumor volume (MTV), and total lesion glycolysis (TLG). TLG, MTV, and SUVp independently predicted both EFS and overall survival with statistical significance on all the preceding 3 ^{18}F-FDG PET/CT assessments suggesting ^{18}F-FDG PET/CT to be a powerful predictor of clinical outcome in osteosarcoma.[33]

The preponderance of the data show ^{18}F-FDG PET/CT to be an important tool in the management of osteosarcoma. Certainly, the data support the use of ^{18}F-FDG PET/CT in the staging and surveillance of osteosarcoma with superior sensitivity and accuracy in the identification of bone metastatic disease as compared with bone scintigraphy. The strength of these data has led some researchers to conclude that ^{18}F-FDG PET/CT should replace bone scintigraphy entirely in the staging and surveillance of patients with osteosarcoma. ^{18}F-FDG PET/CT is similarly emerging as a powerful potential marker of outcome. Several studies have shown that it can be used to not only predict histologic response, but disease-free and overall survival as well (**Fig. 2**). Future studies should consider evaluating ^{18}F-FDG PET/CT as a potential biomarker that can be used to screen for potential targeted agents of interest in osteosarcoma.

EWING SARCOMA
PET with ^{18}F-Fluorodeoxyglucose/Computed Tomography in Staging of Ewing Sarcoma

Ewing sarcoma is a malignant tumor of bone or soft tissue and the second most common malignant tumor of bone in the pediatric patient population. As with other sarcomas, the most common sites of metastatic disease are the lungs and bone. In Ewing sarcoma, however, unlike with osteosarcoma, the tumor can metastasize to other soft tissue sites as well as the bone marrow. At diagnosis, staging includes thorough imaging assessment of the primary tumor, usually with CT scan or MR imaging. Pulmonary metastatic disease is screened for via noncontrast chest CT of the lungs. As with osteosarcoma, bone scintigraphy is typically performed to assess for bone metastasis. Bilateral bone marrow aspirates and biopsies are also performed to complete the staging workup to screen for metastatic spread of disease to the bone marrow. ^{18}F-FDG PET/CT is increasingly being accepted as a potentially strong tool to evaluate patients with Ewing sarcoma and screen for metastatic disease at diagnosis, during and following completion of therapy (**Fig. 3**).

There have been considerable data regarding the utility of ^{18}F-FDG PET/CT in the staging and surveillance of patients with Ewing sarcoma.[34–37] Similar to osteosarcoma, the most immediate benefit of ^{18}F-FDG PET/CT imaging in Ewing sarcoma seems to be in the identification of skeletal and bone metastases. A combined prospective study of osteosarcoma and Ewing sarcoma (sample size 34, of which 23 patients carried a diagnosis of Ewing sarcoma) identified a notably superior sensitivity in the ability of

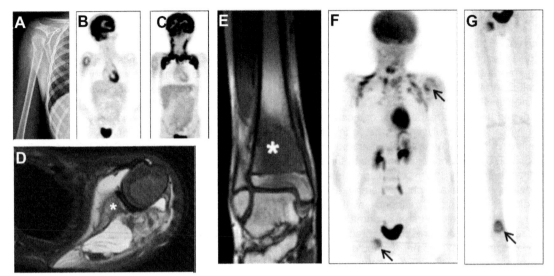

Fig. 2. Recurrent osteosarcoma. A 9-year-old boy presented with acute right shoulder pain in the absence of trauma. (*A*) Radiograph of the right humerus demonstrated a pathologic fracture through a permeative, destructive lesion in the proximal humeral metadiaphysis. (*B*) Coronal image of the torso from the staging whole-body ^{18}F-FDG PET scan demonstrated increased FDG uptake in the centrally necrotic osseous tumor (SUVmax of 4.0). No distant metastases were identified. (*C*) Following 2 cycles of chemotherapy, coronal image from a whole-body ^{18}F-FDG PET scan demonstrated response to therapy with decrease in FDG uptake in the right proximal humeral mass (SUVmax of 2.0). Extensive hypermetabolic brown fat was noted in the neck and upper chest. The patient underwent surgical resection of the primary tumor, placement of an oncologic prosthesis, postsurgical adjuvant chemotherapy, and 2 subsequent thoracotomies for resection of recurrent disease in the lungs. (*D, E*) Two years after the initial diagnosis he underwent MR imaging for evaluation of left shoulder and right ankle pain. Axial short T1 inversion recovery (STIR) MR image of the left shoulder and coronal T1-weighted MR image of the right ankle demonstrated osseous metastases in the left scapula (glenoid, *asterisk* in *D*) and right distal tibial metaphysis (*asterisk* in *E*); there was a soft tissue mass associated with the left scapular lesion. (*F, G*) Anterior MIP images of the torso (*F*) and the lower extremities (*G*) from the restaging ^{18}F-FDG PET scan confirmed multifocal recurrence with FDG-avid lesions in the proximal left scapula, proximal right femur, and distal right tibia (*arrows*). Hypermetabolic brown fat was noted in neck and upper chest.

^{18}F-FDG PET/CT to identify bone metastases (88%) as compared with bone scintigraphy (37%) in patients with Ewing sarcoma, whereas in patients with osteosarcoma, the sensitivity was found to be roughly equivalent (90% vs 81%).[34] In this study, the investigators suggested that the substantial difference in the sensitivities seen with Ewing sarcoma as compared with the minimal differences seen in osteosarcoma lay in the pathophysiology with which osseous metastases may develop in Ewing sarcoma as compared with osteosarcoma. Because Ewing sarcoma can invade the bone marrow. whereas osteosarcoma tends to invade mineralized bone, the suggestion was made that there is likely increased mineral and bone destruction in osteosarcoma that can more easily be identified on bone scintigraphy accounting for the higher sensitivity of this imaging modality in osteosarcoma as compared with Ewing sarcoma.[35] As with other studies of osteosarcoma, this study confirmed improved sensitivity with noncontrast chest CT in the identification

of pulmonary metastases as compared with ^{18}F-FDG PET/CT (100% vs 25%, among both patients with osteosarcoma and patients with Ewing sarcoma).[34] Recent data from a retrospective study of 91 patients with Ewing sarcoma confirmed the ability of ^{18}F-FDG PET/CT to reliably screen for metastatic disease to both bone and bone marrow.[36] This study identified a high concordance rate between bone scintigraphy and ^{18}F-FDG PET/CT, although suggested that specifically in patients with skull-based metastases, bone scintigraphy may have higher accuracy. The investigators highlighted that ^{18}F-FDG PET/CT may be reliably used as a screening tool to identify bone or marrow disease in Ewing sarcoma. However, in certain cases, such as suspected calvarial disease, bone scintigraphy may remain useful in the accurate identification and characterization of lesions adjacent to an area of intense physiologic activity, such as cortical gray matter. Detection of an additional lesion on bone scan not seen on ^{18}F-FDG PET/CT could have

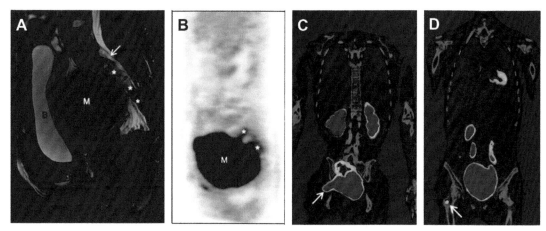

Fig. 3. Metastatic Ewing sarcoma. A 24-year-old woman presented with low back pain and lower extremity weakness. (A) Sagittal T2-weighted fat-saturated MR image demonstrated a large, presacral soft tissue mass (M) anteriorly displacing the urinary bladder (B), involving the adjacent sacrum (*asterisk*), and extending into the epidural space (*arrow*). (B) Corresponding sagittal PET image of the abdomen and pelvis from whole-body ^{18}F-FDG PET confirmed marked FDG uptake in the pelvic mass (M, SUVmax of 13.6) and adjacent osseous sacral involvement (*asterisk*). (C, D) Coronal fused ^{18}F-FDG PET/CT images demonstrated extension of the primary pelvic mass through the right sciatic notch (*arrow* in C) to involve the gluteal muscles. Adjacent sacral bony destruction with increased FDG uptake was confirmed. The pelvic mass caused obstructive hydronephrosis. A hypermetabolic proximal right femoral osseous metastasis was evident (*arrow* in D).

substantial implications with regard to eventual local control with radiation therapy.[36] These results have been confirmed by a recent meta-analysis that similarly confirmed the diagnostic accuracy of ^{18}F-FDG PET/CT in the identification of bone metastases, but again identified gaps in the imaging modality's ability to identify both skull-based and small pulmonary metastases.[37]

PET with ^{18}F-Fluorodeoxyglucose/Computed Tomography in Long-Term Surveillance of Ewing Sarcoma

The data regarding whether ^{18}F-FDG PET/CT can effectively screen patients for future recurrence remain limited at this time; however, a retrospective evaluation of 53 patients suggested a potential role for ^{18}F-FDG PET/CT in the screening for the identification of future skeletal recurrence. Specifically in this study, ^{18}F-FDG PET/CT was found to have high sensitivity (95%), specificity (87%), and accuracy (91.5%) in the identification of bone recurrence or metastases following completion of therapy.[38] This study further concluded that ^{18}F-FDG PET/CT should be included in the screening evaluation for potential Ewing sarcoma recurrence based on high sensitivity (95%), specificity (97%), and positive and negative predictive value (97% and 87.5%, respectively) among patients identified in the study suspected to have had recurrence.[38]

PET with ^{18}F-Fluorodeoxyglucose/Computed Tomography as a Potential Biomarker in Ewing Sarcoma

Multiple studies have evaluated the utility of ^{18}F-FDG PET/CT as a prognostic tool for patients diagnosed with Ewing sarcoma; however, the data from different surveys have been inconsistent. In a recent retrospective survey, 28 patients with Ewing sarcoma of bone were identified who had had ^{18}F-FDG PET/CT imaging both at diagnosis and following induction chemotherapy. In this study, elevated SUVmax at diagnosis and following induction chemotherapy were associated with inferior overall survival. Furthermore in this study, the investigators identified a threshold SUVmax at diagnosis of 11.6 over which patients had both inferior PFS and overall survival.[39] Another older prospective study of patients diagnosed with Ewing sarcoma showed similarly that maximal SUV following neoadjuvant chemotherapy (SUV2) was associated with an inferior 4-year PFS. Specifically, patients who were found to have SUV2 ≥2.5 had a PFS of 27% versus 72% in patients who had SUV2 less than 2.5. These findings were similar when the data were analyzed to include only patients with localized disease (4-year PFS: 33% in patients with SUV2 ≥2.5, 80% in patients with SUV2 <2.5) (**Fig. 4**). This study, however, found equivocal results with SUVmax at diagnosis that was not, in this series of patients, associated with PFS. Furthermore, this study did not find the

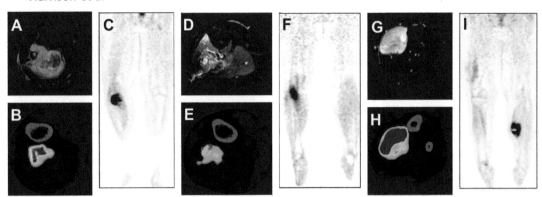

Fig. 4. Localized Ewing sarcoma. A 17-year-old boy presented with a 3-month history of right leg pain. Ultrasound demonstrated a soft tissue mass in the right calf (not shown). (*A*) Axial STIR MR image of the right calf demonstrated increased T2 signal in the proximal fibula associated with a soft tissue mass. (*B, C*) Axial fused PET/CT (*B*) and coronal PET (*C*) images of the lower extremities from a whole-body ^{18}F-FDG PET/CT scan demonstrated increased FDG uptake in the osseous and associated, centrally necrotic soft tissue mass (SUVmax of 10.4). No distant metastatic lesions were identified. (*D–F*) MR imaging and ^{18}F-FDG PET/CT repeated after several cycles of chemotherapy demonstrated response to treatment with decrease in size (axial STIR image, *D*) and FDG avidity of the osseous and associated soft tissue mass (SUVmax of 3.6). (*G–I*) Two and a half years after the initial diagnosis, the patient presented with a lump in the right thigh. On clinical examination, a second mass was palpated in the left calf. Axial STIR MR image (*G*) demonstrated the soft tissue mass in the left calf. The patient underwent excision of the right thigh mass and biopsy of the left calf mass. Pathology confirmed recurrent Ewing sarcoma. Axial fused PET/CT (*H*), and coronal PET images (obtained after excision of the right thigh mass) demonstrated the recurrent soft tissue mass in the left calf (SUV max of 11). PFS was reported as only 33% when SUV2 following neo-adjuvant chemotherapy was greater than 2.5, as occurred in this patient[40].

ratio of SUVmax at diagnosis to SUV2 to be correlated with PFS.[40] These data suggesting that SUV measures following neoadjuvant chemotherapy can be associated with outcome in Ewing sarcoma have been further confirmed in a retrospective analysis of 50 patients with Ewing sarcoma. In this study, patients whose disease progressed had elevated SUV2, defined in this study as median SUV after completion of neoadjuvant chemotherapy. Furthermore, SUV2 was associated with inferior outcome in this study in which patients with elevated SUV II had not only a worse event-free and overall survival but an increased relative risk of relapse and death.[41]

Overall, there is less clarity regarding the role of ^{18}F-FDG PET/CT imaging in the management of pediatric patients with Ewing sarcoma as compared with osteosarcoma. There again is clear utility in the use of ^{18}F-FDG PET/CT at diagnosis and following completion of therapy, particularly in the identification of bone marrow and bone metastases. Furthermore, several studies in Ewing sarcoma continue to support a correlation between elevated SUV following induction chemotherapy and worse overall outcome.

RHABDOMYOSARCOMA
PET with ^{18}F-Fluorodeoxyglucose/Computed Tomography in Staging of Rhabdomyosarcoma

Rhabdomyosarcoma is the second most common sarcoma diagnosis in pediatric patients and the most common soft tissue pediatric sarcoma. Rhabdomyosarcoma can arise in any area of the soft tissue and may metastasize to lungs, bone marrow, bone, soft tissue, and lymph nodes. Initial evaluation of patients with rhabdomyosarcoma includes a thorough evaluation of the primary tumor with MR imaging or CT scan. Staging workup to evaluate for metastatic disease includes imaging of the lungs via noncontrast chest CT, bone scintigraphy, and bilateral bone marrow aspirates and biopsies. Patients with disease that involves a parameningeal site will have a lumbar puncture to rule out spread to the central nervous system. Furthermore, in certain patients, lymph node sampling is undertaken to ensure eventual appropriate local control with radiotherapy. Due to its ability to consistently identify areas of metastatic disease particularly in the lymphatic system, ^{18}F-FDG PET/CT is rapidly becoming standard of care in the evaluation of patients with rhabdomyosarcoma, both at diagnosis and at the time of potential recurrence.

Multiple studies have examined the utility of ^{18}F -FDG PET/CT imaging in the initial evaluation of patients with rhabdomyosarcoma (**Fig. 5**). Investigators at St. Jude Children's Research Hospital retrospectively evaluated the ^{18}F-FDG PET/CT imaging of 30 patients with rhabdomyosarcoma, concluding the imaging modality was particularly efficient in identifying metastatic disease to the lymphatic system, bones, and bone

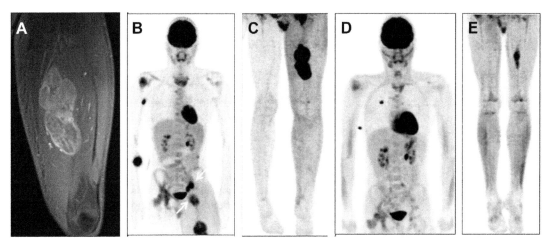

Fig. 5. Metastatic alveolar rhabdomyosarcoma. A 17-year-old boy presented with a 9-month history of swelling and pain in the left thigh. (*A*) Postcontrast, coronal T1-weighted, fat-saturated MR image demonstrated an enhancing soft tissue mass in the anterior thigh muscles. (*B, C*) Anterior MIP images of the upper body (*B*) and the lower extremities (*C*) from a staging ^{18}F-FDG PET/CT demonstrated markedly increased FDG uptake in the left thigh mass (SUVmax of 7.6). FDG-avid, nodal metastases were present in the left pelvic and inguinal lymph nodes (*arrows* in *B*) and bilateral supraclavicular lymph nodes (not shown). Multifocal osseous metastases were present in the right humeral head, manubrium, left scapula, multiple thoracic and lumbar vertebrae, right acetabulum, and right proximal femur. Focal radiotracer in the soft tissues of the right forearm with right axillary lymph node was secondary to partial extravasation of the radiotracer during injection. (*D, E*) Anterior MIP images of the upper body (*D*) and the lower extremities (*E*) from an ^{18}F-FDG PET/CT study obtained after 12 weeks of chemotherapy demonstrated response to treatment with decreased FDG uptake in both the primary and metastatic lesions; however, the lack of a CMR has poor prognostic implications. (*From* Khalatbari H, Paisi MT, Kwatra N, et al. Pediatric Musculoskeletal Imaging: The Indications for and Applications of PET/Computed Tomography. PET Clin. 2019 Jan; 14(1): p145-174; with permission.)

marrow when compared with conventional imaging.[42] The investigators of this study specifically identified ^{18}F-FDG PET/CT to have improved sensitivity and specificity in the identification of nodal disease as compared with conventional imaging. The study similarly found improved sensitivity in the identification of bone marrow and bone disease as compared with bone scintigraphy, leading the investigators to support elimination of bone marrow biopsies and bone scintigraphy in the initial evaluation of a patient with rhabdomyosarcoma, if the ^{18}F-FDG PET/CT does not demonstrate metastatic spread to the bones or bone marrow. The study also evaluated the role of ^{18}F-FDG PET/CT in the evaluation of pulmonary disease, but as in Ewing sarcoma and osteosarcoma, found that noncontrast chest CT to be the preferred assessment.[42] These results were confirmed in a smaller study of patients with rhabdomyosarcoma, which again demonstrated ^{18}F-FDG PET/CT to have high sensitivity in the identification of lymph node metastases and bone metastases (100% in both) when compared with conventional imaging (75% and 66%, respectively).[43] The ability of ^{18}F-FDG PET/CT to detect distant nodal, bone, and bone marrow disease in rhabdomyosarcoma was further confirmed in a recent retrospective review of pediatric and young adult patients diagnosed with rhabdomyosarcoma. This study similarly demonstrated ^{18}F-FDG PET/CT to have a high range of sensitivity and specificity (89%–100% for both) in detecting distant rhabdomyosarcoma nodal metastasis as compared with conventional imaging (sensitivity ranged from 67% to 86%; specificity ranged from 90% to 100%). The study also identified increased sensitivity and specificity in the identification of distant metastatic disease with ^{18}F-FDG PET/CT (range 95%–100% and 80%–100%, respectively), as compared with conventional imaging (range 17%–83% and 43%–100%, respectively).[44]

Although all the data point to a significant role for ^{18}F-FDG PET/CT in the identification of distant metastatic disease in patients with rhabdomyosarcoma, there remain limitations. A recent study examined the concordance rate between tissue sampling via sentinel lymph node biopsy and ^{18}F-FDG PET/CT imaging in patients with pediatric and adolescent soft tissue sarcoma and showed ^{18}F-FDG PET/CT to exhibit only a 29% positive predictive value in the identification of nodal disease.[45] This study suggests that although there remains clear utility in the use of ^{18}F-FDG PET/CT in the identification of distant metastatic disease to bone, bone marrow, and lymph nodes in patients with rhabdomyosarcoma, it should not replace tissue sampling with regard to nodal disease, which may be essential in the planning of effective local control with radiotherapy. The literature does support potential omission of bone marrow biopsy and bone scintigraphy, if ^{18}F-FDG PET/CT does not identify metastatic disease to the bone marrow and skeletal system, respectively.

PET with ^{18}F-Fluorodeoxyglucose/Computed Tomography as a Potential Biomarker in Rhabdomyosarcoma

The data are conflicting regarding whether ^{18}F-FDG PET/CT imaging can be used as a biomarker to predict prognosis in patients with rhabdomyosarcoma. Two studies from Memorial Sloan Kettering Cancer Center support using metabolic response on ^{18}F-FDG PET/CT imaging to predict outcome. In the first study, patients with group 3 rhabdomyosarcoma (patients with nonmetastatic lesions that have not been surgically resected at diagnosis) who sustained a complete metabolic response (CMR) in the primary tumor on ^{18}F-FDG PET/CT imaging after 5 cycles of chemotherapy and radiation therapy were found to have a superior local relapse-free survival (LRFS) over patients who did not achieve CMR (94% vs 75%).[46] This study similarly found a trend toward improved LRFS for patients who achieved a CMR following chemotherapy alone, although these results were not statistically significant. The same group published a follow-up study with a larger sample size, which confirmed the role of ^{18}F-FDG PET/CT in predicting outcome in patients with rhabdomyosarcoma. In this subsequent study, both CMR following chemotherapy as well as following chemotherapy and radiation therapy were found to be associated with an increased 3-year PFS.[47] The investigators of this study were also able to document SUVmax at diagnosis to be correlated with outcome in this subset of patients with rhabdomyosarcoma. Specifically, patients with an SUVmax at diagnosis of ≥9 were found to have a statistically significant inferior 3-year PFS (3-year PFS in patients with SUVmax of <9 at diagnosis: 62%; 3-year PFS in patients with SUVmax of ≥9 at diagnosis: 39%).[47] A recent study from Egypt further suggested a role for maximal SUV at diagnosis in predicting outcome in pediatric rhabdomyosarcoma, demonstrating a superior event-free and overall survival for patients with SUVmax at diagnosis of more than 3.6.[48] Unfortunately, the literature has not been consistent, and other studies do not support using metabolic

response as assessed by ^{18}F-FDG PET/CT to predict outcome in pediatric rhabdomyosarcoma. The Children's Oncology Group has presented results from 2 large cooperative group rhabdomyosarcoma trials that evaluated CMR on ^{18}F-FDG PET/CT imaging in patients with intermediate-risk and high-risk rhabdomyosarcoma. In these studies, no significant difference was seen in 3-year EFS between patients who sustained a CMR on ^{18}F-FDG PET/CT versus patients who did not. Furthermore, unlike in the preceding studies, maximal SUV in the primary tumor at diagnosis did not correlate with 3-year EFS.[49]

The data are conflicting with regard to how best to incorporate ^{18}F-FDG PET/CT in the management of patients with rhabdomyosarcoma. There is certainly a role for the imaging modality in the initial evaluation of patients to screen for distant metastatic disease to lymph nodes, bone, and bone marrow, although recent data suggest that thorough tissue evaluation of nodal disease via sentinel node biopsy remains essential to plan for eventual radiation therapy for local control. Whether ^{18}F-FDG PET/CT can be used to predict outcome in rhabdomyosarcoma remains an ongoing area of controversy, and additional, larger prospective studies are needed to determine whether ^{18}F-FDG PET/CT response can be used as a reliable indicator of eventual outcome in rhabdomyosarcoma.

NON-RHABDOMYOSARCOMA SOFT TISSUE SARCOMA

The data with regard to ^{18}F-FDG PET/CT imaging in the management of pediatric NRSTS are minimal and compromised by the multiple different individual histologies labeled under this generalized classification. Within the adult literature, there are some data supporting the use of ^{18}F-FDG PET/CT in patients with high-grade soft tissue sarcoma (STS). Specifically, a relatively large study of such patients documented that an early metabolic response on ^{18}F-FDG PET/CT defined for the purposes of this study as patients with high-grade STS who sustained a decrease in SUVmax by 26% following 1 cycle of chemotherapy was correlated to a statistically significant improvement in overall survival. The study similarly identified a trend toward improved overall survival seen with patients who sustained a late metabolic response at the end of therapy, although these results were not found to be statistically significant.[50]

The value and utility of ^{18}F-FDG PET/CT imaging in the management of the more common pediatric NRSTS have not been fully established, although there are individual studies in certain histologies

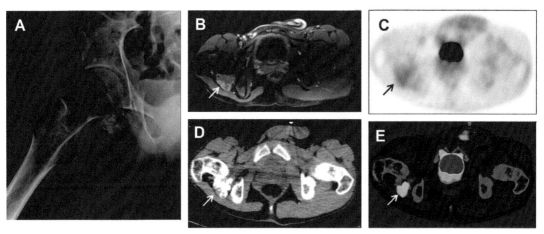

Fig. 6. Synovial sarcoma. A 16-year-old boy presented with a 2-year history of gradually increasing right hip pain associated with decreased range of motion. (*A*) Radiograph of the right hip demonstrated a calcified soft tissue mass posteromedial to the right femoral head. (*B*) Postcontrast, axial T1-weighted fat-saturated MR image demonstrated a heterogeneously enhancing soft tissue mass. (*C–E*) Axial PET, low-dose CT, and fused PET/CT images from a staging ¹⁸F-FDG PET/CT whole-body scan demonstrated mildly increased FDG uptake (SUVmax of 2.7) in this calcified mass (*arrows* in *B–E*). No distant metastases were identified.

that support a role. Synovial sarcoma is the most common malignant STS in the pediatric and adolescent patient population after rhabdomyosarcoma[51] (**Fig. 6**). A few studies have evaluated the use of ¹⁸F-FDG PET/CT in the management of synovial sarcoma, although most examine all patients with synovial sarcoma, regardless of age. One recent prospective study analyzed 44 patients with a diagnosis of synovial sarcoma and documented a worse overall and PFS for patients noted to have increased SUVmax in the primary tumor at diagnosis. Specifically, patients who were noted to exhibit an SUVmax of more than 4.35 on ¹⁸F-FDG PET/CT imaging had a worse overall survival and PFS as compared with patients who exhibited SUV less than 4.35.[52] A second smaller but more recent study has confirmed these findings. This study retrospectively evaluated SUVmax, MTV, and TLG on initial ¹⁸F-FDG PET/CT performed on patients with newly diagnosed synovial sarcoma with the goal of determining whether any of these baseline parameters correlated to eventual outcome. Increased SUVmax, MTV, and TLG were all statistically significantly correlated to poor histologic response to neoadjuvant chemotherapy, as well as to inferior overall survival in this small retrospective study of patients with synovial sarcoma.[53]

Another NRSTS seen predominantly in pediatrics and young adult patients is desmoplastic small round cell tumor (DSRCT), a highly

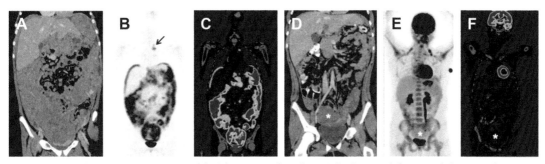

Fig. 7. Metastatic DSRCT. An 11-year-old girl presented with weight loss and fatigue. (*A*) Coronal contrast-enhanced CT image of the abdomen and pelvis demonstrated diffuse mesenteric, omental, and intraperitoneal masses. (*B, C*) Coronal PET and fused PET/CT images from an ¹⁸F-FDG PET PET-CT scan demonstrated that the diffuse mesenteric, omental, and intraperitoneal masses were markedly FDG-avid (SUVmax of 8.9). Left periclavicular (*arrow* in *B*) and right internal mammary (not shown) FDG-avid nodal metastases are also present. (*D, E*) Contrast-enhanced CT and ¹⁸F-FDG PET/CT were repeated after 11 weeks of chemotherapy. Coronal CT and frontal MIP images demonstrated response to therapy with significant decrease in FDG uptake in residual pelvic tumor (*asterisk* in *D–F*, with SUVmax of 4.5) and resolution of FDG uptake in all other sites of disease.

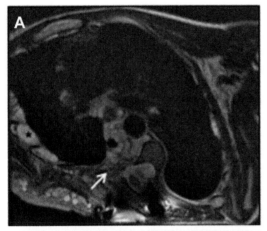

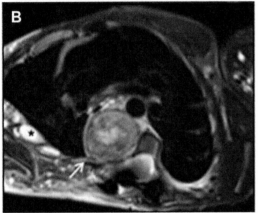

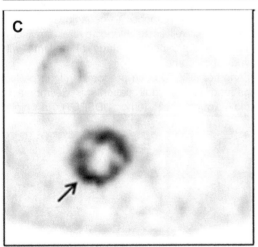

malignant tumor that typically arises in the abdomen and peritoneum and presents with extensive metastatic disease at diagnosis. Outcomes are generally poor despite treatment that typically includes intensive systemic chemotherapy, aggressive surgical resection, and in some cases radiotherapy. In a retrospective study of the imaging findings in patients with DSRCT, 11 of 65 patients evaluated were noted to have had ^{18}F-FDG PET/CT imaging at diagnosis. The study concluded that ^{18}F-FDG PET/CT had exhibited excellent sensitivity (96.1%), specificity (98.6%), and positive and negative predictive value (98.0% and 97.1%, respectively) in the detection and extent of metastatic disease in patients with DSRCT.[54] A smaller retrospective study confirmed the potential utility of ^{18}F-FDG PET/CT in the evaluation of 8 patients with DSRCT. All patients exhibited FDG avidity in the primary tumor, with most exhibiting intense FDG uptake. In addition, and perhaps more significantly, most patients showed decreased uptake of FDG with treatment, suggesting ^{18}F-FDG PET/CT could be used to monitor treatment response (**Fig. 7**). The investigators further demonstrated that ^{18}F-FDG PET/CT continued to be negative in 6 of 7 patients who remained free of disease. The patient who eventually presented with increased uptake in the thoracic cavity was proven to have had histologic recurrence, further suggesting that ^{18}F-FDG PET/CT could potentially aid in the surveillance of patients with DSRCT.[55] Larger prospective studies are needed to fully evaluate how to incorporate ^{18}F-FDG PET/CT into the management of patients diagnosed with DSRCT; however, the preliminary data suggest utility in staging as well as in surveillance of patients for recurrent disease following completion of therapy.

Several studies have examined the use of ^{18}F-FDG PET/CT in identifying potential malignant transformation of benign plexiform neurofibromas into the clinically aggressive NRSTS malignant peripheral nerve sheath tumor (MPNST) in adult patients diagnosed with neurofibromatosis Type 1 (NF1).[56–60] The data from these studies demonstrate a clear association between increased FDG

Fig. 8. MPNST. A 17-year-old boy with NF1, multiple plexiform neurofibromas, and scoliosis presented with interval increase in size of a right paraspinal mass on surveillance MR imaging. (*A, B*) Axial STIR MR images obtained 3 years prior (*A*) and at presentation (*B*) demonstrated interval increase in size of a right paraspinal mass (*arrows*). Plexiform neurofibromas were seen in the chest wall and paraspinal soft tissues (*asterisk*). (*C*) Axial PET image from ^{18}F-FDG PET/CT whole-body scan demonstrated that this

centrally necrotic lesion was hypermetabolic (*arrow*, SUVmax of 11.6). Mass was resected and pathology was consistent with high-grade MPNST. Other benign plexiform neurofibromas along the right posterolateral chest wall were minimally FDG-avid. According to Tsai and colleagues,[61] there was a statistically significant difference in SUVmax between plexiform neurofibromas and MPNSTs with high sensitivity and specificity for diagnosing malignant transformation using a cutoff SUVmax of 4.

avidity seen on ¹⁸F-FDG PET/CT and histologically confirmed malignant transformation to MPNST. In pediatric patients, the role of ¹⁸F-FDG PET/CT in NF1 has not been extensively evaluated, although several of the previously cited studies did include small cohorts of pediatric patients. There has been 1 relatively large cohort of pediatric NF1 that has evaluated the role of ¹⁸F-FDG PET/CT.[61] In this retrospective study, 35 subjects were identified to have had ¹⁸F-FDG PET/CT imaging of a plexiform neurofibroma or lesion concerning for MPNST due to a change in symptoms. Of the 35 patients, 20 were evaluated via surgical biopsy or resection. The investigators demonstrated a statistically significant difference in SUVmax for lesions confirmed to be MPNST as compared with those confirmed to be a benign plexiform neurofibroma, with high sensitivity and specificity for lesions that demonstrated SUVmax of more than 4 (**Fig. 8**).

SUMMARY

Considerable data exist regarding how to fully incorporate ¹⁸F-FDG PET/CT imaging into the management of patients diagnosed with pediatric sarcomas. The literature clearly supports the use of ¹⁸F-FDG PET/CT imaging in the staging and surveillance of osteosarcoma, Ewing sarcoma, and rhabdomyosarcoma, and, indeed, ¹⁸F-FDG PET/CT may be superior to conventional imaging in identifying distant bone metastases in Ewing sarcoma and osteosarcoma. Multiple studies have successfully correlated response on ¹⁸F-FDG PET/CT imaging as well as measures assessed on ¹⁸F-FDG PET/CT, such as SUVmax with outcome, in particular in osteosarcoma and Ewing sarcoma. The data are conflicting with regard to whether response on ¹⁸F-FDG PET/CT imaging is associated with outcome in rhabdomyosarcoma. Because there are multiple different histologic variants of pediatric NRST, how to incorporate ¹⁸F-FDG PET/CT into the management of NRSTS in pediatrics remains an open question, although there are some data in synovial sarcoma, DSRCT, and MPNST. Whereas larger, prospective studies are needed to fully address how best to incorporate this imaging modality into clinical practice, the data are certainly supportive of role for ¹⁸F-FDG PET/CT imaging in pediatric sarcomas.

DISCLOSURE

Supported in part ALSAC, the American Lebanese Syrian Associated Charities, Memphis, TN. (No grant number)

REFERENCES

1. Ries LAG, Smith MA, Gurney JG, et al, editors. Cancer incidence and survival among children and adolescents: United States SEER Program 1975-1995, National Cancer Institute, SEER Program. Bethesda (MD): NIH; 1999. Pub. No. 99-4649.
2. Bielack SS, Kempf-Bielack B, Delling G, et al. Prognostic factors in high-grade osteosarcoma of the extremities or trunk: an analysis of 1,702 patients treated on neoadjuvant cooperative osteosarcoma study group protocols. J Clin Oncol 2002;20:776–90.
3. Meyers PA, Heller G, Healey J, et al. Chemotherapy for nonmetastatic osteogenic sarcoma: the Memorial Sloan Kettering experience. J Clin Oncol 1992;10:5–15.
4. Ferrari S, Bacci G, Picci P, et al. Long-term follow-up and post-relapse survival in patients with non-metastatic osteosarcoma of the extremity treated with neoadjuvant chemotherapy. Ann Oncol 1997;8:765–71.
5. Kempf-bielack B, Bielack SS, Jürgens H, et al. Osteosarcoma relapse after combined modality therapy: an analysis of unselected patients in the Cooperative Osteosarcoma Study Group (COSS). J Clin Oncol 2005;23:559–68.
6. Goorin AM, Harris MB, Bernstein M, et al. Phase II/III trial of etoposide and high-dose ifosfamide in newly diagnosed metastatic osteosarcoma: a Pediatric Oncology Group trial. J Clin Oncol 2002;20:426–33.
7. Gurney JG, Young JL, Roffers SD, et al. Soft tissue sarcomas. In: Ries LAG, Smith MA, Gurney JG, et al, editors. Cancer incidence and survival among children and adolescents: United States SEER Program 1975-1995, National Cancer Institue, SEER Program. Bethesda (MD): NIH; 1999. Pub. No. 99-4649. Available at: https://seer.cancer.gov/archive/publications/childhood/childhood-monograph.pdf.
8. Walterhouse DO, Pappo AS, Meza JL, et al. Shorter-duration therapy using vincristine, dactinomycin, and lower-dose cyclophosphamide with or without radiotherapy for patients with newly diagnosed low-risk rhabdomyosarcoma: a report from the Soft Tissue Sarcoma Committee of the Children's Oncology Group. J Clin Oncol 2014;32:3547–52.
9. Arndt CA, Stoner JA, Hawkins DS, et al. Vincristine, actinomycin, and cyclophosphamide compared with vincristine, actinomycin, and cyclophosphamide alternating with vincristine, topotecan, and cyclophosphamide for intermediate-risk rhabdomyosarcoma: Children's Oncology Group Study D9803. J Clin Oncol 2009;27:5182–8.
10. Breneman JC, Lyden E, Pappo AS, et al. Prognostic factors and clinical outcomes in children and adolescents with metastatic rhabdomyosarcoma—a report from the Intergroup Rhabdomyosarcoma Study IV. J Clin Oncol 2003;21:78–84.

11. Weigel BJ, Lyden E, Anderson JR, et al. Intensive multiagent therapy, including dose-compressed cycles of ifosfamide/etoposide and vincristine/doxorubicin/cyclophosphamide, irinotecan, and radiation, in patients with high-risk rhabdomyosarcoma: a report from the Children's Oncology Group. J Clin Oncol 2016;34:117–22.

12. Grier HE, Krailo MD, Tarbell NJ, et al. Addition of ifosfamide and etoposide to standard chemotherapy for Ewing's sarcoma and primitive neuroectodermal of bone. N Engl J Med 2003;348:694–701.

13. Womer RB, West DC, Krailo MD, et al. Randomized controlled trial of interval-compressed chemotherapy for the treatment of localized Ewing sarcoma: a report from the Children's Oncology Group. J Clin Oncol 2012;30:4148–54.

14. Pratt CB, Pappo AS, Gieser P, et al. Role of adjuvant chemotherapy in the treatment of surgically resected pediatric nonrhabdomyosarcomatous soft tissue sarcomas: a Pediatric Oncology Group Study. J Clin Oncol 1999;17:1219.

15. Luetke A, Meyers PA, Lewis L, et al. Osteosarcoma treatment: where do we stand? A state of the art review. Cancer Treat Rev 2014;40:523–32.

16. Quarticcio N, Treglia G, Salsano M, et al. The role of Fluorine-18-Fluorodeoxyglucose positron emission tomography in staging and restaging of patients with osteosarcoma. Radiol Oncol 2013;47:97–102.

17. Byun BH, Kong CB, Lim I, et al. Comparison of (18) F-FDG PET/CT and (99m) Tc-MDP bone scintigraphy for detection of bone metastasis in osteosarcoma. Skeletal Radiol 2013;42:1673–81.

18. Hurley C, McCarville MB, Shulkin BL, et al. Comparison of (18) F-FDG PET-CT and bone scintigraphy for evaluation of osseous metastases in newly diagnosed and recurrent osteosarcoma. Pediatr Blood Cancer 2016;63:1381–6.

19. Bailly C, Leforestier R, Campion L, et al. Prognostic value of FDG PET indices for the assessment of histologic response to neoadjuvant chemotherapy and outcome in pediatric patients with Ewing sarcoma and osteosarcoma. PLoS One 2017;12:1–14.

20. Cistaro A, Lopci E, Gastaldo L, et al. The role of 18F-FDG PET/CT in the metabolic characterization of lung nodules in pediatric patients with bone sarcoma. Pediatr Blood Cancer 2012;59:1206–10.

21. Chang KJ, Kong CB, Cho WH, et al. Usefulness of increased 18F-FDG uptake for detecting local recurrence in patients with extremity osteosarcoma treated with surgical resection and endoprosthetic replacement. Skeletal Radiol 2015;44:529–37.

22. Sharp SE, Shulkin BL, Gelfand MJ, et al. FDG PET/CT appearance of local osteosarcoma recurrences in pediatric patients. Pediatr Radiol 2017;47:1800–8.

23. Quartuccio N, Fox J, Kuk D, et al. Pediatric bone sarcoma: diagnostic performance of 18F-FDG PET/CT versus conventional imaging for initial staging and follow up. AJR Am J Roentgenol 2015;204:153–60.

24. Hamada K, Tomita Y, Inoue A, et al. Evaluation of chemotherapy response in osteosarcoma with FDG PET. Ann Nucl Med 2009;23:89–95.

25. Denecke T, Hundsdörfer P, Misch D, et al. Assessment of histological response of paediatric bone sarcomas using FDG PET in comparison to morphological volume measurement and standardized MRI parameters. Eur J Nucl Med Mol Imaging 2010;37:1842–53.

26. Byun BH, Kong CB, Lim I, et al. Combination of 18F-FDG PET/CT and diffusion weighted MR imaging as a predictor of histologic response to neoadjuvant chemotherapy: preliminary results in osteosarcoma. J Nucl Med 2013;54:1053–9.

27. Kong CB, Byun BH, Lim I, et al. 18F-FDG PET SUVmax as an indicator of histopathologic response after neoadjuvant chemotherapy in extremity osteosarcoma. Eur J Nucl Med Mol Imaging 2013;40:728–36.

28. Davis JC, Daw NC, Navid F, et al. 18F-FDG uptake during early adjuvant chemotherapy predicts histologic response in pediatric and young adult patients with osteosarcoma. J Nucl Med 2018;59:25–30.

29. Hongtao L, Hui Z, Bingshun W, et al. 18F-FDG positron emission tomography for the assessment of histological response to neoadjuvant chemotherapy in osteosarcomas: a meta-analysis. Surg Oncol 2012;21:e165–70.

30. Costelloe CM, Macapiniac HA, Madewell JE, et al. 18F-FDG PET/CT as an indicator of progression-free and overall survival in osteosarcoma. J Nucl Med 2009;50:340–7.

31. Hawkins DS, Conrad EU 3rd, Butrynski JE, et al. [F-18]-fluorodeoxy-D-glucose-positron emission tomography response is associated with outcome for extremity osteosarcoma in children and adults. Cancer 2009;115:3519–25.

32. Frezza AM, Beale T, Bomanji J, et al. Is [F-18]-fluorodeoxy-D-glucose positron emission tomography of value in the management of patients with craniofacial bone sarcomas undergoing neoadjuvant treatment? BMC Cancer 2014;14:23.

33. Im H, Zhang Y, Wu H, et al. Prognostic value of metabolic and volumetric parameters of FDG PET in pediatric osteosarcoma: a hypothesis generating study. Radiology 2018;287:303–12.

34. Völker T, Denecke T, Steffen I, et al. Positron emission tomography for staging of pediatric sarcoma patients: results of a prospective multicenter trial. J Clin Oncol 2007;25:5435–41.

35. Franzius C, Sciuk J, Daldrup-Link HE, et al. FDG PET for detection of osseous metastases from malignant primary bone tumours: comparison with bone scintigraphy. Eur J Nucl Med 2000;27:1305–11.

36. Newman EN, Jones RL, Hawkins DS. An evaluation of [F-18]-fluorodeoxy-D-glucose positron emission

tomography, bone scan, and bone marrow aspiration/biopsy as staging investigations in Ewing sarcoma. Pediatr Blood Cancer 2013;60:1113–7.

37. Treglia G, Salsano M, Stefanelli A, et al. Diagnostic accuracy of 18F-FDG PET and PET/CT in patients with Ewing sarcoma family tumours: a systematic review and a meta-analysis. Skeltal Radiol 2012;41:249–56.

38. Sharma P, Khangembam BC, Suman KC, et al. Diagnostic accuracy of 18F-FDG PET/CT for detecting recurrence in patients with primary skeletal Ewing sarcoma. Eur J Nucl Med Mol Imaging 2013;40:1036–43.

39. Salem U, Amini B, Chang HH, et al. 18F-FDG PET/CT as an indicator of survival in Ewing sarcoma of bone. J Cancer 2017;8:2892–8.

40. Hawkins DS, Schuetze SM, Butrynski JE, et al. [18F]Fluorodeoxyglucose positron emission tomography predicts outcome for Ewing sarcoma family of tumors. J Clin Oncol 2005;23:8828–34.

41. Raciborska A, Bilska K, Drabko K, et al. Response to chemotherapy estimates by FDG PET is an important prognostic factor in patients with Ewing sarcoma. Clin Transl Oncol 2016;18:189–95.

42. Federico SM, Spunt SL, Krasin MJ, et al. Comparison of PET-CT and conventional imaging in staging pediatric rhabdomyosarcoma. Pediatr Blood Cancer 2013;60:1128–34.

43. Eugene T, Corradini N, Carlier T, et al. 18F-FDG PET/CT in initial staging and assessment of early response to chemotherapy of pediatric rhabdomyosarcoma. Nucl Med Commun 2012;33:1089–95.

44. Norman G, Fayter D, Lewis-Light K, et al. An emerging evidence base for PET-CT in the management of childhood rhabdomyosarcoma: a systematic review. BMJ Open 2015;5:1–8.

45. Wagner LM, Kremer N, Gelfand MJ, et al. Detection of lymph node metastases in pediatric and adolescent/young adult sarcoma: sentinel lymph node biopsy versus fludeoxyglucose positron emission tomography imaging – a prospective trial. Cancer 2016;123:155–60.

46. Dharmarajan KV, Wexler LH, Gavane S, et al. Positron emission tomography (PET) evaluation after initial chemotherapy and radiation therapy predicts local control in rhabdomyosarcoma. Int J Radiat Oncol Biol Phys 2012;84:996–1002.

47. Casey DL, Wexler LH, Fox JJ, et al. Predicting outcome in patients with rhabdomyosarcoma: role of [(18)f]fluorodeoxyglucose positron emission tomography. Int J Radiat Oncol Biol Phys 2014;90:1136–42.

48. El-Kholy E, El Nadi E, Hafez H, et al. Added predictive value of 18F-F-FDG PET/CT for pediatric rhabdomyosarcoma. Nucl Med Commun 2019;40:898–904.

49. Harrison DJ, Parisi MT, Shulkin BL, et al. 18F 2Fluoro-2deoxy-D-glucose positron emission

tomography (FDG PET) response to predict event-free survival (EFS) in intermediate risk (IR) or high risk (HR) rhabdomyosarcoma (RMS): a report from the Soft Tissue Sarcoma Committee of the Children's Oncology Group (COG). Presented at 2016 ASCO Annual Meeting, Chicago, IL, June 3–7, 2016.

50. Hermann K, Benz MR, Czernin J, et al. 18F-FDG PET/CT imaging as an early survival predictor in patients with primary high-grade soft tissue sarcomas undergoing neoadjuvant therapy. Clin Cancer Res 2012;18:2024–31.

51. Ferrari A, Sultan I, Huang TT, et al. Soft tissue sarcoma across the age spectrum: a population-based study from the Surveillance Epidemiology and End Results Database. Pediatr Blood Cancer 2011;57:943–99.

52. Lisle JW, Eary JF, O'Sullivan J, et al. Risk assessment based on FDG PET imaging in patients with synovial sarcoma. Clin Orthop Relat Res 2009;467:1605–11.

53. Chang KJ, Lim I, Park JY, et al. The role of (18)F-FDG PET/CT as a prognostic factor in patients with synovial sarcoma. Nucl Med Mol Imaging 2015;49:33–41.

54. Arora VC, Price AP, Fleming S, et al. Characteristic imaging features of desmoplastic small round cell tumour. Pediatr Radiol 2013;43:93–102.

55. Ostermeier A, McCarville MB, Navid F, et al. FDG PET/CT imaging of desmoplastic small round cell tumor: findings at staging, during treatment and at follow-up. Pediatr Radiol 2015;45:1308–15.

56. Higham CS, Dombi E, Rogiers A, et al. The characteristics of 76 atypical neurofibromas as precursors to neurofibromatosis 1 associated malignant peripheral nerve sheath tumors. Neuro Oncol 2018;20:819–25.

57. Benz MR, Czernin J, Dry SM, et al. Quantitative F18-fluorodeoxyglucose positron emission tomography accurately characterizes peripheral nerve sheath tumors as malignant or benign. Cancer 2010;116:451–8.

58. Treglia G, Taralli S, Bertagna F, et al. Usefulness of whole-body fluorine-18-fluorodeoxyglucose positron emission tomography in patients with neurofibromatosis type1: a systematic review. Radiol Res Pract 2012;2012:1–9.

59. Combemale P, Valeryie-Allanore L, Giammarile F, et al. Utility of 18F-FDG PET with a semiquantitative index in the detection of sarcomatous transformation in patients with neurofibromatosis type 1. PLoS One 2014;9:1–6.

60. Khiewan B, Macapinlac HA, Lev D, et al. The value of 18F-FDG PET/CT in the management of malignant peripheral nerve sheath tumors. Eur J Nucl Med Mol Imaging 2014;41:1756–66.

61. Tsai LL, Drubach L, Fahey F, et al. [18F]-Fluorodeoxyglucose positron emission tomography in children with neurofibromatosis type 1 and plexiform neurofibromas: correlation with malignant transformation. J Neurooncol 2012;108:469–75.

18-F-L 3,4-Dihydroxyphenylalanine PET/Computed Tomography in the Management of Congenital Hyperinsulinism

Lisa J. States, MD[a,b,]*, Sandra Saade-Lemus, MD[a,c],
Diva D. De Leon, MD, MSCE[b,d]

KEYWORDS

- Congenital hyperinsulinism • Hyperinsulinism • F-DOPA • [18F]-FDOPA • Persistent hypoglycemia

KEY POINTS

- 18-F-L 3,4-Dihydroxyphenylalanine ([18F]-FDOPA) PET/computed tomography has become standard of care for the localization of a focal lesion.
- Appropriate selection of patients who can benefit from [18F]-FDOPA-PET is essential.
- Understanding patterns of uptake for diffuse and focal lesions on maximum intensity projection images can improve confidence and diagnostic accuracy.

INTRODUCTION

Congenital hyperinsulinism (HI) is the most common cause of persistent hypoglycemia in neonates, infants, and children. The estimated incidence of HI in the United States is 1 in 25,000 to 50,000 live births, approximately 80 new cases per year.[1] More commonly, affected infants present shortly after birth with severe, persistent hypoglycemia; however, some infants present later with hypoglycemic seizures. Neurologic damage from hypoglycemia is common in children with HI, affecting up to 40% to 50% of them.[2] Prompt diagnosis and treatment can prevent life-threatening complications including death.[1]

HI is a heterogenous disease that can present in isolation or can be part of a more complex syndrome, such as Beckwith-Wiedemann syndrome (BWS). The pathophysiology and molecular genetics of HI are also heterogeneous. Mutations in up to 9 genes encoding proteins that play a key role in the regulation of insulin secretion have been causally linked to HI (**Table 1**). Histologically, HI can be diffuse, affecting all the β cells in the pancreas, focal, affecting only a small, discrete area of the pancreas, or atypical.[1]

The most common type of HI is caused by inactivating mutations in the genes encoding the β-cell K_{ATP} channels located on the chromosome 11p15.1 region, including *KCNJ11*, which encodes the potassium inwardly rectifying channel subunit (Kir6.2), and *ABCC8*, encoding the sulfonylurea receptor 1. Approximately 50% of patients with mutations in one of these 2 genes have focal HI. Focal

[a] Section of Oncologic Imaging, Radiology Department, The Children's Hospital of Philadelphia, 3401 Civic Center Boulevard, Philadelphia, PA 19104, USA; [b] Perelman School of Medicine, University of Pennsylvania, 3400 Civic Center Blvd, Philadelphia, PA 19104, USA; [c] The Roberts Center for Pediatric Research, Room 8255, 2715 South Street, Philadelphia, PA 19146, USA; [d] Division of Endocrinology and Diabetes, Congenital Hyperinsulinism Center, The Children's Hospital of Philadelphia, 3500 Civic Center Boulevard, Philadelphia, PA 19104, USA
* Corresponding author. The Children's Hospital of Philadelphia, 3401 Civic Center Boulevard, Philadelphia, PA 19104.
E-mail address: states@email.chop.edu

PET Clin 15 (2020) 349–359
https://doi.org/10.1016/j.cpet.2020.03.004

Table 1
Genetic mutations linked to hyperinsulinism

Genetic Form	Gene	Chromosome	Inheritance	Clinical Features
Monogenic HI				
K_{ATP}-HI	ABCC8 KCNJ11	11p15	Diffuse: AR or less common, AD Focal: loss of heterozygosity with recessive paternally inherited mutation	Severe hypoglycemia Large birth weight Diazoxide-unresponsive
GDH-HI (HI/HA)	GLUD1	10q	AD	Fasting and protein-induced hypoglycemia Hyperammonemia Diazoxide-responsive
GK-HI	GCK	7p	AD	Variable phenotype in terms of severity and response to diazoxide
HNF4A-HI	HNF4A	20q12-q13.1	AD	Macrosomia; may evolve to MODY1
HNF1A-HI	HNF1A	12q24	AD	May evolve to MODY3
SCHAD-HI	HADH	4q	AR	Mild to moderate hypoglycemia; abnormal acylcarnitine profile
MCT1 (EIHI)	SLC16A1	1p	AD	Exercise-induced hypoglycemia, especially anaerobic exercise
UCP2-HI	UCP2	11q13	AD	Mild to moderate hypoglycemia
Syndromic HI				
BWS	IGF2, H19, CDKN1C	11p15	Sporadic	Macrosomia, macroglossia, hemihypertrophy, visceromegaly, abdominal wall defects, ear creases/pits, embryonal tumors
Kabuki syndrome	KMT2D KDM6A	12q13.12 Xp11.3	AR Sporadic	Postnatal growth restriction, long palpebral fissures with eversion of the lateral third of the lower eyelid, arched and broad eyebrows, large, prominent or cupped ears, persistent fingertip pads, cardiac defects, intellectual disability
Turner syndrome	KDM6A?	X	Sporadic	Short stature, premature ovarian failure, low posterior hairline, congenital heart defects, renal and skeletal abnormalities, autoimmune thyroiditis

Abbreviations: AR, autosomal recessive; AD, autosomal dominant.

K_{ATP}-HI occurs via a "2-hit" mechanism of paternal transmission of a monoallelic recessive mutation in ABCC8 or KCNJ11 followed by a somatic loss of maternal 11p15 compensated by paternal uniparental disomy.[3] The loss of maternally expressed tumor suppressor genes results in an area of focal adenomatosis. Genetic testing is extremely helpful to predict focal HI; the finding of a single heterozygous recessive mutation in either *ABCC8* or *KCNJ11* inherited from the father has 94% positive predictive value for focal disease.[4] There are still some children with a focal lesion who do not have an identifiable pathogenic mutation.

Treatment options for HI are limited. There is only 1 Food and Drug Administration (FDA)-approved drug, diazoxide, a K_{ATP} channel opener, which is ineffective in children with inactivating K_{ATP} channel mutations. Other drugs, particularly somatostatin analogues, are used off-label to treat diazoxide-unresponsive cases. These medications are associated with significant side effects and are frequently ineffective for controlling the hypoglycemia in the most severe cases.[5] For medically unresponsive cases, surgery to remove part or most of the pancreas is sometimes necessary. The objective in medically unresponsive cases is to identify those with focal disease and to localize the lesion before surgery, because these cases can be cured by surgical removal of the lesion.[1]

IMAGING

The investigation of 18-F-L 3,4-dihydroxyphenylalanine ([18F]-FDOPA) PET for detection of a focal lesion of HI began in 2003 with [18F]-FDOPA findings reported by Otonkoski and colleagues[6] in Finland at the European Society for Pediatric Endocrinology in September 2003.[6,7] Otonkoski and colleagues[6] and Ribeiro and colleagues[7] from Finland and France, respectively, were the first to publish the imaging findings [18F]-FDOPA-PET in infants with HI. Multiple published studies with a total of 286 histologically proven cases have found [18F]-FDOPA has sensitivity ranging from 75% to 100% and specificity ranging from 88% to 100% for detecting a focal lesion.[6,8–16] These publications came from established referral centers that provided the on-site radiologists to develop expertise in the interpretation of these studies. Review of the publications shows that when a focal lesion was detected, the accuracy of localization of a focal lesion was greater than 90% and thus provided an important guide to successful surgical resection. Although considered standard of care worldwide, in the United States, [18F]-FDOPA is not approved by the FDA and can only be used under an Investigational New Drug license (IND). A new drug application has been filed in the United States.[17] In October 2019, the FDA approved a new drug application for use of [18F]-FDOPA in adults with Parkinson disease.[18]

In the authors' center, [18F]-FDOPA-PET imaging began at the Hospital for the University of Pennsylvania in 2004 and moved to the Children's Hospital of Philadelphia (CHOP) in 2007 for a combined experience of almost 400 scans. Approximately 60% of infants requiring surgery for management of hypoglycemia have a focal lesion.

HISTOPATHOLOGY

The histopathology of HI can be defined as diffuse, focal, or, less commonly, atypical. During surgery, intraoperative histologic analysis by an experienced pathologist is necessary to confirm a focal lesion of β-cell adenomatosis surrounded by normal pancreatic tissue or diffuse disease characterized by nucleomegaly and abundant cytoplasm of β cells throughout the entire pancreas. A focal lesion of β-cell adenomatosis is histologically distinct from insulinoma. β-Cell adenomatosis is an unencapsulated, irregular-shaped lesion with tentacles extending into normal surrounding tissue with normal islets. Lesions are usually subcentimeter size. The remainder of the pancreatic tissue is normal. An insulinoma is an encapsulated lesion of abnormal cells of varying mitotic index. There are no normal islets. Insulinomas in children are usually benign and can be multifocal in patients with multiple endocrine neoplasia, type 1 syndrome.

Atypical histologic patterns can be seen and include patients with an underlying condition, such as BWS, characterized by an increase of endocrine tissue with variable degrees of islet expansion that can follow a mosaic pattern. Another atypical histologic pattern is characterized by islet cell nucleomegaly (as in diffuse disease) that is confined to a limited region within the pancreas, in a feature that the authors have referred to as localized nuclear enlargement (LINE). Rarely, bifocal, multifocal, and ectopic lesions are discovered.[19,20]

SURGERY

Preoperative localization of a focal lesion using [18F]-FDOPA has become standard of care. Review of 500 pancreatectomies at CHOP revealed 40% with diffuse disease and 49% with focal disease. More than 95% of patients with focal disease who underwent limited resection were cured. A small percentage (7%) had atypical histologic patterns associated with BWS in 4% and LINE in 3%.[21] Patients with diffuse disease who failed medical management underwent 98% pancreatectomy. Of those, approximately 20% were hyperglycemic;

49% had persistent hypoglycemia, and 30% had well-controlled blood glucose levels after surgery. All infants with persistent hypoglycemia require long-term management, including continuous infusion of dextrose through gastrostomy and somatostatin analogues. Nutritional support is essential in children with subtotal pancreatectomy.[21,22]

MECHANISM OF 18-F-L 3,4-DIHYDROXYPHENYLALANINE

Pancreatic cells have the machinery for dopamine metabolism. In the β cell, L-DOPA is transported into cells via a neutral large amino acid transporter, converted to L-dopamine, using the enzyme L-DOPA decarboxylase, and stored in vesicles.[19,20] Radiolabeled L-DOPA, [18F]-FDOPA, is converted to [18F]-dopamine and stored in pancreatic islet vesicles throughout the normal pancreas. Focal lesions have increased activity compared with the background activity in the surrounding normal pancreatic tissue. Detection of a "hot" focal lesion depends on the location, size, and shape of the lesion. Activity in a focal lesion of ß-cell adenomatosis may reflect ß-cell crowding[23] or β-cell overactivity with increased insulin production.[23,24] Carbidopa, a DOPA decarboxylase inhibitor used in the evaluation of other neuroendocrine tumors, blocks the conversion of L-DOPA to dopamine and has been found to block pancreatic uptake of [18F]-DOPA.[7] Carbidopa is currently not recommended in the evaluation of focal HI because of a report by Kauhanen and colleagues[25] showing masking of a focal lesion. Alternatively, the use of carbidopa may be helpful in the evaluation of insulinoma.[26]

PHYSIOLOGIC 18-F-L 3,4-DIHYDROXYPHENYLALANINE UPTAKE

As with all radiotracers, knowledge of the physiologic uptake patterns is essential for interpretation. Physiologic uptake in the liver and kidneys is due to high amounts of DOPA decarboxylase.[24] The kidneys and liver are also sites of excretion of radiotracer. Renal excretion of radiotracer is demonstrated using dynamic imaging protocols. Dynamic protocols can be helpful in the detection of lesions contiguous to the upper pole of the left kidney. If the patient is imaged beyond 50 minutes from infusion of [18F]-FDOPA, uptake can also be seen in the gallbladder, biliary tree, and duodenum because of liver excretion of radiotracer. Because the duodenum and jejunum can be a site of ectopic focal HI lesions, imaging within 60 minutes is recommended to avoid this confounding effect.

Uptake can also be seen in the growth plate cartilage of the spine, ribs, and other bones. A whole-body scan is not a part of the standard recommended protocol, but if performed, it will show uptake in the basal ganglia.

PATIENT SELECTION

Patient selection should be focused on choosing patients with a high likelihood of having a focal lesion. Referral to PET scan should include confirmation of the diagnosis of HI with a critical blood sample obtained during hypoglycemia demonstrating cardinal features of HI: detectable insulin, inappropriately suppressed ketones and free fatty acids, and an inappropriate glycemic response to glucagon at the time of hypoglycemia[27]; genotyping information suggestive of focal disease or inconclusive; phenotyping information demonstrating lack of responsiveness to diazoxide.

Determining the responsiveness to diazoxide is particularly important because lack of response to diazoxide suggests that the KATP channel is defective, and because lack of responsiveness to diazoxide indicates that the child may need surgery. Conversely, responsiveness to diazoxide indicates a functional KATP channel and therefore excludes the possibility of focal HI. The definition of diazoxide responsiveness is thus critical for this determination; a reliable definition of diazoxide-responsiveness is to demonstrate that the cardinal abnormality of HI, that is, fasting hypoketotic hypoglycemia, is corrected while on treatment. Lack of a response to diazoxide initiates the search for a focal lesion. In some cases, the response to diazoxide cannot be appropriately evaluated because of severe side effects; in these cases, FDOPA-PET should be considered when indicated. Genetic testing to exclude diffuse disease is recommended in all patients before FDOPA-PET scanning (**Fig. 1**).

PROTOCOL AND PROCEDURE

In 2006, Mohnike and colleagues[28] published a proposed standard protocol using [18F]-DOPA-PET imaging for the detection of a focal lesion. Since then, publications have used dynamic imaging protocols starting 5 to 20 minutes after injection with 10-minute acquisition times for up to 50 to 60 minutes.[9–16,28] [18F]-FDOPA is manufactured on the day of the scan using established procedures for electrophilic or nucleophilic labeling by a nearby cyclotron facility. Because of the 110-minute half-life of fluorine-18, the delivery time of the radiotracer should be within 2 to 3 hours of production. Depending on the synthesis method

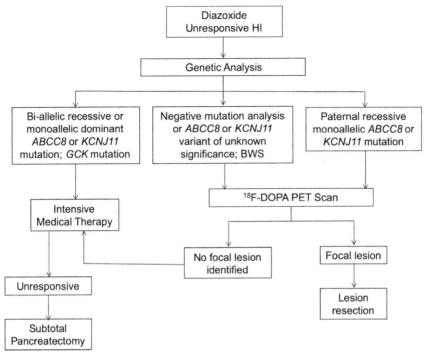

Fig. 1. [18F]-FDOPA patient selection algorithm. (*From* Rayannavar A, De LeonDD. Diazoxide Responsive Forms of Congenital Hyperinsulinism. In: De Leon-Crutchlow DD, Stanley CA (Eds). Congenital Hyperinsulinism: A Practical Guide to Diagnosis and Management. Contemporary Endocrinology, Spinger Nature. Switzerland: Humana Press, 2019. p. 33–47; with permission.)

used, electrophilic versus nucleophilic, the expiration time can vary from 6 hours to 12 hours, respectively. The specific activity of the radiotracer is higher using nucleophilic technique.[29] Typically patients less than 3 years of age undergo general anesthesia with intubation, which requires nothing by mouth for 6 hours before induction. Intravenous (IV) propofol is the most common agent used in the authors' institution. IV glucose is required to maintain plasma glucose levels greater than 70 mg/dL (3.9 mmol/L) before and during the PET scan. Glucagon may be necessary for glycemic control in severe cases and has not been found to interfere with pancreatic uptake in the authors' experience. A point-of-care plasma glucose test is obtained just before injection of radiotracer, 30 minutes into the scan, and at the end of the scan. Anesthesia has been found to increase plasma glucose concentration. Careful titration of the glucose infusion rate should be used to avoid a rapid drop in glucose as anesthesia wears off.[30] IV hydration is used to promote urinary excretion of isotope and decrease radiation dose to the bladder.[9] The radiotracer dose of 3 to 6 MBq/kg (0.08–0.16 mCi/kg) is administered by slow IV injection.[31] In the United States, patients are enrolled in an institutional review board–approved research protocol under an FDA IND and require informed consent.

A typical PET/computed tomographic (CT) protocol will begin with a low-dose noncontrast CT scan of the abdomen, with 3-mm slices, for attenuation correction. PET scanning of the abdomen, at a single bed position, is started within 10 to 15 minutes of injection, and dynamic acquisitions are performed in 10-minute increments over 50 minutes. At the end of the PET acquisition, a low-dose contrast-enhanced CT is performed using 3-mm slice thickness in the portal venous phase for simultaneous opacification of the portal venous system and the arterial system. MR imaging can also be used for image coregistration for anatomic localization. Hybrid imaging with PET/MR imaging is currently limited to a small number of pediatric centers. Protocols using PET/MR imaging can use a similar timing sequence with simultaneous MR imaging acquisitions including volumetric sequences (Dixon T1), T2-weighted fluid-sensitive sequences for visualization of the biliary and pancreatic ducts, and diffusion-weighted imaging for possible lesion detection. Contrast enhancement with gadolinium-based macrocyclic contrast agents may provide added value for surgical planning.

IMAGE INTERPRETATION

Review of images is performed by a nuclear medicine physician or radiologist with experience in nuclear medicine. Images are first reviewed in 3-dimensional (3D) maximum intensity projection (MIP) for the best visualization of the pancreas,

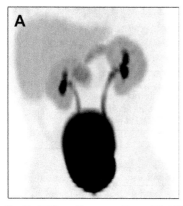 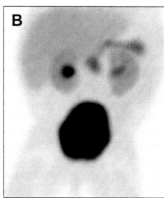 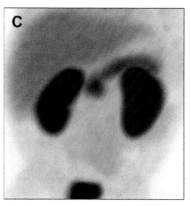

Fig. 2. Diffuse disease pattern: 3D MIP images. (*A*) Homogeneous pattern. (*B*) Heterogeneous pattern with head-body-tail uptake. (*C*) Mild uptake in the pancreatic head, greater than body and tail.

which cannot be viewed in a single plane. This first impression helps to guide review of the fused CT or MR and PET images in 2-dimensions in the axial, coronal, and sagittal planes. The contrast-enhanced images fused to the attenuation-corrected PET images show duodenal, vascular, and ductal anatomy. The duodenum, common bile duct, and splenic artery and vein are key anatomic landmarks, and if in close proximity to the lesion, an alternative surgical approach may be necessary. Thus, identification of these structures is vital for surgical planning.

Lesions not detected by [18F]-FDOPA-PET can be due to the size, shape, or location of the lesion. In Laje and colleagues,[14] lesions that were not identifiable included a flat leaflike lesion on the surface of the pancreas, small lesions, a lesion obscured by activity in the upper pole of the kidney, or a large lesion involving almost the entire pancreas. Depiction of a large pancreas or large

lesion should initiate an evaluation for BWS, which starts with a genetic consultation.

Imaging patterns on the MIP images are incredibly helpful in identification of a focal lesion. A good rule of thumb for interpretation is that a focal lesion is always a single lesion, which is reproducible in multiple frames. Diffuse disease is most often visualized as homogeneous activity throughout the pancreas but can also be heterogeneous with the appearance of multiple focal lesions in the head, body, and tail. The most confounding feature is mild physiologic uptake in the normal tissue of the pancreatic head (**Fig. 2**). This physiologic uptake can be difficult to interpret because up to 55% of focal lesions are found in the head.[21] Focal disease is often visualized as a single, obvious, hot lesion on a background of mild pancreatic activity. An interesting pattern owing to a focal lesion is a "dual pattern" with mild physiologic uptake in the pancreatic head associated

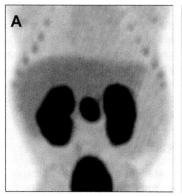 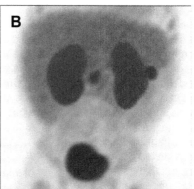 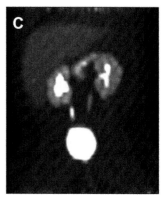

Fig. 3. Focal disease patterns: 3D MIP images. (*A*) Large focal head lesion. (*B*) Dual pattern with physiologic uptake in the pancreatic head and focal uptake in an exophytic pancreatic tail lesion. (*C*) Small focal lesion in the proximal pancreatic body.

Table 2
Patterns on 18-F-L 3,4-dihydroxyphenylalanine PET/computed tomographic scans of 86 evaluable pathology-proven cases of 100 consecutive cases

Pattern	N (%)
Diffuse disease	33 (38)
Homogeneous	20 (61)
Mild increased head	5 (15)
Heterogeneous	8 (24)
Focal lesions	53 (62)
Focal (easy)	39 (74)
Dual head/body or tail	3 (6)
Heterogeneous	4 (7)
Faint uptake	7 (13)

with a focal lesion in the body or tail (**Fig. 3**). A retrospective review of 86 histologically proven cases revealed distinct patterns of uptake provided in **Table 2** (Lisa J. States, M.D.,May, 2013). Review of images using different color scales may increase conspicuity of the lesion and improve the confidence of the interpreting physician.

Fusion with anatomic images such as CT or MR imaging provides detailed anatomy, which allows for an accurate description of the location of a focal lesion (**Fig. 4**). This information is incredibly valuable to the surgeon as a guide for surgical planning. An anterior body lesion may be accessible to laparoscopic resection, and an uncinate lesion may need only a minor resection. A pancreatic head lesion may require a Roux-en-Y pancreaticojejunostomy if the common bile duct is involved or the lesion is large. A lesion in the pancreatic tail at the splenic hilum can be difficult

to resect and puts the patient at risk for a surgically created splenic vein thrombosis. A lesion on the posterior surface of the pancreas may not be visible or palpable by the surgeon; this is where [18F]-FDOPA-PET has the greatest impact (**Fig. 5**).

The most common pitfall of interpretation is due to greater activity in the pancreatic head with respect to the rest of the pancreas. Increased activity in the head may be related to the larger volume of tissue in the pancreatic head compared with the rest of the pancreas. In equivocal cases, any areas of concern should be carefully described and communicated to the surgeon.

ATYPICAL DISEASE IN BECKWITH-WIEDEMANN SYNDROME

In the authors' experience at CHOP, they have used FDOPA-PET to guide pancreatic resection in patients with BWS and persistent life-threatening hypoglycemia. Pancreatic resections vary from 75% to 95%.[14] Patients often have an enlarged pancreas (**Fig. 6**). An enlarged pancreas on an [18F]-FDOPA scan should lead to clinical genetic consultation and include genetic testing for BWS on samples taken from affected tissue,[32] which is incredibly important because BWS has a predisposition to development of embryonal tumors such as wilms' tumor (WT) and hepatoblastoma (HB).[32]

QUANTITATIVE ANALYSIS

Quantitative analysis using the ratio of activity in the lesion to background pancreatic activity has been suggested as an aid to diagnosis of a focal lesion and can be used to increase diagnostic confidence. A standardized uptake value (SUV) ratio can be calculated using SUVmax of the lesion divided by SUVmean of the "normal" pancreatic

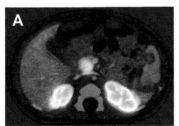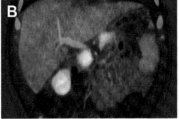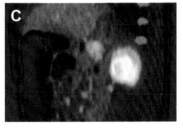

Fig. 4. A 5 week old with HI underwent 5% pancreatectomy of a focal lesion. PET fused with contrast-enhanced CT, reformatted in 3 planes, shows a focal lesion in the pancreatic head. (*A*) Axial fused PET/CT image shows focal lesion in the central pancreatic head. Note the appearance of less intense pancreas surrounding the lesion. (*B*) Coronal fused PET/CT image shows the central location and less intense tissue surrounding the lesion. (*C*) Sagittal fused PET/CT image shows the focal lesion in the superior pancreatic head. Note the portal vein inferior to pancreatic head.

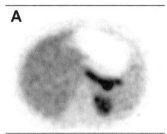
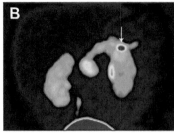

Fig. 5. A 5 month old underwent 2% pancreatectomy for focal lesion along posterior surface of the pancreas. (*A*) Axial PET image shows focal lesion located at the posterior surface of the pancreas at the body-tail junction. (*B*) 3D MIP in color shows the focal lesion (*arrow*) adjacent to the upper pole of the left kidney.

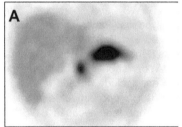
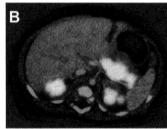
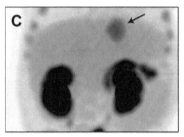

Fig. 6. PET images of 2 babies with BWS. Both underwent 80% pancreatectomy. (*A*) A 3-week-old ex-31-week premature infant with HI unresponsive to diazoxide. 3D MIP shows a large focal lesion involving the entire pancreatic body. (*B*) PET fused with contrast-enhanced CT shows the large focal lesion and enlargement of the pancreatic body. The splenic artery is seen posterior to the lesion. (*C*) A 2-month-old girl with HI and atypical pancreatic histopathology consistent with BWS. 3D MIP shows focal activity in the pancreatic body and bulbous pancreatic tail. Incidental note is made of a round, focal lesion to the left of midline in a known neuroblastoma (*arrow*).

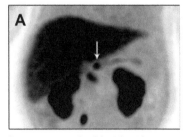
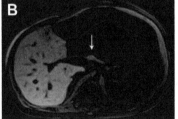
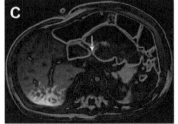

Fig. 7. A 5-week-old girl with HI unresponsive to diazoxide. PET/MR imaging of a focal lesion in the proximal pancreatic body. (*A*) 3D MIP shows a focal lesion (*arrow*) in the proximal pancreatic body/neck region. Note the mild increased activity in the pancreatic head. (*B*) Axial T1-weighted MR image shows the small pancreatic lesion (*arrow*). (*C*) Axial fused PET/T1-weighted image shows the small pancreatic lesion (*arrow*). (*Courtesy of* Royal Children's Hospital Melbourne, Australia; with permission.)

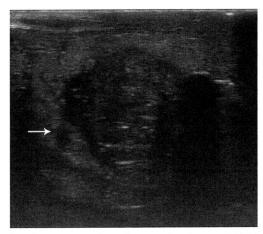

Fig. 8. Intraoperative ultrasound using a 50-MHz transducer. Transverse US image shows a focal lesion hypoechoic to adjacent pancreatic tissue that was not palpable. The common bile duct (arrow) is visualized as a hypoechoic structure at the 8 o'clock position.

tissue. An SUV ratio of $\geq 1.5^6$ or 1.2^{33} has been suggested as diagnostic for a focal lesion. In most cases, visual analysis is adequate for interpretation and localization of a focal lesion.

SAFETY

No adverse events related to the isotope have been seen at CHOP or at Diagnostisch Therapeutisches Zentrum (DTZ) "Berlin-Frankfurter Tor" in more than 550 subjects and therefore is thought to pose little risk to the subjects.[28,34] The [18F]-FDOPA-PET/CT scan involves exposure to radiation. Based on a dose of 3.7 to 5.92 MBq/kg (0.16 mCi/kg) and a patient weight of 10 kg, the estimated effective radiation dose is $0.3 \pm$ mSv/MBq.[35] Because of excretion of radiotracer by the kidneys, the radiation dose to the bladder is 10 times greater than that received by any other organ or tissue. Therefore, adequate hydration is essential for minimizing dose to the bladder.[36,37] The dose of the low-dose CT of the abdomen is 100 mrem, which gives an average dose much lower than 10,000 mrem, the level of radiation known to increase the long-term risk of developing cancer.[38] MR imaging, as an alternative to CT, avoids additional radiation and has been proposed to provide additional visualization of the common bile duct and pancreatic duct to guide surgery in the vicinity of a focal lesion (**Fig. 7**).

In cases where a focal lesion is not detected by [18F]-FDOPA-PET/CT and intraoperative biopsies reveal normal pancreatic tissue (excluding diffuse disease), intraoperative high-resolution sonography may sometimes be helpful in localization of a focal lesion. Characteristic sonographic features include hypoechogenicity or variable homogeneous and in homogenous texture, blurred, irregular margins, filiform or lobular processes, and insular dispersal into the surrounding tissue as well as visualization of the pancreatic duct[39] (**Fig. 8**). Contrast-enhanced ultrasound is also a promising technique that may prove useful in the localization of a focal lesion and evaluation of the pancreatic duct after lesion resection.

SUMMARY

Published data from centers in the United States, Europe, and Japan support the hypothesis that [18F]-FDOPA-PET/CT imaging provides a clinically useful guide to surgical resection of focal lesions. An [18F]-FDOPA-PET scan is indicated in all infants with medically unresponsive HI in whom genetic tests are not consistent with diffuse disease because surgery offers a chance of cure in patients with a focal lesion. Accurate preoperative localization provided by imaging findings on fused PET/CT is essential for successful surgery. An experienced team, including endocrinology, surgery, pathology, nursing, and radiology, is essential for successful and optimal care of this vulnerable patient population.

DISCLOSURE

This article discusses a radiotracer that is not FDA approved for use in children. Dr D. De Leon has received grant/research support from the following companies: Zealand Pharma A/S and Crinetics Pharmaceuticals. She has received consulting fees from Zealand Pharma A/S, Crinetics Pharmaceuticals, Novartis Pharmaceuticals, and Prosciento.

REFERENCES

1. De Leon DD, Stanley CA. Congenital hypoglycemia disorders: new aspects of etiology, diagnosis, treatment and outcomes: highlights of the Proceedings of the Congenital Hypoglycemia Disorders Symposium, Philadelphia April 2016. Pediatr Diabetes 2017;18:3–9.
2. Ludwig A, Enke S, Heindorf J, et al. Formal neurocognitive testing in 60 patients with congenital hyperinsulinism. Horm Res Paediatr 2018;89:1–6.
3. Verkarre V, Fournet JC, de Lonlay P, et al. Paternal mutation of the sulfonylurea receptor (SUR1) gene and maternal loss of 11p15 imprinted genes lead to persistent hyperinsulinism in focal adenomatous hyperplasia. J Clin Invest 1998;102:1286–91.

4. Snider KE, Becker S, Boyajian L, et al. Genotype and phenotype correlations in 417 children with congenital hyperinsulinism. J Clin Endocrinol Metab 2013;98:E355–63.

5. Herrera A, Vajravelu ME, Givler S, et al. Prevalence of adverse events in children with congenital hyperinsulinism treated with diazoxide. J Clin Endocrinol Metab 2018;103:4365–72.

6. Otonkoski T, Nanto-Salonen K, Seppanen M, et al. Noninvasive diagnosis of focal hyperinsulinism of infancy with [18F]-DOPA positron emission tomography. Diabetes 2006;55:13–8.

7. Ribeiro MJ, De Lonlay P, Delzescaux T, et al. Characterization of hyperinsulinism in infancy assessed with PET and 18F-fluoro-L-DOPA. J Nucl Med 2005;46:560–6.

8. Ribeiro MJ, Boddaert N, Bellanne-Chantelot C, et al. The added value of [18F]fluoro-L-DOPA PET in the diagnosis of hyperinsulinism of infancy: a retrospective study involving 49 children. Eur J Nucl Med Mol Imaging 2007;34:2120–8.

9. Hardy OT, Hernandez-Pampaloni M, Saffer JR, et al. Accuracy of [18F]fluorodopa positron emission tomography for diagnosing and localizing focal congenital hyperinsulinism. J Clin Endocrinol Metab 2007;92:4706–11.

10. Barthlen W, Blankenstein O, Mau H, et al. Evaluation of [18F]fluoro-L-DOPA positron emission tomography-computed tomography for surgery in focal congenital hyperinsulinism. J Clin Endocrinol Metab 2008;93:869–75.

11. Capito C, Khen-Dunlop N, Ribeiro MJ, et al. Value of 18F-fluoro-L-DOPA PET in the preoperative localization of focal lesions in congenital hyperinsulinism. Radiology 2009;253:216–22.

12. Masue M, Nishibori H, Fukuyama S, et al. Diagnostic accuracy of [(1)(8)F]-fluoro-L-dihydroxyphenylalanine positron emission tomography scan for persistent congenital hyperinsulinism in Japan. Clin Endocrinol (Oxf) 2011;75:342–6.

13. Zani A, Nah SA, Ron O, et al. The predictive value of preoperative fluorine-18-L-3,4-dihydroxyphenylalanine positron emission tomography-computed tomography scans in children with congenital hyperinsulinism of infancy. J Pediatr Surg 2011;46:204–8.

14. Laje P, States LJ, Zhuang H, et al. Accuracy of PET/CT scan in the diagnosis of the focal form of congenital hyperinsulinism. J Pediatr Surg 2013;48:388–93.

15. Meintjes M, Endozo R, Dickson J, et al. 18F-DOPA PET and enhanced CT imaging for congenital hyperinsulinism: initial UK experience from a technologist's perspective. Nucl Med Commun 2013;34:601–8.

16. Kuhnen P, Matthae R, Arya V, et al. Occurrence of giant focal forms of congenital hyperinsulinism with incorrect visualization by (18) F DOPA-PET/CT scanning. Clin Endocrinol (Oxf) 2014;81:847–54.

17. News: FDA reviews NDA for (18)F-FDOPA in congenital hyperinsulinism. J Nucl Med 2019;60:7n.

18. Center for Drug Evaluation and Research, US Food and Drug Administration. New drug application approval letter (application No. 200655). Maryland: U.S. Food and Drug Administration; 2019.

19. Hussain K, Seppanen M, Nanto-Salonen K, et al. The diagnosis of ectopic focal hyperinsulinism of infancy with [18F]-DOPA positron emission tomography. J Clin Endocrinol Metab 2006;91:2839–42.

20. Peranteau WH, Bathaii SM, Pawel B, et al. Multiple ectopic lesions of focal islet adenomatosis identified by positron emission tomography scan in an infant with congenital hyperinsulinism. J Pediatr Surg 2007;42:188–92.

21. Adzick NS, De Leon DD, States LJ, et al. Surgical treatment of congenital hyperinsulinism: results from 500 pancreatectomies in neonates and children. J Pediatr Surg 2019;54:27–32.

22. Adzick NS, Thornton PS, Stanley CA, et al. A multidisciplinary approach to the focal form of congenital hyperinsulinism leads to successful treatment by partial pancreatectomy. J Pediatr Surg 2004;39:270–5.

23. Sempoux C, Guiot Y, Dahan K, et al. The focal form of persistent hyperinsulinemic hypoglycemia of infancy: morphological and molecular studies show structural and functional differences with insulinoma. Diabetes 2003;52:784–94.

24. de Lonlay P, Simon-Carre A, Ribeiro MJ, et al. Congenital hyperinsulinism: pancreatic [18F]fluoro-L-dihydroxyphenylalanine (DOPA) positron emission tomography and immunohistochemistry study of DOPA decarboxylase and insulin secretion. J Clin Endocrinol Metab 2006;91:933–40.

25. Kauhanen S, Seppanen M, Nuutila P. Premedication with carbidopa masks positive finding of insulinoma and beta-cell hyperplasia in [(18)F]-dihydroxyphenyl-alanine positron emission tomography. J Clin Oncol 2008;26:5307–8 [author reply: 5308–9].

26. Nakuz TS, Berger E, El-Rabadi K, et al. Clinical value of (18)F-FDOPA PET/CT with contrast enhancement and without carbidopa premedication in patients with insulinoma. Anticancer Res 2018;38:353–8.

27. Ferrara C, Patel P, Becker S, et al. Biomarkers of insulin for the diagnosis of hyperinsulinemic hypoglycemia in infants and children. J Pediatr 2016;168:212–9.

28. Mohnike K, Blankenstein O, Minn H, et al. [18F]-DOPA positron emission tomography for preoperative localization in congenital hyperinsulinism. Horm Res 2008;70:65–72.

29. Moerlein S, Bognar C, Gaehle G, et al. Validation of a nucleophilic synthesis platform for clinical application of [18 F]Fluorodopa. J Nucl Med 2017;58(S1): 255.

30. Hardy OT, Litman RS. Congenital hyperinsulinism–a review of the disorder and a discussion of the anesthesia management. Paediatr Anaesth 2007;17: 616–21.

31. Schoder H, Pillarsetty K, Lyashchenko S, et al. Fluorodopa F-18 [18F]FDOPA–Society of Nuclear Medicine and Molecular Imaging. SNMMI PET Center of Excellence and the Center for Molecular Imaging Innovation & Translation; Virginia; 2013.

32. Kalish JM, Doros L, Helman LJ, et al. Surveillance recommendations for children with overgrowth syndromes and predisposition to wilms tumors and hepatoblastoma. Clin Cancer Res 2017;23:e115–22.

33. Arnoux JB, de Lonlay P, Ribeiro MJ, et al. Congenital hyperinsulinism. Early Hum Dev 2010;86:287–94.

34. States LJ, Mohnike K. 18F-DOPA PET. In: De León-Crutchlow DD, Stanley CA, editors. Congenital hyperinsulinism: a practical guide to diagnosis and management. Cham (Swizerland): Springer International Publishing; 2019. p. 85–93.

35. Garg PK, Lokitz SJ, Truong L, et al. Pancreatic uptake and radiation dosimetry of 6-[18F]fluoro-L-DOPA from PET imaging studies in infants with congenital hyperinsulinism. PLoS One 2017;12: e0186340.

36. Harvey J, Firnau G, Garnett ES. Estimation of the radiation dose in man due to 6-[18F]fluoro-L-DOPA. J Nucl Med 1985;26:931–5.

37. Dhawan V, Belakhlef A, Robeson W, et al. Bladder wall radiation dose in humans from fluorine-18-FDOPA. J Nucl Med 1996;37:1850–2.

38. National Research Council, Committee to Assess Health Risks from Exposure to Low Levels of Ionizing Radiation. Health risks from exposure to low levels of ionizing radiation: BEIR VII phase 2. National Academies Press; 2006.

39. von Rohden L, Mohnike K, Mau H, et al. Visualization of the focus in congenital hyperinsulinism by intraoperative sonography. Semin Pediatr Surg 2011;20: 28–31.

PET/Computed Tomography in the Evaluation of Fever of Unknown Origin and Infectious/Inflammatory Disease in Pediatric Patients

Wichana Chamroonrat, MD

KEYWORDS

- FDG • PET/CT • FUO • Fever • Infection • Inflammation • Pediatric

KEY POINTS

- Finding the cause of fever of unknown origin (FUO) in pediatric patients can be challenging for care-givers and parents. 18F-fluorodeoxyglucose (FDG) PET/computed tomography (CT) is a combined imaging tool of both anatomic and functional imaging for localizing possible FUO lesions and guiding for further management.
- FDG is a radiotracer commonly used with PET/CT in evaluation of FUO and is useful for identifying oncologic and infectious/inflammatory disease.
- FDG-PET/CT gives high negative predictive value as well as prognostic value for FUO. If no regional/focal cause is identified by FDG-PET/CT, the fever usually spontaneously resolves.

INTRODUCTION

Fever of unknown origin (FUO) in pediatric population could be defined as fever with core temperature of 38°C or higher, lasting more than a week with negative initial work-up.[1] For children, FUO causes are approximately identified as 40% to 50% infection, 10% to 20% inflammatory disease, 10% to 20% malignancy, and unknown in the rest.[1–3]

In the evaluation of pediatric patients with FUO, a thorough history taking from the patient and parents and comprehensive physical examinations should be done. Possible related signs and symptoms should be documented in case of retrospect review. General initial laboratory work-up includes complete blood count with white blood cell (WBC) differentiation, C-reactive protein (CRP), erythrocyte sedimentation rate (ESR), blood culture and

sensitivity, urine analysis and culture, and chest radiograph for common bases. More targeted, initial work-up includes ultrasonography, antinuclear antibodies, Rh factor, uric acid, antistreptolysin O (for arthritis), cerebrospinal fluid, lymph node aspiration, and bone marrow biopsy (for suspected malignancy).[4]

IMAGING TECHNIQUES

Initial use of imaging in FUO now frequently includes radiograph and/or ultrasonography in appropriate clinical settings; for example, suspected pneumonia using chest radiograph and suspected lesion in internal abdominal organs using ultrasonography. In suspected malignancy, computed tomography (CT) and/or magnetic resonance (MR) imaging could be requested at the

Division of Nuclear Medicine, Department of Diagnostic and Therapeutic Radiology, Faculty of Medicine Ramathibodi Hospital, Mahidol University, Bangkok, Thailand
E-mail address: wichana.cha@mahidol.edu

PET Clin 15 (2020) 361–369
https://doi.org/10.1016/j.cpet.2020.03.002

suspicious region. A disadvantage of CT is radiation, whereas MR imaging is time consuming and commonly requires sedation. Both mainly evaluate anatomic alteration, which is common following functional change.

PET/CT is a tool that combines functional and anatomic evaluation. 18Ffluorodeoxydlucose (FDG), a positron-emitting glucose analogue, is a well-known radiotracer/radiopharmaceutical for malignancy. Because of its nonspecificity, it can be used in active infectious/inflammatory diseases.[5] Therefore, FDG-PET/CT is suitable for FUO evaluation; nevertheless, it still produces radiation. Benefit and radiation risk should be discussed before using FDG-PET/CT.

FDG-PET/CT has proved its superiority over CT alone[6] and other radionuclide imaging using In-111 WBCs or Ga-67 citrate[7–9] in the evaluation of FUO. There have been numerous publications describing the utility of FDG-PET/CT in the evaluation of adult patients with fever of various causes.[10–21] FDG-PET/CT is currently the test that has the best performance, combining single-shot multisystem evaluation[22] with time effectiveness, greater sensitivity, and better image resolution.[7,23,24] Other types of radionuclide imaging might be used if FDG-PET/CT is not feasible.[25] Because of the noninvasive technique of FDG-PET/CT, if FUO is present without suspected hematologic abnormality, it should be done before bone marrow biopsy.[26] Prior adult studies and meta-analyses of FUO suggest that FDG-PET/CT should be the first-line imaging modality[27–29] in order to avoid an unnecessary invasive technique.

18F-FLUORODEOXYGLUCOSE PET/COMPUTED TOMOGRAPHY PROTOCOL

The FDG-PET/CT protocol in FUO or infectious/inflammatory disease seems not significantly different from an oncologic protocol. In general, the preferred preparations are designated to lessen disturbed factors for interpretation, including keeping warm to minimize brown fat, longer fasting to minimize myocardial activity, and withholding strenuous exercise to minimize muscular uptake. In pediatric patients, limiting the length of time the children can spend playing games on mobile devices is also important.[30]

FDG is injected into adult patients who have fasted at least 4 hours; This interval is similar for adolescents and progressively shorter for young children, toddlers, and infants. Blood glucose level before FDG injection should be less than 11.1 mmol/L. After at least 60 minutes, the scan can be obtained.[31,32] Scanning of the whole body length from vertex to feet is also preferred

whenever possible, especially in situations with no diagnostic clues. Limited extremities might be scanned in certain circumstances.

The 2016 update of the North American consensus guideline for pediatric-administered radiopharmaceutical activities recommends FDG doses of 0.1 to 0.14 mCi/kg (3.7–5.2 MBq/kg), with minimal activity of 0.7 mCi (26 MBq).[33]

In FUO, obtaining FDG-PET/CT is suggested while the patient is febrile. Furthermore, positive FDG-PET/CT showed higher yield in patients with fever durations of less than 3 months, abnormal laboratory investigations (high levels of inflammatory factors such as CRP and ESR), and abnormal blood cells (leukocytosis and neutrophilia).[34–36]

18F-FLUORODEOXYGLUCOSE PET/COMPUTED TOMOGRAPHY FINDINGS

A positive FDG lesion on PET/CT could be either a focal or nonfocal abnormality. Nonfocal abnormalities usually present with altered physiologic FDG distribution without a definite focal lesion. In general, focal abnormalities require further investigation in order to reach a conclusion and to change the management. However, altered physiologic FDG distribution in a certain organ or system may imply abnormal behavior or functioning without a true lesion localized in the organ. Diffusely increased bone marrow FDG activity usually results from generalized stimulation of marrow with known ongoing anemia receiving granulocyte colony-stimulating factor; however, in some circumstances, such as FUO, it may be necessary to exclude infiltration of malignancy or infection. Diffuse spleen FDG uptake has higher intensity in autoimmune than infectious disease.[37] Diffusely high subcutaneous fat uptake could be caused by Epstein-Barr virus (EBV) infection.[38] Possibilities of high FDG-avid generalized lymphadenopathy include not only malignancy, commonly in the form of lymphoma, but also benign causes such as viral infection and autoimmune disease.[39–41]

In contrast, if there is no focal abnormality with normal distribution, it would be considered negative FDG-PET/CT. The lesion could not overcome physiologic high FDG activity, particularly located in an organ with high FDG activity such as the brain or the genitourinary system. False-negative FDG-PET/CT in urinary tract infection has been described.[42] The CT portion of PET/CT is better for lesion localization and characterization.

DIAGNOSTIC CRITERIA

In the past 2 decades, there have been more than 31 original articles from more than 15 countries on

6 continents reporting patients with FUO/prolonged fever investigated with FDG-PET/CT.[6,7,17,26,34–36,42–70] Six of these solely studied the pediatric population.[42,50,61,67,69,71] Other studies included a few children among mostly adult patients.[49,52,64] Definitions of FUO in the 6 pediatric articles are broadly similar. Fever should be at least 38°C with initial negative work-up for at least 3 days. The age ranges are between 2 months and 18 years.

Sturm and colleagues[42] reported the first article on pediatric FUO concerning 11 pediatric liver transplant candidates in 2006, all using FDG-PET. Five positive intrahepatic PET findings of cholangitis were all confirmed with bacterial cultures of explant or ascites, whereas 6 negative intrahepatic PET findings showed no proof of cholangitis or liver infection. Urinary tract infection was found in 2 of 6 patients by urinary culture.

Jasper and colleagues[50] reported a slightly larger number of children with FUO using 44 FDG-PET/CT scans. The term "unexplained sign of inflammation" was introduced for an additional 33 FDG-PET/CT findings, similar to inflammation of unknown origin, which was a term used in another article on the adult population[72] in the same year (2009). Both terms were defined as FUO minus fever. Jasper and colleagues[50] found 51% (32 out of 63) of scans helpful from 82% (63 out of 77) of scans that were positive (focus and nonfocus). Helpful scans help in excluding targeted evaluation or allowing targeted evaluation. Between PET and PET/CT, 53% of FDG-PET/CT were considered helpful, whereas 40% of FDG-PET were helpful, indicating that FDG-PET/CT is superior to FDG-PET in the evaluation FUO in pediatric patients. Positive scans correlated to abnormal CRP, neutrophil, and thrombocytes.

Blokhuis and colleagues[61] also reported on a large number of children with FUO using 31 FDG-PET/CT scans and another 12 immune-suppressed children with unexplained fever, and found 75% (10 out of 14) contributory (true-positive) scans from 45% (14 out of 31) abnormal (focal only) scans in children with FUO as well as 88% (7 out of 8) contributory scans from 67% (8 out of 12) abnormal scans in immune-suppressed children with unexplained fever. The same group of investigators also noted that FDG-PET/CT is valuable to identify metastatic infection in pediatric patients.[73]

Chang and colleagues[67] reported 19 children with FUO in intensive care and found 93% (14 out of 15) helpful scans from 79% (15/19) positive scans.

Wang and colleagues[69] reported 14 immuno-compromised children with fever in 2017, all using FDG-PET/CT. High clinical impact of FDG-PET/CT is considered to be when management changes.

Wang and colleagues[69] found 79% (11 out of 14) high clinical impact, but with 57% (8 out of 14) positive scans. In addition, profound neutropenia (neutrophil count <1 cell/μL) seemed not to affect positive scans.

The largest study so far reported was by Pijl and colleagues,[71] which involved 110 children with FUO. FDG-PET/CT identified the cause of the fever in 48% of the patients and changed the treatment plan in 53% of the patients, with a sensitivity of 85.5% and a specificity of 79.2%.[71]

These pediatric articles reported FDG-PET/CT sensitivity of 80% to 100% [50,61,67] and specificity of 66.7% to 79.2%,[61,67,71] similar to the pooled sensitivity of 82.6% and specificity of 57.8% in meta-analysis in the adult population.[74]

DIFFERENTIAL DIAGNOSIS

Lists of final diagnoses of children (up to 20 years old) with fever using and having positive FDG-PET/CT in published case reports, case series, reviews, and original articles categorized as infectious inflammatory diseases, noninfectious inflammatory diseases, and malignancy are detailed here.

Infectious Disease

Infectious thrombosis[50]
Septic pulmonary emboli (*Staphylococcus aureus*)[42,75,76]
Bronchitis[77]
Pneumonia[50,78] (see **Fig. 2**), *Pneumocystis jiroveci*,[77] EBV[67]
Endocarditis[69,76]
Tuberculosis (TB) pericarditis[67]
Left ventricular assist device infection[76]
Colitis[61]
Cholangitis (*Enterococcus*)[79,80]
Chronic appendicitis (**Fig. 1**)
Abscess, intra-abdomen,[78] psoas muscle[50]
Pressure ulcer[61]
Cutaneous granulomatous eruption (primarily on the lower extremities)[81]
Cutaneous infection[67] (*Mycobacterium avium complex*)[81] *Staphylococcus epidermidis*[80]
Osteomyelitis[67,69,78,82,83] (**Fig. 2**)
Occult bacterial infections[83]
Systemic bacterial infection[42]
Invasive fungal infection[69]
Regional and/or disseminated candidiasis[50,61,67,69,77]
Mycobacterium tuberculosis[84]
Mycobacterium kansasii[61]
Clostridium difficile[61]
Herpes virus infection[50]
EBV infection[38,40]
Cytomegalovirus (CMV) infection[77]
Scrub typhus[85]

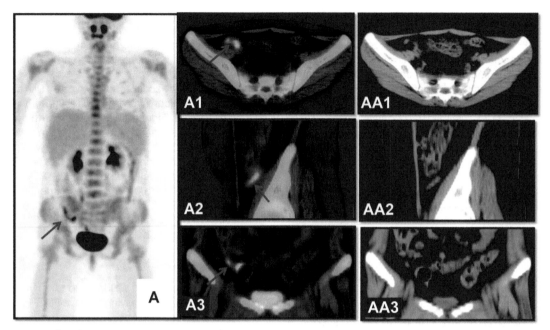

Fig. 1. A female teenager with leukemia after bone marrow transplant presented with fever and abdominal pain. As well as nonspecific diffusely increased bone marrow activity, PET/CT scan showed increased FDG uptake along the appendix (*red arrows*). Maximum intensity projection (MIP): (*A1–A3*) fused axial, sagittal, coronal; and (*AA1–AA3*) CT axial, coronal, sagittal images. Laparoscopic appendectomy was done 2 days after the scan for chronic appendicitis.

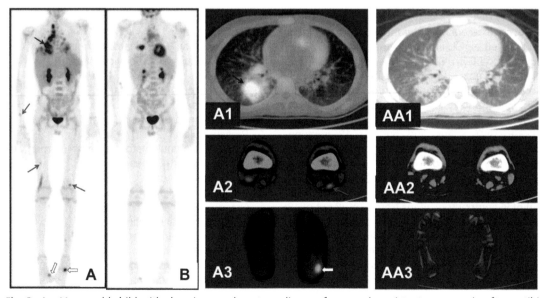

Fig. 2. An 11-year-old child with chronic granulomatous disease, fever, and persistent pneumonia after antibiotics. (*A*) Initial FDG-PET/CT scan (*A, left*) and (*B*) MIP (*A1–A3*) fused axial and (*AA1–AA3*) CT axial images revealed not only active inflammatory changes in the right lung, consistent with pneumonia (*black arrows*) but also multifocal osteomyelitis (*white arrows*) and subcutaneous foci of infections (*red arrows*). Sputum cultures revealed *Candida*. Antifungal medication was added. (*A, right*) Subsequent PET/CT scan MIP image showed some improvement of described lesions.

Noninfectious Inflammatory Disease (Autoimmune and Nonautoimmune)

Crohn disease[86]
Systemic lupus erythematosus[61]
Polyarthritis[50]
Polyarthritis in Henoch-Schönlein vasculitis[87]
Juvenile idiopathic arthritis[50,67]
Still disease or systemic juvenile idiopathic arthritis[50,61,88]
SAPHO (synovitis, acne, pustulosis, hyperostosis, and osteitis) syndrome[61]
Castleman disease[89]
Kawasaki disease[50]
Kikuchi-Fujimoto disease[90]
Chronic granulomatous disease[91]
Nonbacterial osteitis[92]

Malignancy

Acute myeloid leukemia[64]
Hepatosplenic T-cell lymphoma[61]
Peripheral T-cell lymphoma[67]
Primary bone marrow lymphoma[93]
Posttransplant lymphoproliferative disease[50,61,94]
Langerhans cell histiocytosis[95]
Hemophagocytic lymphohistiocytosis[67,78] (secondary to CMV reactivation)[69]
Rosai-Dorfman disease[39,50]
Adrenal cancer[52]
Neuroblastoma[50]
Pheochromocytoma[67]
Multiple endocrine neoplasia type 2[50]

OTHER USES AND CONSIDERATIONS

FDG-PET/CT has been used not only for helping in the diagnosis of FUO and infectious/inflammatory diseases but also in evaluation of treatment response, which is already established in malignancy. Treatment response evaluations for infectious/inflammatory diseases have been shown in extrapulmonary TB,[84,96] antisynthetase syndrome,[97] infective spondylodiscitis,[98] brachiocephalic thrombophlebitis,[99] acute varicella infection,[41] and systemic candidiasis (see **Fig. 2**).

Few children with FUO who had negative FDG-PET/CT results showed spontaneous remission of fever.[67] Similar to adults with FUO, a systematic review and meta-analysis by Takeuchi and colleagues[100] found that adult patients with FUO with negative PET/CT results had a higher probability of spontaneous remission after unsuccessful fever work-up, with cumulative incidence of spontaneous remission ranging from 20% to 78%, compared with 0% to 48% in those with positive results.

SUMMARY

In past few decades, FDG-PET/CT as a combination of functional and anatomic evaluation has been shown to have the best test performance for FUO after the usual initial work-up, not only in adults but also in the pediatric population. The advantages of FDG-PET/CT in the evaluation of FUO and infectious/inflammatory disease in pediatric patients have been discussed, not only for helping diagnosis as listed but also in indicating treatment response. In addition, negative findings in FDG-PET/CT seem to lead to favorable prognostic outcomes.

DISCLOSURE

The author has nothing to disclose.

REFERENCES

1. Antoon JW, Potisek NM, Lohr JA. Pediatric fever of unknown origin. Pediatr Rev 2015;36:380–90 [quiz: 91].
2. Barbi E, Marzuillo P, Neri E, et al. Fever in children: pearls and pitfalls. Children (Basel) 2017;4 [pii: E81].
3. Chien YL, Huang FL, Huang CM, et al. Clinical approach to fever of unknown origin in children. J Microbiol Immunol Infect 2017;50:893–8.
4. Dayal R, Agarwal D. Fever in children and fever of unknown origin. Indian J Pediatr 2016;83:38–43.
5. Zhuang H, Alavi A. 18-fluorodeoxyglucose positron emission tomographic imaging in the detection and monitoring of infection and inflammation. Semin Nucl Med 2002;32:47–59.
6. Rosenbaum J, Basu S, Beckerman S, et al. Evaluation of diagnostic performance of 18F-FDG-PET compared to CT in detecting potential causes of fever of unknown origin in an academic centre. Hell J Nucl Med 2011;14:255–9.
7. Hung BT, Wang PW, Su YJ, et al. The efficacy of (18)F-FDG PET/CT and (67)Ga SPECT/CT in diagnosing fever of unknown origin. Int J Infect Dis 2017;62:10–7.
8. Parisi MT. Functional imaging of infection: conventional nuclear medicine agents and the expanding role of 18-F-FDG PET. Pediatr Radiol 2011;41: 803–10.
9. Seshadri N, Sonoda LI, Lever AM, et al. Superiority of 18F-FDG PET compared to 111In-labelled leucocyte scintigraphy in the evaluation of fever of unknown origin. J Infect 2012;65:71–9.
10. Crouzet J, Boudousq V, Lechiche C, et al. Place of (18)F-FDG-PET with computed tomography in the diagnostic algorithm of patients with fever of unknown origin. Eur J Clin Microbiol Infect Dis 2012; 31:1727–33.

11. Mulders-Manders CM, Simon A, Bleeker-Rovers CP. Rheumatologic diseases as the cause of fever of unknown origin. Best Pract Res Clin Rheumatol 2016;30:789–801.

12. Liu E, Wang S, Lai P, et al. "Hepatic superscan" in a patient with hepatosplenic alphabeta T-cell lymphoma: 18F-FDG PET/CT findings. Clin Nucl Med 2018;43:595–8.

13. Dong A, Bai Y, Wang Y. Focal myositis of the leg presenting as fever of unknown origin detected by FDG PET/CT. Clin Nucl Med 2019;44:251–4.

14. Guhne F, Drescher R, Seifert P, et al. Inflammatory activity of tumoral calcinosis in a patient with fever of unknown origin. Clin Nucl Med 2019;44:e289–90.

15. McCarron EP, Sreenivasan S, Venkatraman L, et al. Kikuchi-Fujimoto disease presenting as post-traumatic pyrexia of unknown origin. Br J Hosp Med (Lond) 2019;80:170–1.

16. Armagan B, Erden A, Beydas O, et al. Is the PET/CT first choice for differential diagnosis of fever of FUO/IUO? Ann Rheum Dis 2018;77:e82.

17. Nazar AH, Naswa N, Sharma P, et al. Spectrum of 18F-FDG PET/CT findings in patients presenting with fever of unknown origin. AJR Am J Roentgenol 2012;199:175–85.

18. Flaus A, Longo MG, Dematons M, et al. 18F-FDG PET/CT in urachal abscess. Clin Nucl Med 2019;44:e349–50.

19. Jinguji M, Kajiya Y, Nakajo M, et al. Increased 18F-FDG uptake in the spleen and multiple lymph nodes in dengue fever. Clin Nucl Med 2016;41:e255–6.

20. Mino N, Yamashita H, Takahashi Y, et al. Polyarteritis nodosa with reversible FDG accumulation in vessels and kidneys. Clin Nucl Med 2019;44:889–91.

21. Hotta M, Minamimoto R, Yashima A, et al. FDG PET/CT findings in TAFRO syndrome. Clin Nucl Med 2018;43:828–9.

22. Watts RA. How to investigate multisystem disease. Best Pract Res Clin Rheumatol 2014;28:831–43.

23. Palestro CJ, Love C. Nuclear medicine imaging in fever of unknown origin: the new paradigm. Curr Pharm Des 2018;24:814–20.

24. Takeuchi M, Dahabreh IJ, Nihashi T, et al. Nuclear imaging for classic fever of unknown origin: meta-analysis. J Nucl Med 2016;57:1913–9.

25. Serrano Vicente J, Parras Castanera E, Infante Torre JR, et al. 67-Gallium SPECT/CT in febrile syndromes of unknown origin. Rev Esp Med Nucl Imagen Mol 2018;37:354–8.

26. Hong FS, Fox LC, Chai KL, et al. Role of bone marrow biopsy for fever of unknown origin in the contemporary Australian context. Intern Med J 2019;49:850–4.

27. Kan Y, Wang W, Liu J, et al. Contribution of 18F-FDG PET/CT in a case-mix of fever of unknown origin and inflammation of unknown origin: a meta-analysis. Acta Radiol 2019;60:716–25.

28. Besson FL, Chaumet-Riffaud P, Playe M, et al. Contribution of (18)F-FDG PET in the diagnostic assessment of fever of unknown origin (FUO): a stratification-based meta-analysis. Eur J Nucl Med Mol Imaging 2016;43:1887–95.

29. Pereira AM, Husmann L, Sah BR, et al. Determinants of diagnostic performance of 18F-FDG PET/CT in patients with fever of unknown origin. Nucl Med Commun 2016;37:57–65.

30. Bai X, Wang X, Zhuang H. Relationship between the elevated muscle FDG uptake in the distal upper extremities on PET/CT scan and prescan utilization of mobile devices in young patients. Clin Nucl Med 2018;43:168–73.

31. Jamar F, Buscombe J, Chiti A, et al. EANM/SNMMI guideline for 18F-FDG use in inflammation and infection. J Nucl Med 2013;54:647–58.

32. Buscombe J. Guidelines for the use of 18F-FDG in infection and inflammation: a new step in cooperation between the EANM and SNMMI. Eur J Nucl Med Mol Imaging 2013;40:1120–1.

33. Treves ST, Gelfand MJ, Fahey FH, et al. 2016 update of the North American consensus guidelines for pediatric administered radiopharmaceutical activities. J Nucl Med 2016;57:15n–8n.

34. Mulders-Manders CM, Kouijzer IJ, Janssen MJ, et al. Optimal use of [18F]FDG-PET/CT in patients with fever or inflammation of unknown origin. Q J Nucl Med Mol Imaging 2019. [Epub ahead of print].

35. Lawal IO, Popoola GO, Lengana T, et al. Diagnostic utility of (18)F-FDG PET/CT in fever of unknown origin among patients with end-stage renal disease treated with renal replacement therapy. Hell J Nucl Med 2019;22:70–5.

36. Okuyucu K, Alagoz E, Demirbas S, et al. Evaluation of predictor variables of diagnostic [18F] FDG-PET/CT in fever of unknown origin. Q J Nucl Med Mol Imaging 2018;62:313–20.

37. Ahn SS, Hwang SH, Jung SM, et al. Evaluation of spleen glucose metabolism using (18)F-FDG PET/CT in patients with febrile autoimmune disease. J Nucl Med 2017;58:507–13.

38. Kong MC, Nadel HR. 18F-FDG PET/CT with diffusely high FDG uptake throughout subcutaneous adipose tissues. Clin Nucl Med 2018;43:762–3.

39. Liu B, Lee NJ, Otero HJ, et al. Rosai-Dorfman disease mimics lymphoma on FDG PET/CT in a pediatric patient. Clin Nucl Med 2014;39:206–8.

40. Thomas DL, Syrbu S, Graham MM. Epstein-Barr virus mimicking lymphoma on FDG-PET/CT. Clin Nucl Med 2009;34:891–3.

41. Sheehy N, Israel DA. Acute varicella infection mimics recurrent Hodgkin's disease on F-18 FDG PET/CT. Clin Nucl Med 2007;32:820–1.

42. Sturm E, Rings EH, Scholvinck EH, et al. Fluorodeoxyglucose positron emission tomography contributes

to management of pediatric liver transplantation candidates with fever of unknown origin. Liver Transpl 2006;12:1698–704.

43. Meller J, Altenvoerde G, Munzel U, et al. Fever of unknown origin: prospective comparison of [18F] FDG imaging with a double-head coincidence camera and gallium-67 citrate SPET. Eur J Nucl Med 2000;27:1617–25.

44. Buysschaert I, Vanderschueren S, Blockmans D, et al. Contribution of (18)fluoro-deoxyglucose positron emission tomography to the work-up of patients with fever of unknown origin. Eur J Intern Med 2004;15:151–6.

45. Jaruskova M, Belohlavek O. Role of FDG-PET and PET/CT in the diagnosis of prolonged febrile states. Eur J Nucl Med Mol Imaging 2006;33:913–8.

46. Bleeker-Rovers CP, Vos FJ, de Kleijn EM, et al. A prospective multicenter study on fever of unknown origin: the yield of a structured diagnostic protocol. Medicine (Baltimore) 2007;86:26–38.

47. Keidar Z, Gurman-Balbir A, Gaitini D, et al. Fever of unknown origin: the role of 18F-FDG PET/CT. J Nucl Med 2008;49:1980–5.

48. Federici L, Blondet C, Imperiale A, et al. Value of (18)F-FDG-PET/CT in patients with fever of unknown origin and unexplained prolonged inflammatory syndrome: a single centre analysis experience. Int J Clin Pract 2010;64:55–60.

49. Ferda J, Ferdova E, Zahlava J, et al. Fever of unknown origin: a value of (18)F-FDG-PET/CT with integrated full diagnostic isotropic CT imaging. Eur J Radiol 2010;73:518–25.

50. Jasper N, Dabritz J, Frosch M, et al. Diagnostic value of [(18)F]-FDG PET/CT in children with fever of unknown origin or unexplained signs of inflammation. Eur J Nucl Med Mol Imaging 2010;37:136–45.

51. Kei PL, Kok TY, Padhy AK, et al. [18F] FDG PET/CT in patients with fever of unknown origin: a local experience. Nucl Med Commun 2010;31:788–92.

52. Ergul N, Halac M, Cermik TF, et al. The diagnostic role of FDG PET/CT in patients with fever of unknown origin. Mol Imaging Radionucl Ther 2011; 20:19–25.

53. Kubota K, Nakamoto Y, Tamaki N, et al. FDG-PET for the diagnosis of fever of unknown origin: a Japanese multi-center study. Ann Nucl Med 2011;25: 355–64.

54. Pelosi E, Skanjeti A, Penna D, et al. Role of integrated PET/CT with [(1)(8)F]-FDG in the management of patients with fever of unknown origin: a single-centre experience. Radiol Med 2011;116: 809–20.

55. Sheng JF, Sheng ZK, Shen XM, et al. Diagnostic value of fluorine-18 fluorodeoxyglucose positron emission tomography/computed tomography in patients with fever of unknown origin. Eur J Intern Med 2011;22:112–6.

56. Solav SV. FDG PET/CT in evaluation of pyrexia of unknown origin. Clin Nucl Med 2011;36:e81–6.

57. Kim YJ, Kim SI, Hong KW, et al. Diagnostic value of 18F-FDG PET/CT in patients with fever of unknown origin. Intern Med J 2012;42:834–7.

58. Pedersen TI, Roed C, Knudsen LS, et al. Fever of unknown origin: a retrospective study of 52 cases with evaluation of the diagnostic utility of FDG-PET/CT. Scand J Infect Dis 2012;44:18–23.

59. Bonilla-Abadia F, Pabon LM, Alvarez AM, et al. Clinical utility of 18F-fluorodeoxyglucose positron emission tomography/computed tomography in Takayasu arteritis – a report of 3 demonstrative cases. J Rheumatol 2013;40:2099.

60. Manohar K, Mittal BR, Jain S, et al. F-18 FDG-PET/CT in evaluation of patients with fever of unknown origin. Jpn J Radiol 2013;31:320–7.

61. Blokhuis GJ, Bleeker-Rovers CP, Diender MG, et al. Diagnostic value of FDG-PET/(CT) in children with fever of unknown origin and unexplained fever during immune suppression. Eur J Nucl Med Mol Imaging 2014;41:1916–23.

62. Buch-Olsen KM, Andersen RV, Hess S, et al. 18F-FDG-PET/CT in fever of unknown origin: clinical value. Nucl Med Commun 2014;35:955–60.

63. Robine A, Hot A, Maucort-Boulch D, et al. Fever of unknown origin in the 2000s: evaluation of 103 cases over eleven years. Presse Med 2014;43: e233–40.

64. Tokmak H, Ergonul O, Demirkol O, et al. Diagnostic contribution of (18)F-FDG-PET/CT in fever of unknown origin. Int J Infect Dis 2014;19:53–8.

65. Gafter-Gvili A, Raibman S, Grossman A, et al. [18F] FDG-PET/CT for the diagnosis of patients with fever of unknown origin. QJM 2015;108:289–98.

66. Singh N, Kumar R, Malhotra A, et al. Diagnostic utility of fluorodeoxyglucose positron emission tomography/computed tomography in pyrexia of unknown origin. Indian J Nucl Med 2015;30: 204–12.

67. Chang L, Cheng MF, Jou ST, et al. Search of unknown fever focus using PET in critically ill children with complicated underlying diseases. Pediatr Crit Care Med 2016;17:e58–65.

68. Tek Chand K, Chennu KK, Amancharla Yadagiri L, et al. Utility of 18 F-FDG PET/CT scan to diagnose the etiology of fever of unknown origin in patients on dialysis. Hemodial Int 2017;21:224–31.

69. Wang SS, Mechinaud F, Thursky K, et al. The clinical utility of fluorodeoxyglucose-positron emission tomography for investigation of fever in immunocompromised children. J Paediatr Child Health 2018;54:487–92.

70. Wang Q, Li YM, Li Y, et al. 18F-FDGPET/CT in fever of unknown origin and inflammation of unknown origin: a Chinese multi-center study. Eur J Nucl Med Mol Imaging 2019;46:159–65.

71. Pijl JP, Kwee TC, Legger GE, et al. Role of FDG-PET/CT in children with fever of unknown origin. Eur J Nucl Med Mol Imaging 2020. [Epub ahead of print].

72. Vanderschueren S, Del Biondo E, Ruttens D, et al. Inflammation of unknown origin versus fever of unknown origin: two of a kind. Eur J Intern Med 2009; 20:415–8.

73. Kouijzer IJ, Blokhuis GJ, Draaisma JM, et al. 18F-FDG PET/CT in detecting metastatic infection in children. Clin Nucl Med 2016;41:278–81.

74. Dong MJ, Zhao K, Liu ZF, et al. A meta-analysis of the value of fluorodeoxyglucose-PET/PET-CT in the evaluation of fever of unknown origin. Eur J Radiol 2011;80:834–44.

75. Mendez-Echevarria A, Coronado-Poggio M, Baquero-Artigao F, et al. Septic pulmonary emboli detected by (18)F-FDG PET/CT in children with S. aureus catheter-related bacteremia. Infection 2017;45:691–6.

76. Meyer Z, Fischer M, Koerfer J, et al. The role of FDG-PET-CT in pediatric cardiac patients and patients with congenital heart defects. Int J Cardiol 2016;220:656–60.

77. Houseni M, Chamroonrat W, Servaes S, et al. Applications of PET/CT in pediatric patients with fever of unknown origin. PET Clin 2008;3:605–19.

78. Yang J, Zhuang H, Servaes S. Fever of unknown origin: the roles of FDG PET or PET/CT. PET Clin 2012;7:181–9.

79. Codreanu I, Zhuang H. Isolated cholangiolitis revealed by 18F-FDG-PET/CT in a patient with fever of unknown origin. Hell J Nucl Med 2011;14:60–1.

80. Yang J, Zhuang H. The role of 18F-FDG PET/CT in the evaluation of pediatric transplant patients. Hell J Nucl Med 2015;18:136–9.

81. Huang Z, Qiu C, Guan Y. 18F-FDG imaging of a rare cutaneous infection by Mycobacterium avium complex. Clin Nucl Med 2014;39:301–4.

82. Chatziioannou S, Papamichos O, Gamaletsou MN, et al. 18-Fluoro-2-deoxy-D-glucose positron emission tomography/computed tomography scan for monitoring the therapeutic response in experimental Staphylococcus aureus foreign-body osteomyelitis. J Orthop Surg Res 2015;10:132.

83. del Rosal T, Goycochea WA, Mendez-Echevarria A, et al. (1)(8)F-FDG PET/CT in the diagnosis of occult bacterial infections in children. Eur J Pediatr 2013; 172:1111–5.

84. A Akdogan R, Halil Rakici AA, Gungor S, et al. F-18 fluorodeoxyglucose positron emission tomography/computed tomography findings of isolated gastric tuberculosis mimicking gastric cancer and lymphoma. Euroasian J Hepatogastroenterol 2018;8: 93–6.

85. Lv J, Liu S, Pan Y, et al. Imaging of scrub typhus by PET/CT. Clin Nucl Med 2015;40:838–9.

86. Wang G, Ma Y, Chen L, et al. Paediatric gastric and intestinal Crohn's disease detected by (18)F-FDG PET/CT. Hell J Nucl Med 2014;17:208–10.

87. Mooij CF, Hermsen R, Hoppenreijs EP, et al. Fludeoxyglucose positron emission tomography-computed tomography scan showing polyarthritis in a patient with an atypical presentation of Henoch-Schonlein vasculitis without clinical signs of arthritis: a case report. J Med Case Rep 2016; 10:159.

88. Meza JC, Munoz-Buitron E, Bonilla-Abadia F, et al. Still's disease in a pediatric patient after liver transplantation. Case Rep Rheumatol 2013;2013: 767684.

89. Fretzayas A, Stasinopoulou A, Moustaki M, et al. Anemia and autoimmunity markers in an adolescent with Castleman disease. Pediatr Int 2015;57: 1199–201.

90. Kim JE, Lee EK, Lee JM, et al. Kikuchi-Fujimoto disease mimicking malignant lymphoma with 2-[(18)F] fluoro-2-deoxy-D-glucose PET/CT in children. Korean J Pediatr 2014;57:226–31.

91. Garg G, DaSilva R, Bhalakia A, et al. Utility of fluorine-18-fluorodeoxyglucose positron emission tomography/computed tomography in a child with chronic granulomatous disease. Indian J Nucl Med 2016;31:62–4.

92. Shimizu M, Saikawa Y, Yachie A. Role of 18-fluoro-2-deoxyglucose positron emission tomography in detecting acute inflammatory lesions of non-bacterial osteitis in patients with a fever of unknown origin: a comparative study of 18-fluoro-2-deoxyglucose positron emission tomography, bone scan, and magnetic resonance imaging. Mod Rheumatol 2018;28:1058–62.

93. Moritani K, Nakano N, Yonezawa S, et al. Usefulness of positron emission tomography-CT for diagnosis of primary bone marrow lymphoma in children. Pediatr Hematol Oncol 2018;35:125–30.

94. Bai X, Yang H, Zhuang H. FDG PET/CT findings of the recurrent posttransplantation lymphoproliferative disorder in a pediatric liver transplant recipient with right leg pain as the only complaint. Clin Nucl Med 2015;40:832–4.

95. Turpin S, Carret AS, Dubois J, et al. Isolated thymic Langerhans cell histiocytosis discovered on F-18 fluorodeoxyglucose positron emission tomography/computed tomography (F-18 FDG PET/CT). Pediatr Radiol 2015;45:1870–3.

96. Arbind A, D'Souza M, Jaimini A, et al. Fluorine-18 fluorodeoxyglucose positron emission tomography/computed tomography imaging in response monitoring of extra-pulmonary tuberculosis. Indian J Nucl Med 2016;31:59–61.

97. Jain TK, Basher RK, Bhattacharya A, et al. 18F-FDG PET/CT in diagnosis and response evaluation in an unusual case of antisynthetase syndrome

presenting as pyrexia of unknown origin. Rev Esp Med Nucl Imagen Mol 2016;35:197–9.

98. Niccoli Asabella A, Iuele F, Simone F, et al. Role of (18) F-FDG PET/CT in the evaluation of response to antibiotic therapy in patients affected by infectious spondylodiscitis. Hell J Nucl Med 2015;18(Suppl 1):17–22.

99. Demirev A, Brans B, Vanmolkot F, et al. Diagnosis of brachiocephalic thrombophlebitis as the cause

of fever of unknown origin by 18F-FDG-PET/CT. Mol Imaging Radionucl Ther 2015;24:25–8.

100. Takeuchi M, Nihashi T, Gafter-Gvili A, et al. Association of 18F-FDG PET or PET/CT results with spontaneous remission in classic fever of unknown origin: a systematic review and meta-analysis. Medicine (Baltimore) 2018;97: e12909.

Pediatric Cardiac PET/CT Imaging

Amol Takalkar, MD, MS, MBA[a,b,*], Miguel Hernandez Pampaloni, MD, PhD[c]

KEYWORDS

- Pediatric cardiac PET • PET/MRI • Hybrid imaging • Molecular imaging • Cardiac PET

KEY POINTS

- Single photon emission computed tomography (SPECT) myocardial perfusion imaging is a proven reliable and cost-effective technique; however, it has several limitations, some specifically related to the pediatric population subgroup.
- Cardiac PET/CT, is now more routinely available and has the least radiation exposure to patients, a very important consideration for pediatric patients.
- Quantification capabilities of cardiac PET/CT and lower radiation dose make it the preferred modality for patients requiring serial scans.
- Cardiac PET/MRI may provide unique advantages in the future.

INTRODUCTION

There has been significant progress in understanding the pathophysiology of various pediatric heart diseases. Moreover, significant progress has been made in the surgical and medical management of these conditions, leading to improved outcomes and an increasing number of children surviving with congenital or acquired heart diseases. These children are at risk for the development of post-treatment myocardial ischemia and hence need to be evaluated periodically to detect this potentially reversible condition.[1,2] Hence, a noninvasive and reliable imaging technique that can accurately assess the pediatric heart (perfusion, function, viability, and structure) would be extremely beneficial in such patient population. Because this patient population is special (pediatric) and is expected to survive long term, any imaging modality that has potential serious adverse effects owing to repeated testing (including cumulative radiation exposure over time) is an obvious concern in this subgroup.

Fortunately, cardiac imaging has also evolved significantly over the past few decades with tremendous advances in nuclear cardiology, computed tomography (CT) and MR imaging of the heart. The phenomenal progress in CT technology now allows us to obtain extremely high-resolution structural images of the heart within a few seconds. This anatomic and structural information provided by CT imaging in exquisite detail is extremely useful in the management of pediatric heart diseases. However, it is associated with significant radiation exposure and there are concerns about the long-term effects of cumulative radiation exposure in children with repeated CT imaging. MR imaging provides a comprehensive cardiac evaluation without any ionizing radiation and with high temporal and contrast resolution. Its spatial resolution is suboptimal compared with CT scans, but is improving. Although it was echocardiography that revolutionized the approach to congenital heart disease, MR imaging has been shown to have tremendous incremental advantages over echocardiography and allows a more robust assessment of cardiac morphology and function (including the

[a] Center for Molecular Imaging & Therapy, Biomedical Research Foundation of Northwest Louisianan, PO Box 38050, Shreveport, LA 71113-8050, USA; [b] Department of Radiology, Louisiana State University Health Sciences Center - Shreveport, 1501 Kings Highway, Shreveport, LA 71103, USA; [c] Department of Radiology & Biomedical Engineering, University of California, San Francisco, 505 Parnassus, M396 San Francisco, CA 94143, USA
* Corresponding author. Center for Molecular Imaging & Therapy, Biomedical Research Foundation of Northwest Louisianan, PO Box 38050, Shreveport, LA 71113-8050.
E-mail address: amol.takalkar@gmail.com

PET Clin 15 (2020) 371–380
https://doi.org/10.1016/j.cpet.2020.03.011

heart, valves, and major vessels). However, despite its considerable advantages, cardiac MR imaging remains a quite labor- and time-intensive procedure, requiring direct hands-on protocol decision making and supervision by a qualified pediatric radiologist experienced in cardiac MR imaging, and intravenous sedation or endotracheal intubation in many pediatric patients.[3] More recently, some concerns have also been raised about the side effects on kidney from MR imaging contrast agents.

Nuclear cardiology has also progressed from simple planar cardiac imaging to more advanced single photon emission CT (SPECT) with electrocardiogram-gating and attenuation correction. For some time SPECT myocardial perfusion imaging remained the unchallenged imaging modality to assess myocardial perfusion noninvasively and is still used routinely in most places. The technique of PET was developed soon after SPECT imaging technique was introduced in the 1970s. However, it took almost 2 decades for PET to come to mainstream clinical imaging. Nevertheless, since the late 1990s, there has been a virtual explosion in the use of PET imaging, especially for oncologic workup. This advance has led to widespread availability of PET instrumentation and decreased the cost of PET imaging. Consequently, other indications, including cardiac applications of PET imaging, have seen increasing use. Presently, there is a lot of literature validating the usefulness and cost effectiveness of cardiac PET imaging for various indications like myocardial perfusion and viability evaluations. However, most of the data in current literature focus on the adult population. Data about the value of cardiac PET imaging in the pediatric population remain sparse, although not completely nonexistent. Because pediatric cardiac conditions are usually addressed in specialized medical centers that have the requisite expertise to effectively treat these complex disease entities, cardiac PET imaging has also remained restricted to such advanced medical and research centers. Although underused, cardiac PET has been proven to be useful in detecting myocardial ischemia and viability in pediatric patients.

ADVANTAGES OF PET OVER SINGLE PHOTON EMISSION COMPUTED TOMOGRAPHY

SPECT myocardial perfusion imaging is a proven reliable and cost-effective technique. However, it has several limitations, some specifically related to the pediatric population subgroup. Compared with CT scans (and also with PET), SPECT has suboptimal spatial resolution. This property assumes more significance in pediatric patients with small hearts. Attenuation correction is also suboptimal with SPECT compared with PET. Owing to dosimetric concerns, the use of thallium radionuclides for SPECT myocardial perfusion and viability studies is limited. Moreover, technetium-based agents suffer from high liver activity that severely affects evaluation of the inferior wall in pediatric patients.[4] SPECT studies also take comparatively longer time to complete during which the child needs to remain still/motionless, necessitating sedation in most patients. Another significant issue with SPECT studies is the inability to provide absolute quantification of regional radiotracer uptake.

In contrast, PET offers superior spatial and temporal resolutions, as well as better attenuation correction. Dosimetric considerations are more favorable with PET because it uses radiopharmaceuticals with significantly shorter half-lives and allows for more efficient protocols.[5,6] Hence, PET protocols are also completed much faster compared with SPECT studies. Radiation exposure to patients undergoing nuclear cardiac imaging is generally less with cardiac PET imaging compared with SPECT cardiac imaging, including with newer SPECT cameras like cadmium zinc telluride SPECT. A recent article by Partington and colleagues,[7] found that the estimated mean effective radiation dose from various myocardial perfusion imaging studies for complex congenital heart disease performed using [99m]technetium sestamibi, [82]rubidium or ^{13}N-ammonia, and sodium iodide (NaI) SPECT, SPECT/CT scans, or cadmium zinc telluride SPECT or PET/CT scanners was the least for ^{13}N-ammonia PET/CT scans (2.1 ± 0.6 mSv) followed by [82]rubidium PET/CT scans (6.1 ± 1.2 mSv), cadmium zinc telluride SPECT (6.3 ± 0.2 mSv), NaI SPECT (8.7 ± 2.3 mSv), and was the most with NaI SPECT/CT scans (12.5 ± 0.9 mSv). This consideration is important in patients requiring repeat or serial imaging, which may very well be the case in pediatric patients. Moreover, it is possible to get absolute quantification of regional radiotracer uptake with PET that facilitates obtaining absolute values of myocardial biochemical processes like regional myocardial blood flow and glucose metabolism. In fact, techniques for obtaining quantification of myocardial blood flow with PET have been validated since the early 1990s.[8–10] The availability of integrated PET/CT scanners makes the studies even shorter with better attenuation correction along with anatomic localization, but adds additional radiation exposure from the CT portion of the study. If the CT scan performed is a dedicated CT scan with contrast enhancement, it is feasible to obtain additional high-resolution structural details, including CT angiography, but adds even more radiation and risks of contrast administration. Therefore, although PET/CT scans (with or without dedicated contrast-enhanced CT studies) offer certain advantages, there is concern over potential long-term consequences with repeated use. To minimize unnecessary radiation exposure in children, the dedicated PET scanner at Children's Hospital in Philadelphia has the unique capability of using either CT scans or regular transmission scanning for attenuation correction, so that the CT portion is applied only when absolutely essential. On most PET/CT scanners, there is no alternative capability for attenuation correction other than the CT scan, which may not be absolutely essential/advisable in all pediatric PET imaging studies.

PET INSTRUMENTATION

A typical PET scanner is a cylindrical assembly of numerous block detectors in a ring configuration for optimal spatial resolution. Several scintillators such as NaI, bismuth germanium oxide, lutetium oxyorthosilicate, gadolinium oxyorthosilicate, and the newer lutetium-yttrium oxyorthosilicate can detect the radioactive events occurring in PET imaging. PET radiopharmaceuticals contain a positron emitter that undergoes positron (β^+) decay, emitting a positron (β^+), and a neutrino (ν). The emitted positron travels a very short distance in surrounding tissue and then combines with an electron to annihilate and release a pair of 511 KeV photons at almost exactly 180° apart. It is these photons (and not the actual positrons) that are nearly simultaneously detected by the scintillation detectors in PET scanners as coincidence events and millions of such coincidences are acquired and stored in sinogram form as lines of response that basically connects the detector pair in which the coincidence occurs. These emission data are then digitally reconstructed and attenuation correction algorithms are applied to generate high-resolution tomographic images depicting the radiopharmaceutical biodistribution.

CARDIAC PET RADIOPHARMACEUTICALS

Several PET radiopharmaceuticals have been evaluated to assess various myocardial biochemical parameters, including perfusion, glucose and oxidative metabolism, hypoxia, autonomic innervation, and others. Currently, Rb-82 chloride and N-13 ammonia are approved by the US Food and Drug Administration and used clinically for myocardial perfusion studies and F-18 fluorodeoxyglucose (FDG) is used for evaluating myocardial glucose metabolism. Other PET radiopharmaceuticals are not routinely used clinically, but are widely used in the research realm. These include O-15 water for evaluating myocardial perfusion (which is considered an ideal perfusion agent because it is freely diffusible and metabolically inert; however, it requires complex mathematical algorithms and generates images that are too noisy for visual interpretation) and C-11 acetate (which can reliably assess myocardial oxidative metabolism, but is not useful in ischemic myocardium and use is further hampered by difficulty in optimal delivery/distribution from cyclotron site to imaging center owing to its short half-life and relatively long synthesis time). Several other agents to assess cardiac autonomic nervous system, cardiac receptors, cardiac hypoxia, and cardiac gene therapy assessment are also in the research or translational environment.

N-13, a cyclotron produced radioisotope, has relatively optimal physical characteristics and biologic properties to generate excellent PET images (a 9.9-minute half-life, 1.19 MeV average positron energy, and about 0.4-mm average positron range). It shows prolonged myocardial retention owing to its high extraction rate and metabolic trapping via the glutamine synthetase pathway. Although it is feasible to perform exercise stress perfusion studies with N-13 ammonia in contrast with Rb-82 chloride (which allows only pharmaceutical stressing), this advantage is not substantial in the pediatric population (especially younger children).

Rb-82, a generator produced radioisotope, has slightly less favorable physical characteristics (higher positron energy of 3.15 MeV and longer average positron range of about 2.8 mm) somewhat impairing its inherent spatial resolution. Its ultrashort half-life of 75 seconds enables the study to be completed very fast (within 1 hour or less), but also necessitates the administration of higher doses of the radiopharmaceutical. The extremely short half-life of Rb-82 also allows (or actually necessitates) imaging almost during effect of the pharmacologic stressing agent, thus acquiring "pure" stress images (and not post-stress images) not contaminated by residual radiotracer from the rest injection and with minimal background activity. Although Rb-82 does not require an in-house cyclotron because it is generator produced and each generator can be used for up to a month, the generator itself is quite expensive, dictating a certain number of minimum studies to justify its use financially. Rb-82 chloride shows pharmacologically similar behavior to potassium and thallium-201 and needs an active Na/K-ATPase pump for intracellular transport.

F-18 FDG by far remains the most widely used PET radiopharmaceutical. F-18 is a cyclotron produced radioisotope with a half-life of 110 minutes. This factor obviates the need for an on-site cyclotron, because it is feasible to transport the radiopharmaceutical to imaging centers located 2 to 3 hours away from the cyclotron site. The half-life also eases time frame restrictions on study protocols, but is low enough not to cause prolonged exposure. Moreover, its optimal physical characteristics (0.63 MeV average positron energy and 0.3-mm average positron range) produce high resolution PET images. Because FDG is a glucose analogue, the images represent a map of glucose metabolism in the body. Glucose transporters (mainly GLUT-1 and GLUT-4) are responsible for intracellular transport of FDG wherein it undergoes phosphorylation to FGD-6-phosphate by the enzyme hexokinase. However, FDG-6-phosphate is not a good substrate for enzymes phosphohexose isomerase or glucose-6-phosphate dehydrogenase and hence it does not undergo further metabolism. Because FDG-6-phosphate cannot diffuse out of the cells, it remains metabolically trapped within the cells (**Fig. 1**). Cells and tissues with higher rates of glucose metabolism show upregulation of glucose transporters and increased glucose (and consequently FDG) uptake. Because there is no further metabolism or radioactive decay to daughter molecules, all the activity on FDG PET imaging represents FDG-6-phosphate alone and areas with increased FDG uptake represent areas with high glucose metabolism (like cancer cells, inflammatory cells or other cells with high glucose metabolism like gray matter cells in brain or cardiac myocytes under certain circumstances). The substrate preferred by myocardium for its energy needs is highly variable and several factors, including the hormonal milieu and available substrate concentration affect it substantially. A fasting environment with low plasma glucose as well as insulin levels but high plasma free fatty acid levels promotes free fatty acid as the preferred myocardial substrate. In contrast, in a postprandial setting with increased plasma glucose and consequently insulin levels, as well as under ischemic and hypoxic conditions, glucose is favored over free fatty acid as the preferred substrate by the myocytes.[11–19] This is the underlying basis for using FDG to assess myocardial glucose metabolism (and C-11 acetate to assess myocardial oxidative metabolism). **Table 1** summarizes the commonly used cardiac PET radiopharmaceuticals in pediatric population.

CARDIAC PET PROTOCOLS

The PET imaging protocol depends on the indication for the study and the radiopharmaceutical being used. PET myocardial perfusion imaging protocol is slightly different using Rb-82 chloride versus N-13 ammonia. With N-13 ammonia, typically a rest–stress protocol is followed, consisting of a transmission scan followed by an initial set of rest emission images of the heart obtained 5 minutes after the intravenous administration of N-13 ammonia. After an interval of about 50 to 60 minutes during which the tracer is allowed to decay completely, either pharmacologic (more common) or exercise (technically challenging but feasible; may not be practical in infants and small children) stressing is performed and a subsequent set of stress emission images of the heart are obtained 5 minutes after another intravenous administration of N-13 ammonia followed by a second

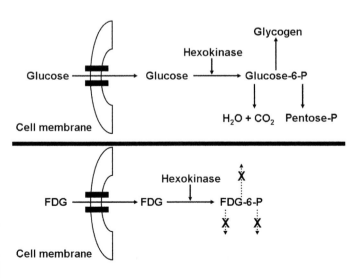

Fig. 1. Schema for FDG metabolic-trapping in cardiac myocytes.

Table 1
Commonly used cardiac PET radiopharmaceuticals

Radio-Pharmaceutical	Radioisotope	Source	Half-Life	Usefulness
C-11 acetate	C-11	Cyclotron	20 min	Cardiac oxidative metabolism
F-18 FDG	F-18	Cyclotron	110 min	Glucose metabolism
N-13 ammonia	N-13	Cyclotron	9.9 min	Myocardial perfusion
Rb-82 Chloride	Rb-82	Generator	75 s	Myocardial perfusion

transmission scan. The protocol using Rb-82 is largely similar, except that there is almost no delay between the rest and stress studies in view of the extremely short half-life of Rb-82. Also, the emission images are obtained very shortly (about 1–3 minutes) after radiopharmaceutical administration and only pharmacologic stress is feasible with Rb-82 chloride as the perfusion agent.

Absolute quantification of regional myocardial perfusion/blood flow is feasible and validated with PET. This process requires the ability to accurately measure the rapid initial changes of radiopharmaceutical occurring in the tissue of interest immediately after radiopharmaceutical administration till a steady-state situation is achieved. The high temporal and spatial resolution of PET imaging coupled with the short half-life of PET radioisotopes allows dynamic acquisition of PET data and, using various tracer kinetic models, absolute quantification of regional myocardial blood flow is derived.[8,9] However, this testing is not routinely practiced in the standard clinical setting (usually only static images are obtained) and is more labor intensive, requiring rigorous data reprocessing. The calculated regional myocardial blood flow is generally provided in terms of milliliters per minute per 100 g of myocardial tissue.

The protocol to assess myocardial glucose metabolism requires some additional preparation. Because cardiac glucose uptake can be highly variable, patients are usually asked to fast for at least 4 hours (preferably overnight) before study. The fasting blood sugar level is expected to be less than 110 mg/dL in most patients in this patient population and, after checking the fasting blood sugar level, an oral glucose loading dose is given (except in neonates) about 60 minutes before FDG administration to facilitate high FDG uptake by the cardiac myocytes. However, older children with known diabetes may require additional insulin supplementation with the glucose loading dose to maintain a blood sugar level between 110 and 140 mg/dL. After 60 more minutes, dedicated PET images of the heart are obtained. To assess myocardial viability, a myocardial glucose metabolism study (rest only is adequate) is routinely coupled with a myocardial perfusion study, if one has not been performed recently or is not available for direct comparison with the metabolism images.

Although the pediatric cardiac PET protocols are similar to adult cardiac PET imaging protocols, there are a few special considerations. An important issue is the dose of the administered radiopharmaceuticals. This dose usually needs to be adjusted for the child's body weight rather than a standard dose that is usually prescribed in adults. Moreover, because the protocols last for a relatively long time, sedation is necessary for most patients. Several sedation protocols are in clinical use, including chloral hydrate, fentanyl, and midazolam,[20,21] and it is best to collaborate with a pediatric anesthesiologist to achieve optimal sedation and acquire high-quality images. In addition to sedation, familiarity and experience with handling pediatric concerns and providing an environment that will ease the child's nervousness and keep him or her calm and cooperative also help significantly to achieve optimal results.

CLINICAL APPLICATIONS OF PEDIATRIC CARDIAC PET STUDIES

The major indications for pediatric cardiac PET studies include assessing myocardial perfusion for ischemia as well as coronary flow reserve and assessing myocardial viability in several congenital and acquired cardiac diseases in children.[22–24] Accurate assessment of myocardial perfusion is important in therapeutic planning as well as the post-treatment follow-up of various congenital and acquired heart diseases in this patient population. As described elsewhere in this article, PET offers several advantages over SPECT and can potentially detect myocardial abnormalities earlier, allowing earlier therapeutic intervention and facilitating a better outcome. In addition, absolute quantification of regional myocardial blood flow allows assessment of coronary flow reserve that provides supplemental information to aid in the clinical decision making process and long-term follow-up strategies.

A common indication for cardiac perfusion imaging in children is to detect perfusion abnormalities in patients after corrective surgery for congenital heart disorders like transposition of great arteries (TGA) or anomalous origin of left coronary artery from the pulmonary artery. TGA is now usually corrected by the arterial switch operation (ASO) and about 10% of such patients suffer from adverse events related to coronary perfusion abnormalities (myocardial infarction and sudden death owing to coronary occlusion).[25,26] Perfusion defects in patients who had undergone ASO were reported by Vogel and colleagues[27] using isoproterenol stress thallium-201 computed scintigraphy. Weindling and colleagues[1] reported regional myocardial ischemia in patients with history of ASO by demonstrating reversible perfusion defects on exercise stress myocardial perfusion imaging with 99m-technetium–labeled sestamibi SPECT technique. Subsequently, several investigators evaluated myocardial perfusion with cardiac PET imaging in this patient population and detected perfusion abnormalities in asymptomatic patients without evidence for contractile dysfunction. Although the incidence of reversible perfusion defects was slightly lower on PET imaging compared with SPECT imaging, there was diminished coronary flow reserve as suggested by lower adenosine-induced hyperemic myocardial blood flow.[28,29] Myocardial flow reserve was also found to impaired with adenosine stress N13-ammonia PET myocardial perfusion imaging in patients who underwent the earlier Mustard or atrial switch repair for TGA.[30] Bengel and colleagues[27] attributed the impaired coronary flow reserve to possible altered vasoreactivity or endothelial dysfunction, but the long-term prognostic significance of this remained unclear at that time. However, subsequently, Hauser and colleagues[29] reported reduced coronary flow reserve as detected by PET myocardial perfusion imaging correlated significantly with impaired ventricular function in the absence of coronary stenosis by angiography in children late after Fontan-like operations and this was felt to be risk factor for long-term outcome.[31] Singh and colleagues have also reported diminished myocardial flow reserve in long term survivors of anomalous origin of left coronary artery from the pulmonary artery repair using adenosine stress N13-ammonia PET myocardial perfusion imaging and suggested that this may limit cardiac output reserve and impair exercise tolerance.[32] In most of these studies, along with the diminished coronary flow reserve, the resting myocardial blood flow was mostly found to be increased. Donnelly and colleagues[33] compared the resting myocardial blood flow and coronary flow reserve in infants who had anatomic repair of a congenital heart lesion with infants who had Norwood palliation for hypoplastic left heart syndrome. Using adenosine stress PET myocardial perfusion imaging with N-13 ammonia, they reported increased resting myocardial blood flow with diminished coronary flow reserve in infants after anatomic repair of a congenital heart lesion but decreased resting as well as maximal (adenosine stimulated) myocardial blood flow leading to diminished coronary flow reserve in infants after Norwood palliation for hypoplastic left heart syndrome. The authors proposed that decreased coronary flow reserve along with reduced oxygen delivery to the ventricular myocardium may partly be responsible for the unfavorable outcome seen after Norwood palliation.

Hernandez and colleagues[21] have reported good correlation between PET myocardial perfusion and metabolism imaging and echocardiography, angiography as well histopathology in infants and children with suspected coronary abnormalities. They confirmed that PET perfusion metabolism imaging can reliably and accurately assess myocardial viability in pediatric population. Rickers and colleagues[34] used information from PET myocardial viability evaluation using gated FDG PET to determine treatment approach for infants and children with suspected infarction after ASO for TGA. They detected viable myocardium in akinetic or hypokinetic regions with corresponding coronary stenosis/occlusion and chose revascularization as the preferred treatment in this setting and follow-up revealed recovery of full function in these infants. Patients with impaired glucose metabolism indicating scarring did not undergo revascularization and were steered toward medical management. A few patients had normal glucose metabolism in areas that were akinetic or dyskinetic on echocardiography and were also found to have to have no coronary stenosis or occlusion angiographically. These areas were felt to represent myocardial stunning. **Figs. 2** and **3** demonstrate myocardial viability with PET perfusion metabolism imaging after ASO in patients with TGA.

Another condition that has been relatively well-evaluated with cardiac PET imaging is Kawasaki disease. Also known as mucocutaneous lymph node syndrome, it is a disease of unknown etiology characterized by acute vasculitis of mostly medium-sized arteries, including the coronaries. Cardiac manifestation of Kawasaki disease are by far the most clinically significant and are generally due to involvement of the coronaries that can

NH$_3$

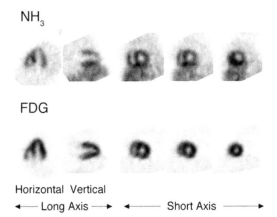

FDG

Horizontal Vertical
◄——— Long Axis ——► ◄——— Short Axis ———►

Fig. 2. Viable myocardium on PET perfusion metabolism viability imaging in an infant with history of ASO for TGA. N-13 ammonia perfusion PET demonstrates perfusion defects in the lateral wall, apex, and anterior wall with preserved glucose metabolism in those areas indicating myocardial viability.

progress from vasculitis to aneurysms to stenosis or occlusion leading to myocardial infarction and scarring. In untreated cases, coronary manifestations can occur in up to 40% of patients. Cardiac PET imaging has been shown to be useful in assessing the various coronary manifestations of Kawasaki disease during its natural history of the disease progression. Ohmochi and colleagues[35] demonstrated diminished myocardial flow reserve in the presence of coronary aneurysms associated with Kawasaki disease. Yoshibayashi and colleagues[36] assessed the significance of newly

NH$_3$

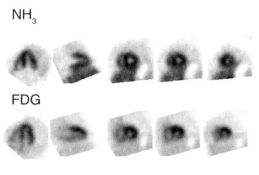

FDG

Horizontal Vertical
◄——— Long Axis ——► ◄——— Short Axis ———►

Fig. 3. Nonviable myocardium/scarring on PET perfusion metabolism viability imaging in an infant with history of ASO for TGA. PET perfusion metabolism viability imaging in an infant with history of ASO for TGA. N-13 ammonia perfusion PET demonstrates perfusion defects in the lateral and inferior walls with decreased glucose metabolism in those areas as well indicating nonviable myocardium/scarring.

appearing abnormal Q waves and their disappearance in patients with Kawasaki disease with PET perfusion metabolism myocardial viability imaging and found that the new appearance of abnormal Q waves in patients with Kawasaki disease indicates myocardial injury but a large number of them are associated with metabolically active myocardium and their early disappearance is usually associated with viable myocardium. Moreover, myocardial viability evaluation using PET perfusion metabolism imaging has shown value in assessing treatment. Hwang and colleagues[37] found PET abnormalities in about 60% of patients with acute and subacute phases of Kawasaki disease and in about 40% of patients in the convalescent phase of Kawasaki disease. Different therapies during the acute phase of Kawasaki disease were not significantly effective in avoiding or diminishing myocardial injury, notwithstanding the absence of coronary arterial abnormalities. However, the 5-day regimen of intravenous immunoglobulin therapy resulted in significantly lower incidence of PET abnormalities compared with the single-day regimen. Iemura and colleagues[38] investigated the long term consequences of regressed aneurysms after Kawasaki disease and found persisting abnormal vascular wall morphology and vascular dysfunction at the site of regressed coronary aneurysms in patients with previous Kawasaki disease. Because ischemic perfusion defects have been reported on scintigraphic imaging even with normal coronary angiography,[39,40] long-term follow-up is recommended in these patients because they seem to be at risk for developing coronary abnormalities including atherosclerosis in adult life. Because PET myocardial perfusion imaging can detect even a small degree of perfusion abnormalities, it can play a central role in the follow-up of myocardial perfusion status in this setting. In fact, several investigators have confirmed decreased hyperemic-induced myocardial blood flow and diminished coronary flow reserve in patients with a history of Kawasaki disease with angiographically normal coronary arteries.[41–44] This finding is believed to be related to endothelial dysfunction with residual damage in the coronary microcirculation and impaired coronary vasoreactivity. Thus, in addition to being useful in assessing the cardiac perfusion and viability manifestations of the various coronary manifestations occurring in Kawasaki disease, cardiac PET is also valuable in monitoring the consequences of coronary involvement with Kawasaki disease, and long-term follow-up.

Thus, cardiac PET imaging provides a safe, reliable, and accurate means of assessing various myocardial processes, including perfusion, flow reserve, and metabolism in a wide range of congenital and acquired heart conditions, such as Kawasaki disease, coronary artery anomalies, cardiac transplant vasculopathy, valvular heart disease, and postsurgical correction of various congenital heart diseases like TGA and anomalous origin of left coronary artery from the pulmonary artery, among others. It also offers precise assessments of the coronary blood flow and flow reserve over time for long-term follow-up and has the least radiation exposure compared with SPECT cardiac studies.

Other potential applications of PET/CT in pediatric cardiac imaging include but are not limited to evaluating cardiovascular inflammation or infection[45] such as vasculitis,[46] endocarditis,[47–49] and ventricular assist device-associated infection.[50,51]

PEDIATRIC CARDIAC PET/MR IMAGING

PET/MR imaging has recently emerged as an interesting noninvasive imaging technique with potential applications in a variety of fields including neurology, oncology, and cardiology. This technique takes advantage of a simultaneous data acquisition that combines structural, functional, and molecular imaging information; this could be the substrate to disclose new information for a better characterization and understanding of the pathophysiology of the ill heart muscle. In particular, the tissue characterization offered by MR techniques with and without contrast agents allows for functional parameters, including left and right ventricular ejection fraction, myocardial perfusion, and the assessment of intravascular and extravascular volumes. The exquisite PET tracers that are able to detect and monitor biochemical processes with high sensitivity and specificity provides supplemental valuable information to the functional characterization of the cardiovascular processes. Although definite clinical applications are yet to be clearly identified, and despite the already intrinsic benefit of reduced radiation exposure by using MR imaging compared with CT protocols, the functional characterization of morphologic abnormalities and the monitoring of cardiac interventions in the spectrum of congenital heart diseases could be an attractive platform for these patients. Moreover, the radiation dose from a PET/MR imaging study is lower compared with a PET/CT study, further making it more favorable method, especially for pediatric patients.[52–54] Nevertheless, a generally longer imaging time is required by PET/MR imaging than PET/CT and should be considered in ordering the study because in pediatric patients

sedation or general anesthesia is more frequently necessary to obtain high-quality MR images.

However, more prospective clinical trials would be necessary to provide scientific evidence to support the application of PET/MR imaging in pediatric patients. Especially in pediatric imaging, the completion of such studies is a challenge owing to the often limited number of patients and high ethical demands. One possible approach to generate reliable data would be the implementation of pediatric PET/MR imaging registries pooling examinations from different sites and providing the necessary data to answer central clinical questions.

SUMMARY

Cardiac PET imaging can play a significant role in assessing and managing children with congenital and acquired heart disorders, but remains largely underused for multiple reasons not related to the accuracy or usefulness of the modality. PET offers several advantages over other imaging modalities in the evaluation of cardiac perfusion and metabolism. The technique for cardiac PET imaging has been validated by several investigators. There is sufficient literature to establish the usefulness of this imaging modality in the pediatric population and this finding merits larger prospective studies to confirm the long-term clinical significance of the findings from these highly sophisticated studies. Specifically, the implications of decreased coronary flow reserve and perfusion abnormalities after surgical correction of a congenital heart lesion in the absence of demonstrable coronary stenosis on angiography remain unclear. However, further work with cardiac PET may provide a broader understanding of myocardial perfusion and coronary flow reserve in infants. Myocardial perfusion assessment (with SPECT or PET) in combination with myocardial glucose metabolism with FDG PET is the gold standard for evaluating myocardial viability.[45] Current work focusing on evaluation of cardiac innervation, cardiac receptor function, and noninvasive cardiac gene therapy assessment with PET imaging has tremendous potential to revolutionize cardiac evaluation. Awareness and widespread availability of PET systems is expected to increase the use of cardiac PET applications in the pediatric population. The advent of integrated PET/CT systems with advanced CT technology and the upcoming integrated PET/MR imaging systems lead us to hope for even more promising future possibilities for cardiac evaluation in a 1-stop approach.

DISCLOSURE

The authors have nothing to disclose.

REFERENCES

1. Weindling SN, Wernovsky G, Colan SD, et al. Myocardial perfusion, function and exercise tolerance after the arterial switch operation. J Am Coll Cardiol 1994;23:424–33.
2. Bonhoeffer P, Bonnet D, Piéchaud JF, et al. Coronary artery obstruction after the arterial switch operation for transposition of the great arteries in newborns. J Am Coll Cardiol 1997;29:202–6.
3. Krishnamurthy R. Pediatric cardiac MRI: anatomy and function. Pediatr Radiol 2008;38(Suppl 2):S192–9.
4. Machac J. Gated positron emission tomography for the assessment of myocardial perfusion and function. In: Germano G, Berman DS, editors. Clinical gated cardiac SPECT. 2nd edition. Malden (MA): Blackwell Futura; 2006. p. p285–316.
5. ICRP Committee 2. Radiation dose to patients from radiopharmaceuticals. A report of a Task Group of Committee 2 of the International Commission on Radiological Protection. Ann ICRP 1987;18:1–377.
6. Hernandez-Pampaloni N. Cardiovascular applications. In: Charron M, editor. Practical pediatric PET imaging. New York: Springer; 2006. p. 407–27.
7. Partington SL, Valente AM, Bruyere J Jr, et al. Reducing radiation dose from myocardial perfusion imaging in subjects with complex congenital heart disease. J Nucl Cardiol 2019. https://doi.org/10.1007/s12350-019-01811-y.
8. Hutchins GD, Schwaiger M, Rosenspire KC, et al. Noninvasive quantification of regional blood flow in the human heart using N-13 ammonia and dynamic positron emission tomographic imaging. J Am Coll Cardiol 1990;15:1032–42.
9. Kuhle WG, Porenta G, Huang SC, et al. Quantification of regional myocardial blood flow using 13N-ammonia and reoriented dynamic positron emission tomographic imaging. Circulation 1992;86:1004–17.
10. Liedtke AJ. Alterations of carbohydrate and lipid metabolism in the acutely ischemic heart. Prog Cardiovasc Dis 1981;23:321–6.
11. Schelbert HR, Henze E, Phelps ME, et al. Assessment of regional myocardial ischemia by positron-emission computed tomography. Am Heart J 1982;103(4 Pt 2):588–97.
12. Schwaiger M, Fishbein MC, Block M, et al. Metabolic and ultrastructural abnormalities during ischemia in canine myocardium: noninvasive assessment by positron emission tomography. J Mol Cell Cardiol 1987;19:259–69.
13. Kalff V, Schwaiger M, Nguyen N, et al. The relationship between myocardial blood flow and glucose uptake in ischemic canine myocardium determined with fluorine-18-deoxyglucose. J Nucl Med 1992;33:1346–53.
14. Marwick TH, MacIntyre WJ, Lafont A, et al. Metabolic responses of hibernating and infracted myocardium to revascularization: a follow-up study of regional perfusion, function, and metabolism. Circulation 1992;85:1347–53.
15. Vanoverschelde JL, Wijns W, Depre C, et al. Mechanisms of chronic regional postischemic dysfunction in humans: new insights from the study of noninfarcted collateral-dependent myocardium. Circulation 1993;87:1513–23.
16. Liedtke AJ, Renstrom B, Hacker TA, et al. Effects of moderate repetitive ischemia on myocardial substrate utilization. Am J Physiol 1995;269(1 Pt 2):H246–53.
17. Liedtke AJ, Renstrom B, Nellis SH, et al. Mechanical and metabolic functions in pig hearts after 4 days of chronic coronary stenosis. J Am Coll Cardiol 1995;26:815–25.
18. Liedtke AJ. The origins of myocardial substrate utilization from an evolutionary perspective: the enduring role of glucose in energy metabolism. J Mol Cell Cardiol 1997;29:1073–86.
19. American Academy of Pediatrics Committee on Drugs. Guidelines for monitoring and management of pediatric patients during and after sedation for diagnostic and therapeutic procedures. Pediatrics 1992;89(6 pt 1):1110–5.
20. Practice guidelines for sedation and analgesia by nonanesthesiologists. Anesthesiology 2002;96:1004–17.
21. Hernandez-Pampaloni M, Allada V, Fishbein MC, et al. Myocardial perfusion and viability by positron emission tomography in infants and children with coronary abnormalities: correlation with echocardiography, coronary angiography, and histopathology. J Am Coll Cardiol 2003;41:618–26.
22. Singh TP, Muzik O, Forbes TF, et al. Positron emission tomography myocardial perfusion imaging in children with suspected coronary abnormalities. Pediatr Cardiol 2003;24:138–44.
23. Chhatriwalla AK, Prieto LR, Brunken RC, et al. Preliminary data on the diagnostic accuracy of rubidium-82 cardiac PET perfusion imaging for the evaluation of ischemia in a pediatric population. Pediatr Cardiol 2008;29:732–8.
24. Tanel RE, Wernovsky G, Landzberg MJ, et al. Coronary artery abnormalities detected at cardiac catheterization following the arterial switch operation for transposition of the great arteries. Am J Cardiol 1995;76:153–7.
25. Wernovsky G, Mayer JE Jr, Jonas RA, et al. Factors influencing early and late outcome of the arterial switch operation for transposition of the great arteries. J Thorac Cardiovasc Surg 1995;109:289–301.
26. Vogel M, Smallhorn JF, Gilday D, et al. Assessment of myocardial perfusion in patients after the arterial switch operation. J Nucl Med 1991;32:237–41.

27. Bengel FM, Hauser M, Duvernoy CS, et al. Myocardial blood flow and coronary flow reserve late after anatomical correction of transposition of the great arteries. J Am Coll Cardiol 1998;32:1955–61.

28. Yates RW, Marsden PK, Badawi RD, et al. Evaluation of myocardial perfusion using positron emission tomography in infants following a neonatal arterial switch operation. Pediatr Cardiol 2000;21:111–8.

29. Hauser M, Bengel FM, Kühn A, et al. Myocardial blood flow and flow reserve after coronary reimplantation in patients after arterial switch and Ross operation. Circulation 2001;103:1875–80.

30. Singh TP, Humes RA, Muzik O, et al. Myocardial flow reserve in patients with a systemic right ventricle after atrial switch repair. J Am Coll Cardiol 2001;37:2120–5.

31. Hauser M, Bengel FM, Kühn A, et al. Myocardial perfusion and coronary flow reserve assessed by positron emission tomography in patients after Fontan-like operations. Pediatr Cardiol 2003;24:386–92.

32. Singh TP, Di Carli MF, Sullivan NM, et al. Myocardial flow reserve in long-term survivors of repair of anomalous left coronary artery from pulmonary artery. J Am Coll Cardiol 1998;31:437–43.

33. Donnelly JP, Raffel DM, Shulkin BL, et al. Resting coronary flow and coronary flow reserve in human infants after repair or palliation of congenital heart defects as measured by positron emission tomography. J Thorac Cardiovasc Surg 1998;115:103–10.

34. Rickers C, Sasse K, Buchert R, et al. Myocardial viability assessed by positron emission tomography in infants and children after the arterial switch operation and suspected infarction. J Am Coll Cardiol 2000;36:1676–83.

35. Ohmochi Y, Onouchi Z, Oda Y, et al. Assessment of effects of intravenous dipyridamole on regional myocardial perfusion in children with Kawasaki disease without angiographic evidence of coronary stenosis using positron emission tomography and H2(15)O. Coron Artery Dis 1995;6:555–9.

36. Yoshibayashi M, Tamaki N, Nishioka K, et al. Regional myocardial perfusion and metabolism assessed by positron emission tomography in children with Kawasaki disease and significance of abnormal Q waves and their disappearance. Am J Cardiol 1991;68:1638–45.

37. Hwang B, Liu RS, Chu LS, et al. Positron emission tomography for the assessment of myocardial viability in Kawasaki disease using different therapies. Nucl Med Commun 2000;21:631–6.

38. Iemura M, Ishii M, Sugimura T, et al. Long term consequences of regressed coronary aneurysms after Kawasaki disease: vascular wall morphology and function. Heart 2000;83:307–11.

39. Hamaoka K, Onouchi Z, Ohmochi Y. Coronary flow reserve in children with Kawasaki disease without angiographic evidence of coronary stenosis. Am J Cardiol 1992;69:691–2.

40. Muzik O, Paridon SM, Singh TP, et al. Quantification of myocardial blood flow and flow reserve in children with a history of Kawasaki disease and normal coronary arteries using positron emission tomography. J Am Coll Cardiol 1996;28:757–62.

41. Furuyama H, Odagawa Y, Katoh C, et al. Assessment of coronary function in children with a history of Kawasaki disease using (15)O-water positron emission tomography. Circulation 2002;105:2878–84.

42. Furuyama H, Odagawa Y, Katoh C, et al. Altered myocardial flow reserve and endothelial function late after Kawasaki disease. J Pediatr 2003;142:149–54.

43. Hauser M, Bengel F, Kuehn A, et al. Myocardial blood flow and coronary flow reserve in children with "normal" epicardial coronary arteries after the onset of Kawasaki disease assessed by positron emission tomography. Pediatr Cardiol 2004;25:108–12.

44. Bax JJ, Visser FC, van Lingen A, et al. Metabolic imaging using F18-fluorodeoxyglucose to assess myocardial viability. Int J Card Imaging 1997;13:145–55.

45. Subramaniam RM, Janowitz WR, Johnson GB, et al. ACR-SPR-STR practice parameter for the performance of cardiac Positron Emission Tomography - computed Tomography (PET/CT) imaging. Clin Nucl Med 2017;42:918–27.

46. Soliman M, Laxer R, Manson D, et al. Imaging of systemic vasculitis in childhood. Pediatr Radiol 2015;45:1110–25.

47. Chau A, Renella P, Arrieta A. Multimodality cardiovascular imaging in the diagnosis and management of prosthetic valve infective endocarditis in children report of two cases and brief review of the literature. Cardiol Young 2019;29:1526–9.

48. Dixon G, Christov G. Infective endocarditis in children: an update. Curr Opin Infect Dis 2017;30: 257–67.

49. Domingues CM, Ferreira MJ, Silva R, et al. 18F-FDG-PET/CT in diagnosis of Q fever endocarditis. J Nucl Cardiol 2019. https://doi.org/10.1007/s12350-019-01750-8.

50. Absi M, Bocchini C, Price JF, et al. F-fluorodeoxyglucose-positive emission tomography/CT imaging for left ventricular assist device-associated infections in children. Cardiol Young 2018;28:1157–9.

51. Meyer Z, Fischer M, Koerfer J, et al. The role of FDG-PET-CT in pediatric cardiac patients and patients with congenital heart defects. Int J Cardiol 2016; 220:656–60.

52. Robson PM, Dey D, Newby DE, et al. MR/PET imaging of the cardiovascular system. JACC Cardiovasc Imaging 2017;10(10 Pt A):1165–79.

53. Gatidis S, Bender B, Reimold M, et al. PET/MRI in children. Eur J Radiol 2017;94:A64–70.

54. Barton GP, Vildberg L, Goss K, et al. Simultaneous determination of dynamic cardiac metabolism and function using PET/MRI. J Nucl Cardiol 2019;26: 1946–57.

Printed and bound by CPI Group (UK) Ltd, Croydon, CR0 4YY

03/10/2024

01040371-0014